D0850433

An Atlas of
HISTOPATHOLOGY OF SKIN DISEASES

THE ENCYCLOPEDIA OF VISUAL MEDICINE SERIES

An Atlas of
HISTOPATHOLOGY OF
SKIN DISEASES

David T. Shum, MB, FRCPC

Director, Surgical Pathology, London Health Sciences Center
Associate Professor, Department of Pathology, Division of Dermatology
The University of Western Ontario, London, Ontario, Canada

and

Lyn C. Guenther, MD, FRCPC

Professor and Chair, Division of Dermatology
The University of Western Ontario, London, Ontario, Canada

with

Ann Utovac, MD, FRCPC and Kenneth W. Alanen, MD

Residents, Department of Pathology
The University of Western Ontario, London, Ontario, Canada

and

James E. Rasmussen, MD

Professor of Dermatology and Pediatrics, Department of Dermatology
The University of Michigan Medical Center, Ann Arbor, Michigan, USA

The Parthenon Publishing Group
International Publishers in Medicine, Science & Technology

NEW YORK   LONDON

Library of Congress Cataloging-in-Publication Data
Shum, David T.
   An atlas of histopathology of skin diseases / David T. Shum and Lyn C.
Guenther
      p.   cm.   --   (The Encyclopedia of visual medicine series)
   Includes bibliographical references and index.
   ISBN 1-85070-929-7
   1. Skin--Histopathology--Atlases.   I. Guenther, Lyn C.
II. Title.   III. Series.
   [DNLM: 1. Skin Diseases--pathology atlases.   WR 17S562a 1998]
RL81.S47   1998
616.5'07--dc21
DNLM/DLC
for Library of Congress   98-30129
                                                               CIP

British Library Cataloguing in Publication Data
Shum, D. T.
   An atlas of histopathology of skin diseases. - (The encyclopedia of visual
   medicine series)
   1. Skin - Diseases 2. Skin - Histopathology 3. Dermatology
   I. Title II. Guenther, Lyn C.
   616.5'07
   ISBN 1-85070-929-7

Published in the USA by
The Parthenon Publishing Group Inc.
One Blue Hill Plaza
PO Box 1564, Pearl River
New York 10965, USA

Published in the UK and Europe by
The Parthenon Publishing Group Limited
Casterton Hall, Carnforth
Lancs. LA6 2LA, UK

Copyright ©1999
Parthenon Publishing Group

Printed and bound in Great Britain by
Butler & Tanner Ltd, Frome and London

Contents

Preface

Although a clinical diagnosis based on history and clinical appearances is possible for most dermatologic diseases, the skin biopsy remains the most practical, cost-effective and reliable procedure in the work-up of a patient with ambiguous disease. Histopathologic features are often disease-specific and tissue examination can be used to confirm a diagnosis or exclude other possibilities. In addition, histopathologic diagnosis is the gold standard for neoplastic disease and a tissue diagnosis is absolutely essential for all cutaneous malignancies. It is therefore not difficult to understand why dermatohistopathology has always been, and will remain, an indispensable part of pathology and dermatology residency training.

Recognition of basic histopathologic changes and an appreciation of the associated clinical implications are a truly challenging task, given the large number of diseases affecting the skin. Indeed, it may be viewed as both an art and a science. This book has been designed to be a practical, easy-to-use, pictorial guide for residents and practicing pathologists and dermatologists. However, no book can replace the practical experience of examining slides under the microscope.

The book is organized into 36 chapters, each of which lists and illustrates entities with similar diagnostically important architectural and cytologic features. A visual and text-based differential diagnostic approach was chosen after the repeated observation that many trainees were good at identifying major microscopic changes, but were often unable to appreciate the subtle findings which distinguish a particular entity from others with similar major changes. Awareness and identification of the major abnormalities, and knowledge of the differential diagnoses for these abnormalities and their key differentiating features, are essential for arriving at the most appropriate diagnosis.

Basic histopathologic features are the building blocks for a complex picture of diseases. An atlas that is rich in illustrations is especially suited to demonstrate these features. This book contains more than 600 illlustrations of histologic features. Individual diseases are indexed at the end of the book. As many diseases are characterized by multiple prominent changes, these are discussed in more than one chapter; for example, dermatofibroma is included in the chapters on epidermal hyperplasia, giant cells, and connective tissue tumors. Such 'multireferencing' not only emphasizes the overlapping histopathologic changes and differential diagnoses, but also results in a synopsis of individual diseases, thereby rendering this book a practical reference for microscopic examination.

All illustrations are placed to one side of the page, and each is accompanied by a text providing a description and diagnostic hints. This arrangement is easy to read and, in addition, allows the book to be used for self-assessment exercises by covering the side with the text.

Clinicopathologic correlation is often essential for an accurate diagnosis. Some conditions (for example, lichen planus and lichenoid keratosis; various dermatitides and photoeruptions; and seborrheic keratoses and linear epidermal nevi) are histologically so similar that clinical input is required for a definitive histopathologic diagnosis. Because the clinical features are so important, clinical descriptions and differential diagnoses for each photomicrograph have been included.

An understanding of dermatopathology is important not only for pathologists, but also for practicing dermatologists. If a histopathologic diagnosis does not 'fit' clinically, the proper diagnosis may often be reached by understanding that some conditions which present rather different clinical appearances, may in fact look similar under the microscope. Thus, if a typical linear epidermal nevus were to be removed and the histologic diagnosis of seborrheic keratosis returned on the pathology report, the dermatologist's clinical diagnosis would still be correct as the two conditions may have an identical appearance on histology.

Most of the material included in this atlas was taken from the files of the London Health Sciences Centre in London, Ontario, Canada. The micrographs are taken from actual cases, and the text and diagnostic hints offered are based on our own personal experience. References to individual diseases are not cited as they are readily available from any standard dermatopathology and dermatology textbook such as Lever's *Histopathology of the Skin*, Ackerman's *Histologic Diagnosis of Inflammatory Skin Diseases*, McKee and Marsdan's *Pathology of the Skin with Clinical Correlation*, Mehregan and Pinkus' *Guide to Dermatohistopathology*, Farmer and Hood's *Pathology of the Skin*, Fitzpatrick *et al.*'s *Dermatology in General Medicine* and Rook *et al.*'s *Textbook of Dermatology*.

David T. Shum
Lyn C. Guenther
London, Ontario

Acknowledgments

I am most grateful to my two residents, Dr Ann Utovac and Dr Ken Alanen, for their inspiration, encouragement, and assistance in the preparation of the material for this atlas. Their involvement has ensured that the contents of this book are presented in a concise and practical format, and are useful to trainees as well as consultants. In addition, to obtain a global perspective, Dr Jim Rasmussen, University of Michigan at Ann Arbor, MI, USA, kindly reviewed all of the material.

Dr A.B. Ackerman graciously reviewed a sample chapter and made some excellent suggestions; I applaud his help and appreciate his informed advice.

This work would not have been possible without the support of all my colleagues in pathology and dermatology. I am expecially indebted to the pathology staff of the now defunct Victoria Hospital, London, Ontario, who gave me access to an extensive archive of dermatopathological cases dating back to the 1920s.

I am also grateful to Dr G. Wysocki and Dr M. Joseph, University of Western Ontario, London, Ontario, and to Dr Philip E. Le Boit and Dr Timothy McCalmont, University of California, San Francisco, CA, for kindly lending me their cases of mucosal lichen planus, erythema toxicum neonatorum, and sclerema neonatorum for inclusion in this atlas.

I thank Dr Marvin S. Smout, Dr W.E. Pace, and Dr J.T. Headington for their guidance and teaching in pathology and dermatology.

Finally, Mr John Regan, Regan Photography, Dorchester, Ontario, and Ms Ineke Van Turnhout, photographer, London Health Sciences Centre, Ontario, expertly developed and printed thousands of photographs, and my best friend and wife Annie, patiently sorted through these photographs for final inclusion in this book. Mrs M. Hickling also assisted in the typing of the manuscript.

David T. Shum
London, Ontario

Section I Laboratory Methods

Biopsies

Biopsies should be planned to yield maximal information. When taking a biopsy from a patient with a skin eruption, intact, non-excoriated lesions should be sampled. Trauma and secondary impetiginization may alter and obscure the histologic findings. If there are lesions at different stages of evolution, more than one sample may be helpful.

Biopsies should be generous, of a sufficient depth to assess the pathology, and technically well done. Fat must be included if a panniculitis is suspected and fascia for fasciitis. These diagnoses cannot be made with superficial shave biopsies. A full-thickness punch biopsy that is at least 4 mm in diameter or an elliptiform incisional biopsy are preferable for sampling skin eruptions. The tissue should be handled with care, not crushed with forceps, and promptly placed in the appropriate fixative or transport medium. It is important to make sure that the specimen is completely covered by the fixative and not adherent to the side of the bottle or crushed in the lid.

Shave biopsy

A thin slice of skin is cut. This type of biopsy is easy and quick to perform; healing is rapid and scarring minimal. It is useful for sampling skin tumors such as seborrheic keratoses, actinic keratoses, and basal and squamous cell carcinomas. It is not appropriate for melanomas.

Punch biopsy

Punches cut cylindrical pieces of tissue. A properly executed punch biopsy should include tissue from the stratum corneum down to the subcutaneous tissue. Unlike a shave biopsy, the entire dermis is examined. When biopsying alopecia, the punch should be tangential to the skin in straight-haired individuals so as to follow the direction of the hair. In those with curly hair, the punch should be perpendicular to the skin surface. Active rather than scarred areas of alopecia should be biopsied.

Wedge incisional biopsy

An elliptiform full-thickness piece of tissue is excised. A larger scar is produced than with either shave or punch biopsy, but a wedge incisional may be necessary under the following circumstances:

When the pathology occurs primarily in the subcutaneous tissue or fascia;

When the pathologic process is patchy and areas of normal skin occur between abnormal areas;

When examination of disease progression from involved to non-involved skin is helpful;

When additional tissue is required for bacterial and / or fungal cultures.

Tissue for microbiologic culture should be transported to the laboratory on sterile gauze moistened with normal saline without preservatives.

Excisional biopsy

The entire lesion is removed in an excisional biopsy. Benign and malignant skin tumors, particularly pigmented lesions, are removed with excisional biopsies. Small lesions may be completely removed with a punch whereas larger lesions may require an elliptiform scalpel excision.

Suspected melanomas should be excised completely when possible. As the prognosis and treatment of melanoma depend on the maximum depth as measured by an ocular micrometer, a punch biopsy or wedge incisional biopsy should be done and the darkest and / or thickest area included. However, sampling errors may occur with punch and wedge biopsies.

A control biopsy may be necessary for comparison in suspected cases of anetoderma, atrophoderma, and morphea. Control biopsies should be taken from the same body site because skin thickness varies with different body areas.

If the clinical and pathologic diagnoses diverge, the clinician and pathologist should discuss their findings. Additional biopsies from other lesions at different sites may help to sort out difficult cases.

Tissue processing

Fixation

For routine histology: 10% neutral buffered formalin or formol-alcohol (one part 40% formaldehyde to nine parts 95% ethyl alcohol) to prevent freezing during transport in the winter months;

For immunofluorescence: Michel's solution;

For electron microscopy: 10 % glutaraldehyde.

Gross examination

Punch biopsies < 4 mm do not require trimming and may be placed directly into cassettes;

Larger punch biopsies may be halved slightly off-center and both pieces should be submitted;

Excisional biopsies wider than 4 mm require trimming so that the tissue can be fitted 'end-on' in the cassette and sectioned perpendicular to the skin surface;

If margins require evaluation, India ink should be applied to them with a cotton swab, followed by the application of Bouin's fixative to prevent running of ink;

Submit the closest margins and representative sections at the deepest extension of the tumor.

Processing

Formalin-fixed specimens are submitted in labeled cassettes;

Tissue processor passes specimens through graded solutions of alcohol (50% to absolute) to dehydrate the tissue;

Tissue is then passed through two or three changes of xylol and two or three changes of paraffin wax to allow the wax to infiltrate the tissue to provide internal support for sectioning;

This is usually an overnight process.

Embedding

Processed tissue infiltrated with paraffin wax is removed from cassettes;

Epidermis is identified and the tissue is oriented in a mould with the epidermis at 90° to the knife when the tissue block is mounted on a microtome.

Cutting

Blocks are cooled with ice water to harden the wax;

They are placed on the microtome so that the knife hits the epidermis first, the area of greatest resistance;

This prevents artificial separation of the dermis which occurs when the epidermis is cut last;

Routine tissue sections are cut at 4–5°F, and a tissue ribbon comprising multiple tissue sections may be prepared and floated on the surface of a water bath;

The tissue ribbon is place onto a glass slide and is ready to be stained after the slides are dried in an oven.

Stains

Alcian blue

Acid mucins such as sulfated glycosaminoglycans stain intensely blue at very low pH (0.5);

Most glycosaminoglycans stain best at pH 2.5;

Also highlights blood vessel walls, eccrine and apocrine cells and mast cells.

Bismarck brown

Metachromatic stain similar to Giemsa and toluidine blue stains;

Cytoplasmic granules of mast cells are stained brown;

Preferred stain for mast cells because staining is not as intense as with other metachromatic stains.

Colloidal iron

Good stain for sialomucins and glycosaminoglycans.

Giemsa

Highlights bacteria, which appear deep blue;

May be used to stain mast cells.

Gram

Useful for highlighting bacteria and differentiating as Gram-positive or Gram-negative;

Both stain purple when crystal violet is applied initially, but the outer membrane of Gram-negative (but not Gram-positive) organisms is removed with alcohol;

A second dye, often carbolfuchsin, may be added, staining Gram-negative organisms pink.

Grocott–methenamine–silver (GMS)

Commonly used stain to highlight bacteria and fungi, which appear black;

Necrotic debris also stains black and may obscure organisms when the condition is extensive.

Hematoxylin and eosin (H & E)

Most widely used for routine sections;

Nuclei are stained blue or purple;

Cytoplasm appears pink;

Keratohyalin granules appear dark-purple;

Collagen is eosinophilic (pink-staining).

Leder

Highlights neutrophilic myeloid cells and mast cells, which stain scarlet.

Masson–Fontana

Stains melanin, but is not specific for it, as any reducing substance produces precipitation of metallic silver.

Mucicarmine

Stains mucin of epithelial derivation; stain of choice to highlight the capsule of *Cryptococcus neoformans*.

Periodic acid–Schiff (PAS)

Positive reaction is deep-pink or magenta;

Many substances are positive, including glycogen, neutral and weakly acidic mucin, and basement membrane;

Glycogen is removed by diastase digestion;

The preferred stain for fungal organisms and tissue, sections should first be digested with diastase to remove glycogen particles, which may cause too much background staining.

Prussian blue

Common stain for iron, which stains blue;

Helpful if required to differentiate 'brown pigment' as iron or melanin;

Does not stain iron in ferrous form or when incorporated into hemoglobin.

Steiner

Similar to Warthin–Starry stain, stains spirochetes, bacteria in bacillary angiomatosis and Legionnaire's disease, and Donovan's bodies black.

Verhoeff

Stains elastic tissue black.

Warthin–Starry

Classical stain for spirochetes, but considered by some to be less reproducible and more difficult to control than Steiner stain.

Ziehl–Neelsen

Traditional stain for acid-fast bacilli, which are stained red;

For atypical mycobacteria and *Mycobacterium leprae*, Fite's modification, in which sunflower seed oil is added to help penetration of the stain into the fatty cell wall of acid-fast bacilli, is recommended.

Immunohistochemical stains

bcl-2 protein

Related to t(14;18) translocation, overproduction of *bcl*-2 protein may be seen in most nodal follicular lymphomas in North America, but staining for *bcl*-2 protein is of dubious diagnostic value with cutaneous follicular lymphomas and SALTomas.

Carcinoembryonic antigen (CEA)

Typically found in benign and malignant glandular tumors;

Positive in mammary and extramammary Paget's disease.

Chromogranin

Family of peptides located within neuroendocrine cells, often used as a 'panendocrine marker';

Positive in tumor cells of Merkel cell carcinoma.

Cytokeratin

There are many cytokeratins; they are present in all epithelial cells and in most epithelial cell-derived tumors (carcinomas);

Often, a 'cocktail' of keratins is used (such as AE1 / AE3) to determine whether a poorly differentiated neoplasm is a carcinoma.

CD1a (OKT6)

Antigen present on Langerhans cells; should be used in addition to S100 protein, peanut agglutinin and electron microscopy (for Birbeck granules) if a diagnosis of Langerhans cell histiocytosis is being considered.

CD34

Antigen found in endothelial cells, and Kaposi's sarcoma, angiosarcoma, and other soft tissue tumors, including dermatofibrosarcoma protuberans.

CD43

T-cell marker which may be expressed by malignant lymphocytes in a SALToma.

CD68 (KP-1)

Glycosylated transmembranous protein found in lysosomes of macrophages;

Expression of CD68 has been reported in malignant fibrous histiocytoma, atypical fibroxanthoma, histiocytosis X, and melanoma.

Desmin

Intermediate filament associated with smooth muscle, skeletal muscle and, to a lesser extent, myofibroblasts.

Factor XIIIA

Enzyme involved in homeostasis;

Found in dermal dendrocytes, dermatofibromas and some cases of juvenile xanthogranuloma and xanthoma disseminatum.

HMB-45

More specific, but less sensitive, for melanoma than S100 protein; also seen in some nevi and in angiomyolipomas;

Often negative in desmoplastic melanomas;

S100 protein and HMB-45 should both be ordered when a diagnosis of metastatic melanoma is being considered.

Immunoglobulin heavy chain IgG, IgM, and IgA

Accurate and consistent demonstration of immunoglobulin deposits in tissue, such as IgG anti-BMZ antibodies in bullous pemphigoid and lupus band in lupus erythematosus, requires non-fixed frozen tissue or tissue stored in Michel's solution and direct immunofluorescence microscopy.

Ki-1

Activation marker found on some T cells, Reed–Sternberg (RS) cells of Hodgkin's disease and RS-like cells of lymphomatoid papulosis, and anaplastic large cell lymphoma.

LCA (leukocyte common antigen)

As its name suggests, present on most lymphocytes (but not plasma cells) and lymphomas.

Leu M1

Also known as CD15; present on Reed–Sternberg cells and on cells of some adenocarcinomas.

Light chains (κ and λ)

Predominance of either κ or λ light chains usually indicates clonality;

Light chain restriction is suggestive of either B-cell lymphoma or myeloma;

λ, in contrast to κ, light chain is often expressed in cutaneous mantle cell lymphoma.

Neuron-specific enolase

Glycolysis-associated enzyme fairly specific for cells and tumors of neuroectodermal / neuroendocrine origin, including melanocytes;

Positive in tumor cells of Merkel cell carcinoma.

Pan B (L26)

Stains most mature B cells and well-to-moderately differentiated B-cell lymphomas.

S100 protein

Acute protein found in melanocytes, nevus cells, chondrocytes, Schwann cells and glial cells;

Sensitive, but not specific, for melanoma.

Smooth muscle actin

Intermediate filament found in most contractile cells;

Anti-smooth muscle actin is useful for identifying smooth muscle tumors.

UCHL-I

Also known as 'pan-T-cell' marker because it stains both CD4 and CD8 cells, and T-cell tumors (such as mycosis fungoides).

Vimentin

Intermediate filament most commonly found in mesenchymal tissues, and mesenchymal and melanocytic tumors;

Unfortunately, this has a low specificity (often found in epithelia).

Section 2 Histopathology of Skin Diseases Illustrated

EPIDERMIS

HYPERKERATOSIS AND PARAKERATOSIS

Because the keratin layer varies in thickness and compactness according to anatomic site, the biopsy site must be known before making an assessment based on the thickness and degree of **hyperkeratosis**. The stratum corneum of palmar and plantar skin is particularly thick and compact in contrast to that of the upper back, which is relatively thin with a basket-weave appearance.

The 'spaces' in the normal keratin layer responsible for the basket-weave appearance are retraction artifacts of the keratinized cells when the tissue is fixed in formalin and routinely processed for light microscopy. The compact keratin layer of the palm and sole probably reflects the slightly different composition of soft keratin in different body sites.

Histologic changes of the keratin layer alone are seldom diagnostic. **Hyperkeratosis** and **parakeratosis** are signs of disturbed epidermal growth. They are non-specific changes that are common to many inflammatory and neoplastic skin diseases. Nevertheless, certain conditions typically show characteristic changes of the stratum corneum (for example, parakeratosis in psoriasis, compact hyperkeratosis in lichen planus, and alternating foci of hyperkeratosis and parakeratosis in lichen simplex chronicus

and pityriasis rubra pilaris). The absence of characteristic keratin layer changes in these cases should raise doubts as to the diagnosis.

Orthokeratosis (from the Greek word *ortho* meaning 'correct') refers to a keratin layer composed of flattened anucleate cells in the usual basket-weave array. Compact hyperkeratosis, on the other hand, refers to a thickening of the stratum corneum with loss of the basket-weave appearance of the keratin layer.

Parakeratosis refers to the retention of pyknotic nuclei in the keratin layer. Parakeratosis is usually accompanied by underlying hypogranulosis. This contrasts with compact hyperkeratosis, which often overlies hypergranulosis.

Hyperkeratosis and **parakeratosis** manifest clinically as scaling. Papulosquamous eruptions are a group of morphologically similar diseases that have scaly papules and include psoriasis, pityriasis rubra pilaris, parapsoriasis, pityriasis lichenoides, lichen planus, pityriasis rosea, superficial fungal infections, secondary syphilis and mycosis fungoides. Scaling is also seen in eczematous conditions (including atopic dermatitis, contact dermatitis, seborrheic dermatitis, photodermatitis, and stasis dermatitis), ichthyoses, collagen vascular conditions (such as lupus erythematosus, dermatomyositis), and skin tumors (for example, seborrheic keratosis and squamous cell carcinoma).

The color and distribution of the scales may help to distinguish these various conditions. In psoriasis, the scales are usually thick and silvery-white. In pityriasis rubra pilaris, scales may be fine to thick, and the palms and soles orange-red with diffuse thickening. In pityriasis lichenoides, the scale is fine and mica-like. In lichen planus, hyperkeratosis is manifested as fine, lacy, reticulated lines called 'Wickham's striae'. In pityriasis rosea, the scale is peripheral, forming a 'collarette'. Peripheral scaling is also seen in dermatophytic fungal infections. In tinea versicolor, however, fine scaling involves the entire lesion. In seborrheic dermatitis, the scales are often large, yellow, and waxy. In discoid lupus erythematosus, the scale is adherent and extends into dilated hair follicles. When the scale is removed, it has the appearance of a carpet tack due to the retained follicular keratin spikes. In subacute lupus erythematosus, the lesions are often annular with slight scaling. In actinic keratoses, the scales are adherent and feel like fine sandpaper whereas the scales are usually thicker in squamous cell carcinomas. Lesions of porokeratosis are sharply demarcated with raised scaly borders – the 'cornoid lamellae' – which have an easily recognizable microscopic appearance.

Normal skin from the back	1.1
Normal palmar skin	1.2
Hyperkeratosis	1.3
Parakeratosis	1.4

Differential diagnoses

Hyperkeratosis

Lichen planus	1.5
Lichen sclerosus	1.6
Acanthosis nigricans / epidermal nevus / seborrheic keratosis / acanthosis papulosa nigra	1.7
Keratinizing well-differentiated squamous cell carcinoma	1.8
Epidermolytic hyperkeratosis	1.9

Parakeratosis

Psoriasis	1.10
Porokeratosis	1.11
Actinic keratosis	1.12
Verruca vulgaris	1.13
Necrolytic migratory erythema	1.14

Combined hyperkeratosis and parakeratosis

Lichen simplex chronicus	1.15
Subacute and chronic dermatitis	1.16
Seborrheic dermatitis	1.17
Pityriasis lichenoides et varioliformis acuta	1.18
Pityriasis lichenoides chronica	1.19
Pityriasis rubra pilaris	1.20
Pityriasis rosea	1.21
Lupus erythematosus	1.22
Dermatophytosis	1.23
Ichthyosis	1.24

HYPERKERATOSIS

1.1 Normal skin from the back

♦ basket-weave appearance of the normal stratum corneum is an artifact of fixation and processing

♦ keratohyaline granules (arrow), a precursor of 'soft keratin', are seen in the keratinocytes of the granular layer

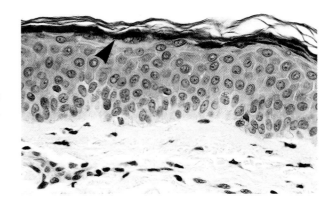

1.2 Normal palmar skin

♦ thick compact stratum corneum is normal in palmar and plantar skin

♦ thin eosinophilic zone (large arrow) below the keratin layer is the stratum lucidum, present only in skin with a thick stratum corneum

♦ exaggerated rete ridges (small arrow)

♦ epidermis of plantar skin is approximately four times thicker than that of the eyelids

♦ absence of hair follicles, and sebaceous and apocrine glands (unlike skin elsewhere on the body)

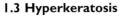

1.3 Hyperkeratosis

♦ thickened horny layer secondary to accelerated keratinization and abnormal retention of keratinized anucleate squamous cells

♦ increased keratin formation in the epidermis is reflected by hypergranulosis (arrow), a constant finding in compact hyperkeratosis

♦ hyperkeratosis is considered to be marked when the stratum corneum is as thick as the underlying layers of epidermis

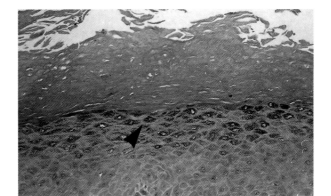

1.4 Parakeratosis

♦ retention of pyknotic nuclei in the keratin layer

♦ sign of accelerated epidermal cell growth

♦ parakeratosis is evident in this example of actinic keratosis in which dysplastic squamous cells are proliferating at an increased rate

♦ increased epidermal turnover in psoriasis results in confluent parakeratosis

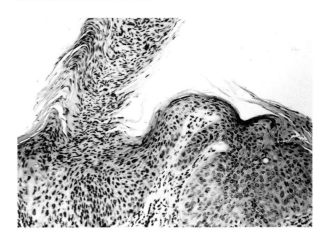

1.5 Lichen planus

♦ compact hyperkeratosis and wedge-shaped hypergranulosis are characteristic

♦ parakeratosis may be seen in mucosal lichen planus; however, if seen in glabrous skin, its presence suggests excoriations or alternate diagnoses, such as lichenoid dermatitis and benign lichenoid keratosis

♦ hyperplastic or atrophic epidermis

♦ band-like lymphocytic infiltration of the basal cell layer and basal cell necrosis are constant features

♦ clinically characterized by pruritic, polygonal, purple, planar papules with lacy reticulated Wickham's striae

♦ lower extremities, flexor wrists, forearms; may be generalized; oral and genital involvement common; may show nail changes

♦ hypertrophic lesions may clinically mimic psoriasis and lichen simplex chronicus

♦ atrophic lesions may mimic lichen sclerosus

♦ lichen amyloidosus, with its discrete, small, itchy papules which coalesce to form hyperkeratotic plaques typically on the shins, may be confused clinically with lichen planus

♦ lichen planus and discoid lupus erythematosus (LE; erythematous to violaceous plaques with hyperkeratosis and central atrophy most commonly on the face and scalp) are usually not confused clinically, but may be misdiagnosed histologically

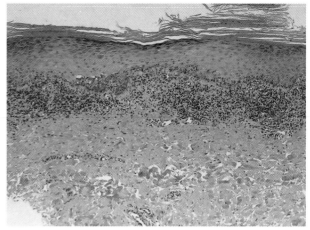
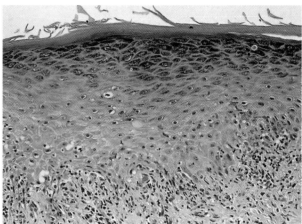

1.6 Lichen sclerosus

♦ marked hyperkeratosis associated with epidermal atrophy

♦ few degenerated basal cells, but lacks lichenoid infiltrate

♦ unique edematous and eosinophilic changes (homogenization) of the superficial dermal collagen fibers which become homogenized and amorphous

♦ lymphocytic infiltrate seen deep to the altered collagen

♦ commonly presents as 'figure-of-eight' whiteness and itching of the vulva and perineal area in middle-aged women; may occur on the penis

♦ extragenital lesions are flat-topped white papules (often with follicular plugs) that coalesce to form plaques, which may clinically resemble morphea; morphea and lichen sclerosus may coexist

♦ lichen sclerosus has been associated with Lyme disease

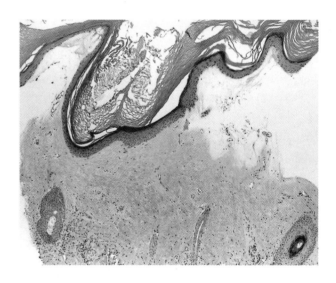

1.7 Acanthosis nigricans

♦ despite its name, there is minimal acanthosis, but considerable hyperkeratosis and papillary hyperplasia

♦ note the relative thinning of the epidermis, with papillomatosis, in contrast to normal epidermis (right-hand margin of specimen)

♦ clinical correlation is required for histologic diagnosis because the microscopic appearance may be identical to **epidermal nevus**, hypertrophic **seborrheic keratosis** and **acanthosis papulosa nigra**

♦ presents as a velvety brown plaque on the nape of the neck, axillae, groin and inner aspects of the thighs; diagnosis usually made clinically

♦ brownish discoloration is largely due to hyperkeratosis and papillomatosis; epidermal hyperpigmentation is usually minimal

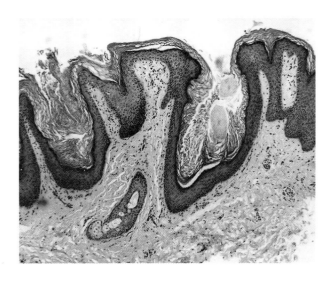

1.8 Keratinizing well-differentiated squamous cell carcinoma

♦ majority of squamous cell carcinomas on sun-exposed skin are well-differentiated and produce keratin

♦ tumor surface is covered by a thick layer of keratin

♦ biopsy needs to be deep enough to demonstrate the architecture and any reticular dermal invasion by atypical neoplastic squamous cells

♦ clinically and histologically, squamous cell carcinoma may be confused with keratoacanthoma; lesions showing infiltrative deep and lateral margins, marked dysplasia and mitotic activity without the typical keratoacanthoma crater-like architecture, are best categorized as squamous cell carcinoma

♦ indurated reddish-brown scaly tumor nodule with or without ulceration

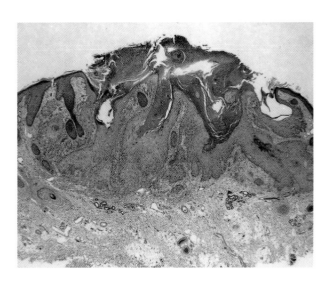

1.9 Epidermolytic hyperkeratosis

♦ compact hyperkeratosis associated with vacuolization of the superficial squamous cells

♦ keratohyaline granules are coarse and irregular, and may be mistaken for human papillomavirus inclusions

♦ this change is often encountered incidentally in biopsies of other lesions (such as dermatitis, benign and malignant tumors)

♦ a main feature of the rare autosomal-dominant disease bullous congenital icthyosiform erythroderma, which presents shortly after birth with erythema and blisters, followed by generalized, brown, warty scaling particularly on the flexural surfaces of the extremities

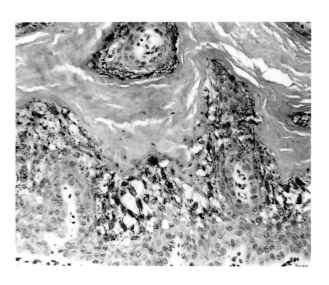

PARAKERATOSIS

1.10 Psoriasis

♦ confluent parakeratosis without hyperkeratosis is uncommon, but characteristic of psoriasis

♦ granular layer is inconspicuous (hypogranulosis)

♦ regular psoriasiform epidermal hyperplasia with club-shaped dermal papillae

♦ exocytosis of neutrophils and microabscesses within the parakeratotic cell layer and superficial epidermis are other characteristic features to look for under higher magnification

♦ dermal infiltrate surrounds vessels and does not extend into the reticular dermis

♦ well-defined, erythematous, scaly plaques on elbows, knees, sacrum, and scalp; nail changes and arthritis are common

♦ usually diagnosed clinically; biopsy is usually not necessary

♦ clinical differential diagnosis: dermatophytosis (positive fungal culture and PAS staining); pityriasis rosea (focal parakeratotic mounds, but no microabscesses); lichen simplex chronicus (irregular epidermal hyperplasia and no microabscesses); Bowen's disease (dysplastic squamous cells); squamous cell carcinoma; secondary syphilis (positive VDRL and plasma cell infiltration); LE (basal cell degeneration and keratin plugging of hair follicles); and mycosis fungoides (atypical T-cell infiltrate)

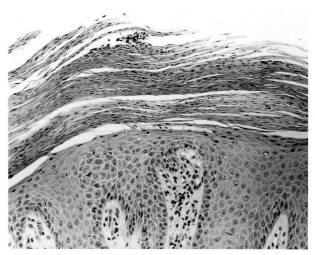

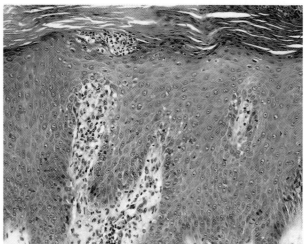

1.11 Porokeratosis

♦ an angulate column of parakeratotic cells, the 'cornoid lamella', forms the raised keratotic border of porokeratosis

♦ the cornoid lamella arises from an epidermal invagination, the apex of which points away from the center of the lesion (left-hand side of section)

♦ hypogranulosis is seen at the base with a few dyskeratotic and vacuolated squamous cells

♦ surrounding stratum corneum is orthokeratotic

♦ when biopsying lesions suspected of porokeratosis, it is essential that the edge of the lesion be included so that the characteristic cornoid lamella can be seen

♦ cornoid lamella is typical, but not diagnostic, of porokeratosis; it may also be seen in actinic keratosis

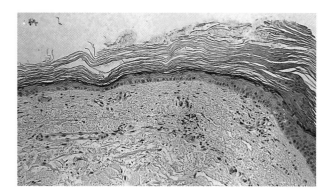

(continued next page)

♦ biopsy from the center shows an atrophic epidermis, pigmentary incontinence, and mild dermal lymphocytic infiltration

♦ clinically, one or more annular, sharply demarcated, lesion(s) with a scaly border

♦ variants include: plaque type (Mibelli), disseminated superficial actinic porokeratosis (DSAP) on sun-exposed skin, porokeratosis plantaris, palmaris et disseminata, punctate, linear, and reticulate

♦ DSAP may be confused clinically with, but differentiated histologically from, actinic keratoses, flat seborrheic keratoses, and flat warts

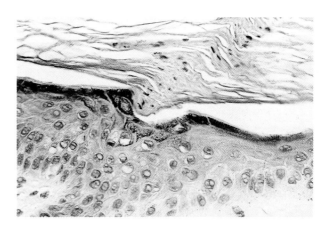

1.12 Actinic keratosis

♦ parakeratosis is usually present on the surface and spares the follicular epithelium (involvement of follicular epithelium in Bowen's disease)

♦ parakeratosis in this setting displays larger, crowded, irregular nuclei, reflecting the underlying dysplasia

♦ epidermis may be atrophic or hyperplastic

♦ dysplasia of the lower squamous layers; note the large hyperchromatic nuclei of the keratinocytes (arrow)

♦ grading of dysplasia is unimportant, but marked full-thickness epidermal squamous dysplasia is called bowenoid actinic keratosis

♦ reddish-brown, rough, scaly macules on sun-exposed skin, especially the face and dorsum of the hands

♦ usually not difficult to identify clinically, but may mimic seborrheic keratosis, basal cell carcinoma, porokeratosis, and squamous cell carcinoma

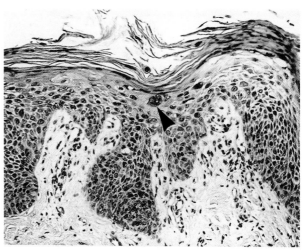

1.13 Verruca vulgaris

♦ parakeratotic nuclei are enlarged, round, and hyperchromatic

♦ vertical columns of parakeratosis from the tips of the papillae

♦ this plantar wart shows eosinophilic cytoplasmic inclusions, which should not be confused with molluscum bodies

♦ firm papule with a rough horny surface due to human papillomavirus

♦ diagnosis of verrucous squamous carcinoma should be considered and a biopsy performed when 'warts' are persistent

♦ occasionally, filiform warts may be confused clinically with skin tags; plantar warts with calluses or corns, genital warts with condyloma lata of secondary syphilis, or squamous cell carcinoma

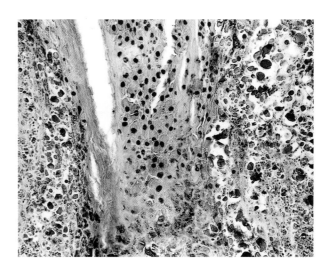

1.14 Necrolytic migratory erythema

♦ diffuse parakeratosis is seen overlying the eosinophilic and pale-staining superficial epidermal cell layers
♦ pallor and eosinophilia of the upper layers of epidermis are due to cell necrosis, hence the term 'necrolytic'
♦ some vacuolated keratinocytes are seen in this case
♦ lesions of some duration may show exocytosis of neutrophils and subcorneal vesiculation
♦ circinate and configurate lesions are present most commonly on the face, perineum, trunk, and lower extremities
♦ usually associated with glucagonoma

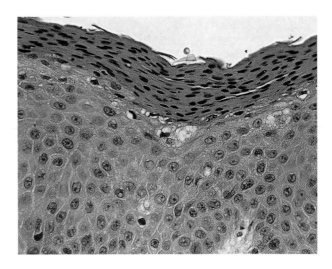

COMBINED HYPERKERATOSIS AND PARAKERATOSIS

1.15 Lichen simplex chronicus

♦ compact hyperkeratosis with focal parakeratosis
♦ marked irregular epidermal hyperplasia which may mimic squamous cell carcinoma histologically, but rarely clinically
♦ absence of cytologic atypia in contrast to squamous cell carcinoma
♦ prominent vertically oriented collagen fibers and telangiectatic vessels in dermal papillae
♦ slight perivascular lymphocytic infiltrate
♦ results from repeated scratching and rubbing
♦ presents as one or more lichenified, erythematous, scaly plaques
♦ common on the neck, wrists, ankles, palms, and anogenital area
♦ may be confused clinically with psoriasis

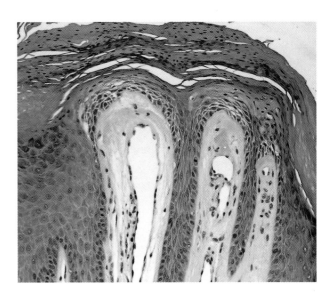

1.16 Subacute and chronic dermatitis

♦ longer-standing dermatitis shows focal hyperkeratosis and parakeratosis
♦ depending on the intensity of the inflammation, there are varying degrees of spongiosis and exocytosis of lymphocytes
♦ this shows a lesion with ongoing active inflammation, as suggested by the foci of spongiosis (arrows) and exocytosis of lymphoctes
♦ there is a moderate degree of lymphocytic infiltration of the superficial dermal vessels

(continued next page)

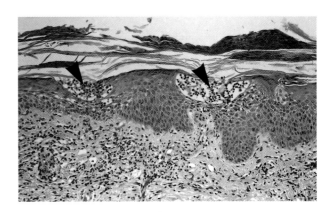

♦ this is a more chronic lesion lasting several months

♦ there is compact hyperkeratosis and the epidermis is markedly thickened

♦ although a lymphocytic infiltrate of the superficial dermal vessels is present, there is a minimal degree of spongiosis or exocytosis

♦ clinically manifests as redness, scaling, pruritus, and papulovesicles

♦ a biopsy is usually not indicated, but should be considered in persistent and recalcitrant cases to rule out the possibility of mycosis fungoides

♦ clinical differential diagnosis: psoriasis; Bowen's disease; discoid LE; and superficial basal cell carcinoma

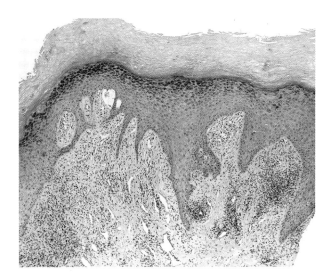

1.17 Seborrheic dermatitis

♦ focal parakeratosis and hyperkeratosis with neutrophilic exudate similar to psoriasis

♦ may show a predilection for follicular ostia

♦ spongiosis and a slight degree of epidermal hyperplasia are features more typical of seborrheic dermatitis than psroiasis

♦ diagnosis is difficult to make solely on the basis of the histologic findings; clinical correlation is required

♦ scaly dermatitis with a predilection for the scalp, face, chest, axillae, and groin

♦ clinical differential diagnosis: psoriasis; tinea versicolor; pityriasis rosea; atopic dermatitis; contact dermatitis; and impetigo

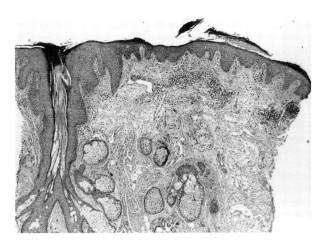

1.18 Pityriasis lichenoides et varioliformis acuta (PLEVA)

♦ also known as Mucha–Habermann disease

♦ focal parakeratosis and hyperkeratosis

♦ diffuse extravasation of red cells in dermis in acute lesions (arrows); erythrocytes may be entrapped within parakeratotic cell layers

♦ colloid bodies in the squamous cell layers; basal cell degeneration

♦ marked lymphocytic vasculitis involving superficial and deep dermal vessels; biopsy is diagnostic in full-blown lesions

♦ generalized eruption with abrupt onset of crops of reddish-brown scaly papules, which may become vesicular and necrotic, and ulcerate

♦ clinical differential diagnosis: varicella; leukocytoclastic vasculitis; and insect bites

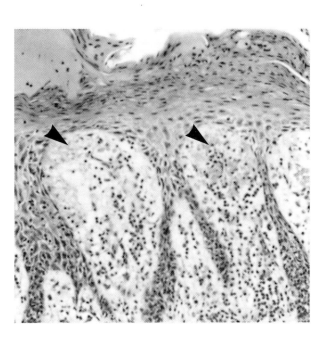

1.19 Pityriasis lichenoides chronica

♦ slight hyperkeratosis and parakeratosis (non-specific changes)
♦ neutrophils and red cell extravasation are slight or absent
♦ basal cell necrosis and colloid bodies are subtle
♦ pigmentary incontinence
♦ may begin *de novo* or evolve from PLEVA
♦ reddish-brown scaly papules which heal with hyper-pigmentation
♦ clinical differential diagnosis: guttate psoriasis; pityriasis rosea; and secondary syphilis
♦ clinical correlation often required for histologic diagnosis

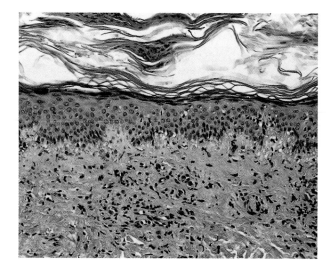

1.20 Pityriasis rubra pilaris

♦ fully developed lesions show epidermal acanthosis with thick, rather than thin, suprapapillary epidermis, short rete ridges, and alternating foci of hyperkeratosis and parakeratosis
♦ keratin plugging of hair follicles
♦ slight perivascular lymphoid cellular infiltrate in superficial dermis
♦ no neutrophils or microabscesses as seen in psoriasis
♦ histologic changes are most prominent around follicles, which should thus be included in biopsy sample
♦ rare chronic condition characterized by orange scaly plaques with 'island sparing' and keratotic papules
♦ often confused clinically with psoriasis, but no micro-abscesses
♦ clinical correlation often required for histologic diagnosis

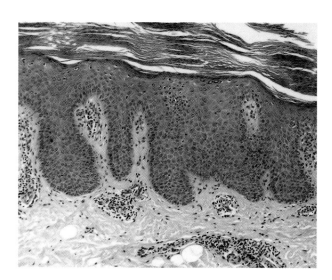

1.21 Pityriasis rosea (PR)

♦ usually well-defined parakeratotic cell mounds with spongiosis and exocytosis in underlying epidermal cell layers
♦ slight lymphoid infiltrate in superficial dermis; 'herald patch' may show heavier inflammation in deeper dermis
♦ clinical correlation usually required as histology is non-specific
♦ often onsets clinically with a herald patch with a collarette of fine scale attached at the periphery and free at the center, followed by multiple smaller lesions in a Christmas tree-like arrangement on the trunk, thighs and arms; self-limited eruption in young adults
♦ clinical differential diagnosis: dermatophytosis; nummular dermatitis; psoriasis; secondary syphilis; viral exanthema; drug eruption; and tinea versicolor

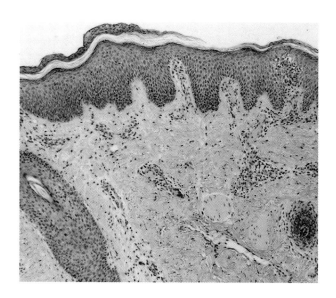

1.22 Lupus erythematosus (LE)

♦ compact hyperkeratosis, focal parakeratosis and keratin plugging of hair follicles; perivascular and peri-adnexal lymphocytic infiltrate

♦ basal cell vacuolar degeneration and hyaline thickening of epidermal basement membrane in chronic lesions

♦ discoid lesions are reddish-brown to violaceous plaques with hyperkeratosis and central atrophy, typically on the face and scalp

♦ in subacute LE, the lesions are often annular with a slight scale

♦ clinical differential diagnosis: benign lymphocytic infiltrate; psoriasis; seborrheic dermatitis; photodermatoses; dermatophyte fungal infections; and sarcoidosis

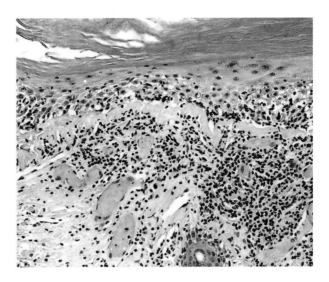

1.23 Dermatophytosis

♦ slight non-specific hyperkeratosis and/or parakeratosis resembling dermatitis

♦ a few neutrophils and/or eosinophils with spongiosis may be present

♦ diagnosis should be suspected in any dermatitic lesions; the keratin layer should always be examined under high magnification (×400) for the presence of hyphae and spores (arrows)

♦ presence of dermatophytes may be confirmed by PAS staining after diastase digestion

♦ classically, a circular, red, scaly patch that spreads peripherally and has central clearing

♦ on the feet, scaling and maceration in the lateral web space may extend onto the sole, resulting in the so-called moccasin foot

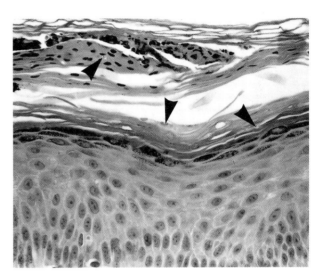

1.24 Ichthyosis

♦ a slight degree of hyperkeratosis is usually seen in ichthyosis vulgaris and X-linked ichthyosis whereas hyperkeratosis is often marked in lamellar ichthyosis

♦ this is an example of focal parakeratosis in congenital ichthyosiform erythroderma

♦ a group of diseases with persistent, usually generalized, non-inflammatory scaling

♦ most cases are inherited, but may be acquired (for example, in association with Hodgkin's disease)

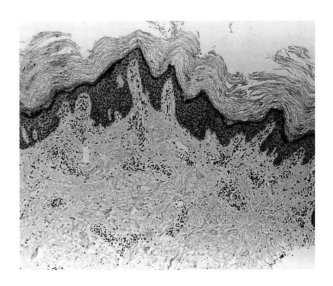

HYPERPLASIA AND ACANTHOSIS

Hyperplasia of the epidermis implies increased thickness secondary to an increased number of cells. **Acanthosis** (from the Greek word *akantha* which means 'thorn' or 'prickle') refers to thickening of the epidermis due to an increase in the number of cells in the spinous layer. The two terms are often used interchangeably. Hyperplasia is seen in both inflammatory and neoplastic condi-

tions. Its presence should alert the observer to look for epidermal dysplastic changes. Alternatively, it may hint at an underlying dermal tumor such as a dermatofibroma.

Papillomatosis (from the Latin word *papula*, which means 'nipple') refers to the upward projections of the dermal papillae. Papillomatosis is a consequence of epidermal hyperplasia. It may result in undulations of the epidermal surface.

Hyperplastic / acanthotic epidermis	2.1

Differential diagnoses

With squamous dysplasia

Hypertrophic actinic keratosis	2.2
Bowen's disease	2.3
Bowenoid papulosis	2.4
Condyloma acuminatum	2.5
Squamous cell carcinoma	2.6
Keratoacanthoma	2.7

Without squamous dysplasia

Seborrheic keratosis, acanthotic type	2.8
Epidermal nevus	2.9
Clear cell acanthoma (Degos' acanthoma)	2.10

With inflammatory infiltrate

Subacute and chronic dermatitis	2.11
Mycosis fungoides	2.12
Deep fungal infection	2.13
Chondrodermatitis nodularis chronica helicis	2.14
Psoriasis	2.15
Lichen planus	2.16

With dermal tumor

Dermatofibroma (fibrous histiocytoma)	2.17
Granular cell tumor	2.18
Eccrine poroma / hidroacanthoma simplex	2.19
Nevocellular nevus	2.20
Melanoma	2.21

2.1 Hyperplastic / acanthotic epidermis

♦ in psoriasis, the acanthosis is regular and marked in established lesions

♦ elongated, club-shaped, dermal papillae are seen projecting upwards into the thickened epidermis

♦ small round 'islands' of dermis (arrows) represent cross-sections of dermal papillae and their presence is indicative of papillomatosis

WITH SQUAMOUS DYSPLASIA

2.2 Hypertrophic actinic keratosis

♦ epidermal thickening and parakeratosis in hypertrophic lesions

♦ squamous cells show nuclear enlargement (increased nuclear:cytoplasmic ratio), nuclear pleomorphism, hyperchromasia, dyskeratosis, and increased and abnormal mitoses

♦ actinic keratoses are precancerous, rough, scaly, reddish-brown macules and papules on sun-exposed skin

♦ induration at the base suggests malignant change

2.3 Bowen's disease

♦ dysplastic squamous cells are confined to the epidermis and adnexal epithelium

♦ dermis is not invaded (squamous carcinoma in situ)

♦ Bowenoid features include nuclear enlargement, hyperchromasia, and pleomorphism of epidermal cells, dyskeratosis, increased mitotic activity, and presence of numerous abnormal mitotic figures

♦ clinically, a slowly enlarging, erythematous, sharply demarcated patch with serrated 'notched' margins, typically on the trunk and extremities

♦ clinical differential diagnosis: dermatophytosis; psoriasis; nummular dermatitis; and discoid LE

2.4 Bowenoid papulosis

♦ identical microscopic features to Bowen's disease, but on genital skin

♦ multiple, small, red- to tan-colored papules on the penis and vulva give a cobblestone appearance

♦ associated with the human papillomavirus

♦ bowenoid papulosis may spontaneously regress

♦ distinguished from Bowen's disease by clinical appearance and occurrence in a younger age group

♦ clinical differential diagnosis includes condyloma, skin tags, and seborrheic keratoses (rarely on genitalia)

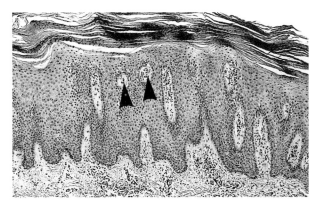

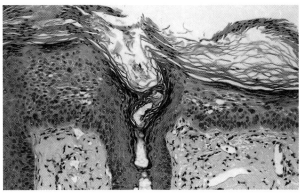

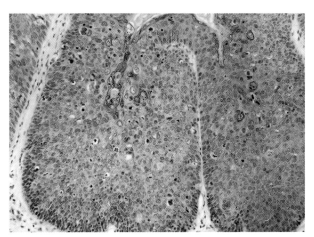

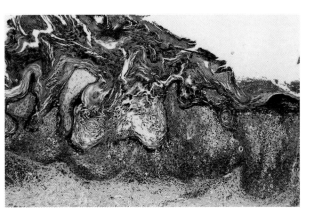

2.5 Condyloma acuminatum

♦ verrucous epidermal hyperplasia is marked
♦ papillomatosis
♦ focal parakeratosis and some degree of hypergranulosis are usually present
♦ in contrast to cervical condylomata, koilocytosis (enlarged vacuolated nuclei) may be subtle
♦ a condyloma is a warty lesion on genital skin caused by the human papillomavirus (usually types 6, 11, 18, 45 or 56)
♦ clinical differential diagnosis: seborrheic keratoses (uncommon in this area); skin tags; and condylomata lata from secondary syphilis

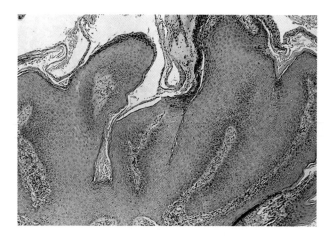

2.6 Squamous cell carcinoma

♦ thickening of the epidermis due to proliferation of malignant squamous cells
♦ cytologic atypia is accompanied by infiltrative growth (ragged margins) of squamous cells into the reticular dermis
♦ 'keratin pearls' (arrow) are common in well-differentiated tumors
♦ macroscopically, there is an indurated flesh-colored to reddish-brown, hyperkeratotic, scaly papule or nodule which may be ulcerated

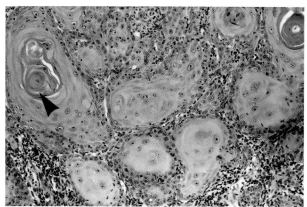

2.7 Keratoacanthoma

♦ rapidly growing, benign squamous tumor that mimics squamous cell carcinoma clinically and histologically
♦ architecture is important for diagnosis, so the entire lesion should be biopsied; if not possible, then a wedge biopsy from the center of the lesion, including the edge on at least one side, should be taken
♦ epidermis extends around a central keratin-filled crater
♦ squamous cells have abundant eosinophilic 'ground-glass' cytoplasm
♦ 'pushing' smooth margins in contrast to a squamous cell carcinoma
♦ single and small groups of apoptotic keratinocytes with pyknotic nuclei and condensed cytoplasm are often present, especially in involuting lesions
♦ necrotic keratinocytes are associated with a neutrophilic infiltrate
♦ heavy inflammatory cellular infiltration of the dermis
♦ fibrous dermal scarring in regressing lesion
♦ clinically, it presents on areas of chronic sun-exposure as a rapidly growing, firm, dome-shaped nodule with a central keratotic plug

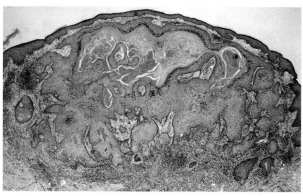

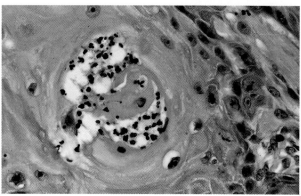

WITHOUT SQUAMOUS DYSPLASIA

2.8 Seborrheic keratosis, acanthotic type
- a benign tumor of keratinocytes resulting in marked thickening of the epidermis
- squamous cells and smaller basaloid cells
- keratin tunnels are 'pseudohorn cysts', formed by papillomatous epidermal hyperplasia
- hyperkeratosis is common
- when the lesion is irritated, parakeratosis is present
- brown warty papules and plaques commonly seen in people age > 50 years on the trunk, limbs, and face
- clinical differential diagnosis: melanocytic nevi; flat warts; lentigines; and actinic keratosis

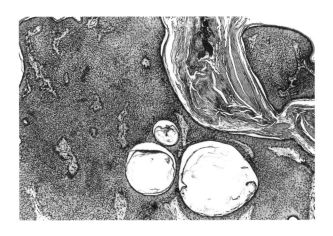

2.9 Epidermal nevus
- also known as hard nevus of Unna, soft epidermal nevus, verrucous nevus, linear nevus, and systematized nevus
- histologically similar to hyperkeratotic seborrheic keratosis and acanthosis nigricans
- lymphocytic infiltrate in inflammatory linear verrucous epidermal nevus
- flesh-colored, yellow, or brown linear or swirled papules and plaques with a warty or velvety surface presenting at birth or in childhood
- association with skeletal deformities, epilepsy, mental retardation
- diagnosis usually made clinically; biopsy rarely required; on the head, may be confused with a nevus sebaceus, which shows abnormal follicular structures

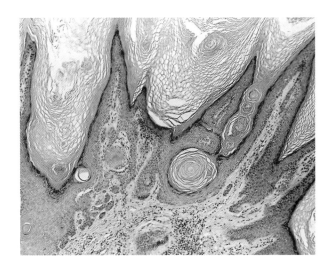

2.10 Clear cell acanthoma (Degos' acanthoma)
- acanthotic epidermis is due to the abnormal presence of well-demarcated masses of keratinocytes with pale-staining cytoplasm
- the clear cytoplasm of these abnormal keratinocytes is due to accumulation of glycogen; the cells are thus PAS-positive and diastase-sensitive (stain disappears after diastase treatment)
- neutrophilic exocytosis is often observed in this benign tumor
- moist, solitary, red, nodular tumor 1–2 cm, with a thin crust, commonly located on the shin in adults
- diagnosis is rarely made clinically; may be mistaken clinically for an amelanotic melanoma

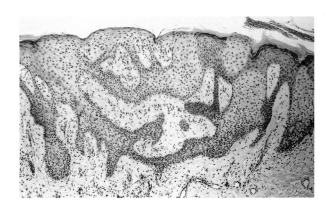

WITH INFLAMMATORY INFILTRATE

2.11 Subacute and chronic dermatitis
♦ dermatitis of several weeks' duration, especially if excoriated, shows epidermal hyperplasia
♦ uniform squamous cells, but with parakeratosis, spongiosis, and exocytosis of lymphocytes
♦ slight perivascular lymphocytic infiltration of the superficial dermal vessels

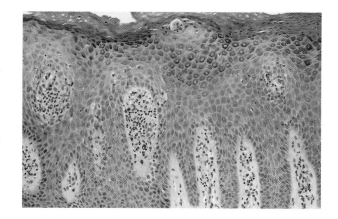

2.12 Mycosis fungoides
♦ epidermis may be acanthotic rather than atrophic
♦ epidermotropic lymphocytes with perinuclear halos along the basal epidermis
♦ Pautrier's abscess refers to clusters of three or more of these lymphocytes
♦ minimal spongiosis
♦ recalcitrant eczematous patches, plaques, tumors, or generalized erythroderma

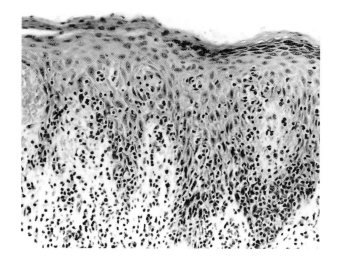

2.13 Deep fungal infection
♦ irregular or so-called pseudoepitheliomatous epidermal hyperplasia is common with deep fungal infections
♦ infiltrative downgrowth of epidermis mimics squamous cell carcinoma
♦ critical evaluation for dysplastic cytologic and nuclear changes, and differentiation from inflammatory atypia is required to rule out squamous cell carcinoma
♦ granulomatous reaction (multinucleated giant cell, arrow) and suppuration in dermis favor infection, although keratin in squamous cell carcinomas may also incite a granulomatous inflammatory response
♦ clinicopathologic correlation is helpful, but the finding of fungal organisms is diagnostic

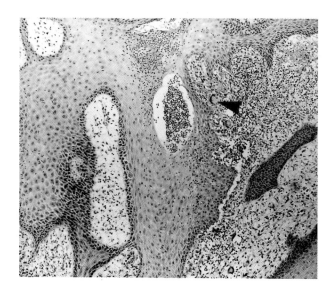

2.14 Chondrodermatitis nodularis chronica helicis

♦ hyperkeratosis and irregular hyperplasia of epidermis

♦ epidermal ulcer usually present with degenerated cartilage (arrow)

♦ increased vascularity of dermis and presence of dilated vessels with aggregates of glomus cells

♦ lymphocytic and neutrophilic infiltrates, especially if ulcerated

♦ presents as an inflammatory, painful, scaly or crusted, firm, small nodule, usually on the upper pole of the helix

♦ squamous cell carcinoma is both a gross and microscopic differential diagnosis

♦ clinically must also be differentiated from basal cell carcinomas, actinic keratoses, seborrheic keratoses, keratoacanthoma, and warts

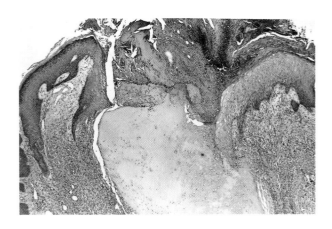

2.15 Psoriasis

♦ acute lesions may not show the typical uniform hyperplasia and elongation of epidermal rete ridges

♦ thinning of the suprapapillary epidermis explains the clinical Auspitz sign (when scales are removed, small bleeding points arise where the thin suprapapillary epithelium is torn off)

♦ congested, prominent, vertically oriented vessels in the club-shaped dermal papillae; exocytosis of neutrophils and microabscesses

♦ well-defined, erythematous, scaly plaques typically on elbows, knees, sacrum, and scalp

♦ clinical differential diagnosis: dermatophytosis; pityriasis rosea; lichen simplex chronicus; Bowen's disease; squamous cell carcinoma; secondary syphilis; LE; and mycosis fungoides

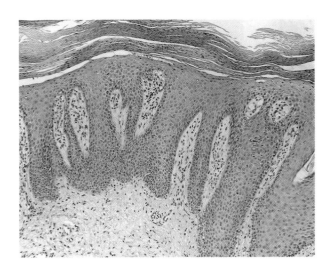

2.16 Lichen planus

♦ except for the ulcerative and atrophic types, there is typical 'saw-tooth' epidermal hyperplasia

♦ band-like lymphocytic infiltrate obscures the epidermodermal junction; colloid bodies are present

♦ clinically, purple polygonal, pruritic, planar papules with white, lacy, Wickham's striae on lower extremities, and flexor aspects of the wrists and forearms; may be generalized; oral and genital involvement common; may show nail changes

♦ clinically may mimic psoriasis, lichen simplex chronicus, lichen amyloidosus, and lichen sclerosus

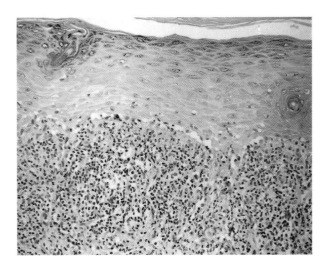

WITH DERMAL TUMOR

2.17 Dermatofibroma (fibrous histiocytoma)

♦ epidermal acanthosis and basal hyperpigmentation often present

♦ elongated hyperpigmented rete ridges (arrow) have been compared to 'dirty fingers'

♦ these features differentiate dermatofibroma from dermatofibrosarcoma protuberans

♦ occasionally, basaloid hyperplasia in acanthotic epidermis may histologically mimic a superficial basal cell carcinoma (reddish-brown scaly patch); however, clinical appearances of these two conditions differ

♦ fibrohistiocytic cellular proliferation in dermis

♦ presents most commonly on the lower legs as firm reddish-brown papules or nodules with ill-defined borders that fade into normal skin

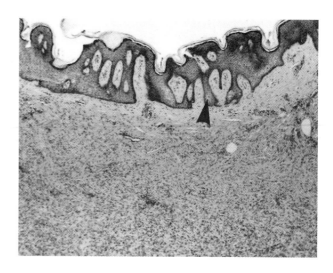

2.18 Granular cell tumor

♦ epidermal hyperplasia may be marked in some lesions; thus, a superficial biopsy may erroneously suggest a squamous cell carcinoma, especially with a mucosal lesion

♦ benign tumor of Schwann cell origin, S100 protein-positive

♦ cytoplasmic granules are secondary lysosomes which are PAS-positive and diastase-resistant

♦ rounded, uniform, central nuclei

♦ ubiquitous tumor that is almost always benign, and may present on the tongue and skin

♦ solitary or multiple, firm, pink to brown nodule(s)

♦ may have a warty and/or ulcerated surface

♦ multiple lesions may have an autosomal-dominant inheritance

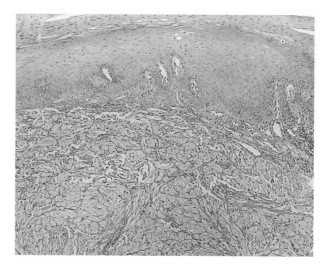

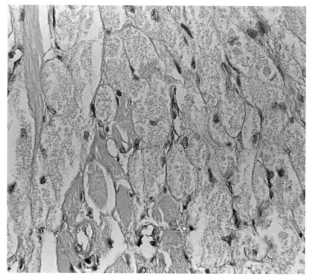

2.19 Eccrine poroma

♦ adenoma of the intraepidermal portion of the eccrine duct
♦ originates from the epidermis, causing apparent epidermal thickening
♦ there are broad columns of uniform squamoid cells expanding the epidermis, and islands of similar cells in the dermis
♦ if the proliferation is entirely intraepidermal, it is referred to as **hidroacanthoma simplex**
♦ as in any eccrine gland adenoma, ductular and cystic structures lined by PAS-positive cuticle may be seen
♦ usually a flesh-colored or erythematous solitary tumor on the sole, but may be seen wherever there are eccrine glands

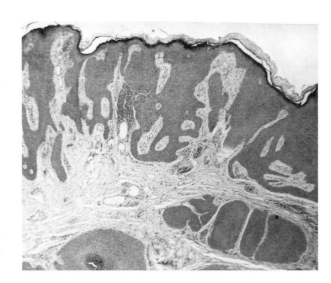

2.20 Nevocellular nevus

♦ papillomatosis and papillary epidermal hyperplasia are very common in compound and intradermal nevi, and Spitz nevi
♦ hyperkeratosis and keratin tunnels are sometimes present
♦ melanocytic nevic cell nests often surrounded by hyperplastic epidermis
♦ intradermal nevi are well-demarcated, flesh-colored to brown, uniform papules

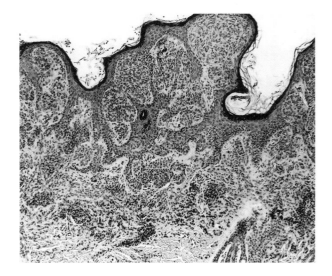

2.21 Melanoma

♦ epidermal hyperplasia is often seen with malignant melanoma
♦ irregular pseudoepitheliomatous epidermal hyperplasia is seen with a spindle cell malignant melanoma
♦ unlike ulceration, the epidermal hyperplasia has no prognostic relevance
♦ atypical melanocytes with hyperchromatic nuclei are seen infiltrating the dermis (arrow)
♦ clinically, asymmetric papule or nodule with irregular borders and variegated color

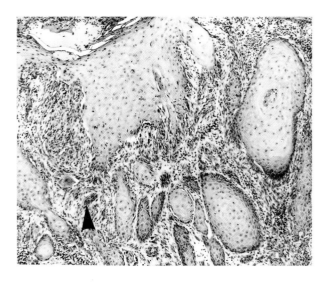

ATROPHY AND ULCER

Atrophy of the epidermis refers to a decrease in the number and / or size of the cells in the spinous layer. This results in thinning of the epidermis and is often accompanied by shortening or even absence of the rete ridges. An atrophic epidermis may be transparent; fine wrinkling may be present and the normal skin lines may or may not be retained. Attenuation of the epidermis is common with many benign and malignant tumors of the dermis. Atrophy may be a consequence of preceding inflammation (for example, discoid LE), injury (such as radiation), or ischemia.

An **ulcer** is the loss of the epidermis and at least part of the superficial dermis. If only the superficial layers or all of the epidermis are lost, it is referred to as an **erosion**. Regenerative epidermal hyperplasia is often seen at the edges of an ulcer.

An atrophic epidermis is more prone to ulceration, especially if the atrophy is a consequence of a rapidly growing tumor. Malignancy should always be considered, in addition to infectious, inflammatory, vascular or traumatic causes, when assessing ulcers.

ATROPHY

3.1 Atrophic epidermis
♦ atrophic epidermis overlying recent fibrous and vascular scar tissue
♦ thickness of squamous cell layer is only one or two cells thick
♦ note also the hyperkeratosis and parakeratosis on the skin surface

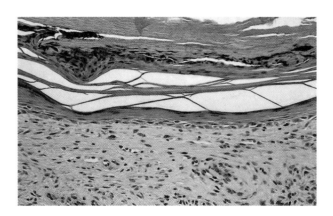

3.2 Ulcer
♦ loss of entire epidermis in a chronic ischemic skin ulcer
♦ layers of necrotic cellular debris, inflammatory exudate, granulation tissue, and underlying fibrous tissue form the base of the ulcer
♦ epidermal hyperplasia and parakeratosis are common features of the ulcer edge

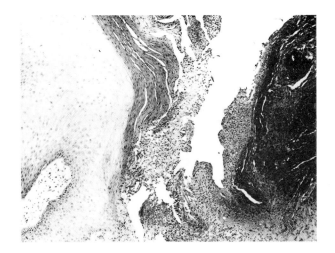

WITH INFLAMMATION

3.3 Atrophic actinic keratosis
♦ focal parakeratosis is common in actinic keratoses
♦ thinned epidermis with squamous dysplasia is evident
♦ squamous cells in the lower epidermis are in disarray and may have enlarged nuclei
♦ amorphous dermal solar elastosis and dilated blood vessels are evident

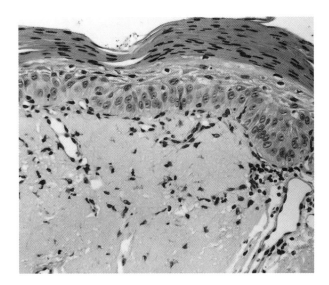

3.4 Atrophic lichen planus
♦ thinned epidermis rather than the characteristic saw-tooth hyperplasia typical of lichen planus; may be ulcerated
♦ hyperkeratosis and hypergranulosis may not be striking
♦ basal cell degeneration, pigmentary incontinence, and band-like lymphocytic infiltrate are present
♦ neutrophil and plasma cell infiltration with secondary infection commonly seen in mucosal **erosive lichen planus**, a chronic painful condition primarily involving the oral mucosa and tongue
♦ lichen planus, particularly the erosive type, may be associated with hepatitis C infection
♦ biopsy rules out squamous cell carcinoma and differentiates from vesiculobullous conditions, such as pemphigus and cicatricial pemphigoid

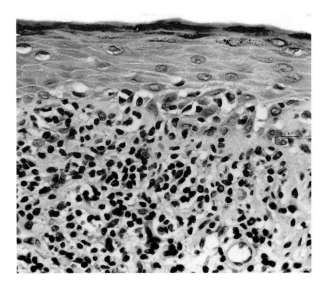

3.5 Lichen nitidus

♦ overlying epidermis is atrophic centrally
♦ compact hyperkeratosis
♦ an epidermal collarette is sometimes present
♦ vacuolar degeneration of the basal cell layer
♦ lichenoid inflammatory cell infiltrate with giant cells
  (giant cells are not seen in lichen planus)
♦ clinically manifested as pinpoint-sized (1–2 mm in diameter), shiny, flat-topped, flesh-colored papules that
  are the result of the nodular infiltrate in the superficial dermis
♦ usually, multiple asymptomatic papules on the penis,
  flexor aspects of arms, and lower abdomen
♦ clinical differential diagnosis: lichen planus (larger size,
  no giant cells); flat warts (vacuolated cytoplasm of
  keratinocytes and eosinophilic cytoplasmic inclusions); bowenoid papulosis (dysplastic squamous
  cells); keratosis pilaris (dilated hair follicle with
  keratotic plug and sometimes a twisted hair); lichen
  spinulosus (patches of keratotic follicular papules,
  dilated hair follicle with keratotic plug); lichen striatus (linear eruption in children, dermatitic histologic appearance without acanthosis); lichen amyloidosus (Congo red staining of amyloid deposits);
  sarcoidosis (granulomas)

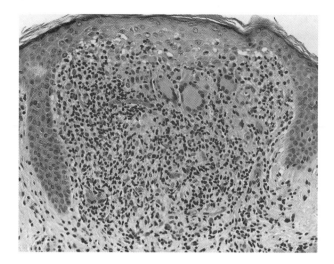

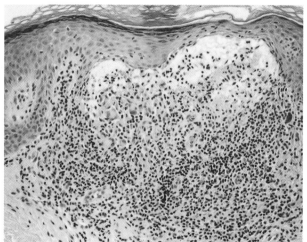

3.6 Lichen sclerosus et atrophicus

♦ hyperkeratosis, epidermal atrophy, basal cell degeneration and follicular plugging
♦ eosinophilic homogenization of the superficial dermis
  is characteristic
♦ hyperkeratotic, flat-topped, white, polygonal papules
  with follicular plugging on female or male genitalia,
  or extragenital sites
♦ may coalesce to form plaques resembling morphea
♦ atrophy with 'cigarette-paper wrinkling' is common in
  chronic lesions; erosions are common in atrophic
  lesions
♦ vulvar 'figure-of-eight' distribution in middle-aged
  women and children
♦ biopsy is usually taken to differentiate the condition
  from squamous cell carcinoma or morphea

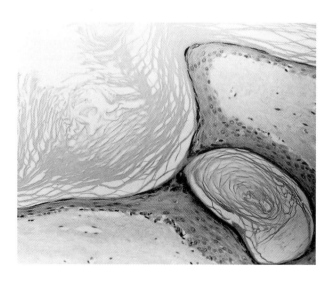

3.7 Lupus erythematosus (LE)

♦ most lesions, especially chronic ones, show hyper-keratosis, epidermal atrophy, and hyaline thickening of the basement membrane (arrow)

♦ atrophy is usually seen centrally in chronic lesions

♦ epidermal changes are similar to those observed in lichen planus and lichen sclerosus

♦ lymphocytic infiltrate is perivascular and periadnexal, and may be band-like

♦ discoid lesions are reddish-brown to violaceous plaques with hyperkeratosis and central atrophy; they occur most commonly on the face and scalp

♦ subacute cutaneous LE lesions are annular with a slight scale

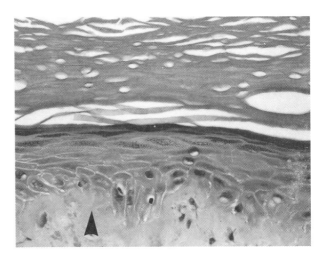

3.8 Chronic radiation dermatitis

♦ epidermal atrophy is irregular and may alternate with hyperplastic, hyperkeratotic areas; ulceration may be present in severe cases

♦ squamous dysplastic change is common

♦ there is hyaline change of superficial dermal collagen with reactive stellate fibroblasts

♦ superficial telangiectatic vessels; endothelial cells may have foamy cytoplasm and enlarged nuclei

♦ thrombi may be seen

♦ risk of invasive carcinoma is well documented, and a biopsy is usually taken to rule out malignant degeneration

♦ clinical features: thinned, hairless skin; hyper- and hypopigmentation; scaling; induration; and telangiectasia

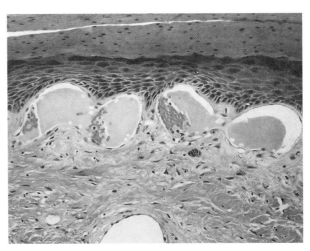

3.9 Porokeratosis

♦ center is atrophic whereas the advancing edge shows a parakeratotic cell column, the 'cornoid lamella'

♦ biopsy from the center shows epidermal atrophy, pigmentary incontinence, and mild lymphocytic infiltration of the dermis

♦ clinically, one or more annular, sharply demarcated lesion(s) with a peripheral wafer-like horny ridge

♦ disseminated superficial actinic porokeratosis may be confused clinically with, but differentiated histologically from, actinic keratosis, flat seborrheic keratosis, or flat warts

♦ when sampling lesions suspected of porokeratosis, it is essential that the edge of the lesion be included so that the characteristic 'cornoid lamella' may be seen

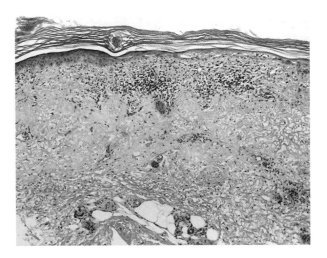

WITH DERMAL TUMOR

3.10 Benign fibrous papule of the face

♦ overlying atrophic epidermis with slight hyperkeratosis is shown here

♦ stellate and plump fibroblasts are seen with dilated dermal vessels

♦ perivascular and periadnexal fibrous tissue replaces normal collagen fibers

♦ solitary, firm, dome-shaped, flesh-colored papule 2–3 mm in diameter, seen commonly on the nose

♦ clinical differential diagnosis: basal cell carcinoma; sebaceous hyperplasia; and intradermal nevus

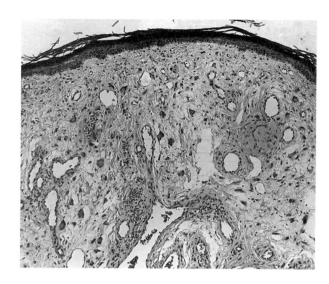

3.11 Nodular basal cell carcinoma (BCC)

♦ an ulcer is shown here overlying nodules of basal cell carcinoma, which infiltrate the dermis and extend to the bottom margin

♦ inflammatory exudate is present at the ulcer base and tumor surface

♦ pink translucent papule or nodule with telangiectasia

♦ ulceration is common in larger BCCs

♦ common on sun-exposed skin, BCCs may also occur on genitalia and on non-sun-exposed skin

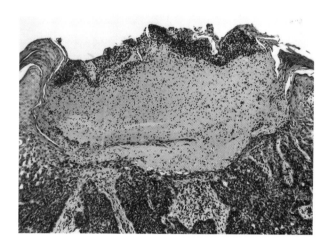

3.12 Capillary hemangioma

♦ overlying atrophic epidermis

♦ a collarette (epidermal downgrowth at the periphery) is often seen, but has little diagnostic significance

♦ endothelial proliferation with some capillary lumina, nuclear enlargement, and mitoses are not uncommon in actively growing lesions

♦ satellite nodules of capillaries may be seen around the main tumor and a few lesions may recur after local excision; these features should not be taken as signs of malignant change

♦ absence of ulceration and inflammation suggests capillary hemangioma instead of **pyogenic granuloma**, a histologically similar benign vascular proliferation occurring in children and adults, often following trauma

♦ capillary hemangiomas are present at birth or onset in infancy, grow rapidly for the first year, then involute in most cases

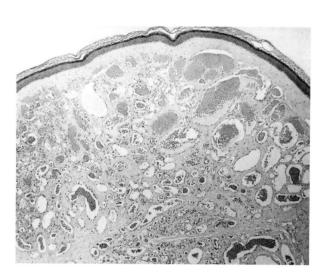

ACANTHOLYSIS

Acantholysis refers to the separation of spinous cells due to dissolution of desmosomal junctions. Pemphigus vulgaris and Hailey–Hailey disease are the prototypical acantholytic dermatoses. The former is due to autoantibody-mediated destruction of the desmosomes whereas the latter is due to a genetic defect of the desmosomal complex. The result is the formation of flaccid vesicles and bullae. Within these blisters, free-floating rounded eosinophilic cells with central nuclei are seen, referred to as 'acantholytic cells', which may be seen on Tzanck smear preparations: the floor of the vesicle is gently scraped; the scrapings are placed on a glass slide, and stained with Wright's or Giemsa stain before examination.

Loss of cell cohesion may also be due to cell necrosis, as seen in herpetic vesicles. This has been referred to as secondary acantholysis. Typical acantholytic cells with rounded eosinophilic cell bodies are not observed in secondary acantholysis.

Identification of the level of acantholysis within the epidermis is the key to the differential diagnosis of these disorders. When taking a biopsy from a blistering dermatosis, it is preferable to biopsy a complete intact blister. If the lesions are large, the biopsy should be taken from the edge of the blister so that the roof of the blister and level of the split can be seen. It is more difficult to make a diagnosis if only the floor of the blister is seen, especially if there is secondary infection and / or regeneration.

Some of the blistering diseases are associated with specific antibody and complement deposition. Immunofluorescent studies of perilesional skin (direct immunofluorescence) and serum (indirect immunofluorescence) may be of help in the diagnosis of these conditions. Biopsy specimens for direct immunofluorescence should be transported in Michel's medium, not in formalin.

Acantholytic cells	4.1

Differential diagnoses

Acantholysis involving all layers of the epidermis

Hailey–Hailey disease (familial benign pemphigus)	4.2
Grover's disease (transient acantholytic dermatosis)	4.3

Acantholysis confined to the superficial epidermis

Pemphigus foliaceus, fogo selvagem	4.4
Subcorneal pustular dermatosis (bullous impetigo, staphylococcal scalded skin syndrome)	4.5

Acantholysis confined to the suprabasilar layers

Pemphigus vulgaris	4.6
Pemphigus vegetans	4.7
Darier's disease (keratosis follicularis)	4.8
Warty dyskeratoma (isolated dyskeratosis follicularis)	4.9
Actinic keratosis	4.10
Adenoid (acantholytic) squamous cell carcinoma	4.11
Incidental focal acantholytic dyskeratosis	4.12

4.1 Acantholytic cells

♦ acantholytic vesicles form as a result of squamous cell separation

♦ keratinocytes of the prickle cell layer lose their intercellular bridges and desmosomal cell junctions

♦ acantholytic cells are rounded with central nuclei and a rim of condensed eosinophilic cytoplasm

♦ unlike spongiosis, the space between acantholytic cells is prominent, and inflammatory cells are sparse

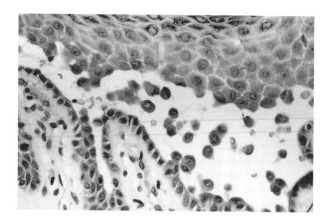

ACANTHOLYSIS INVOLVING ALL LAYERS OF THE EPIDERMIS

4.2 Hailey–Hailey disease (familial benign pemphigus)

♦ acantholysis of the squamous cell layer is usually extensive and often involves the full thickness of epidermis

♦ resembles a dilapidated brick wall

♦ blister is intraepidermal

♦ rounded acantholytic cells with condensed eosinophilic cytoplasm are numerous within the blister

♦ dyskeratotic keratinocytes (corps ronds and grains) are rarely seen compared with Darier's disease

♦ inflammation is present only with superimposed bacterial infection

♦ autosomal-dominant with flaccid blisters and crusts in intertriginous areas and neck

♦ clinical differential diagnosis: impetigo (positive bacterial culture); pemphigus vulgaris or vegetans; and Darier's disease

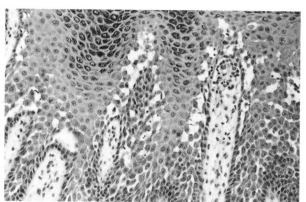

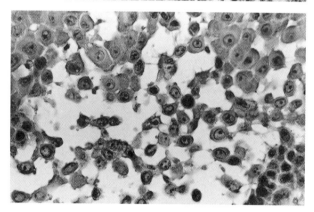

4.3 Grover's disease (transient acantholytic dermatosis)

♦ as the name implies, acantholysis is the characteristic finding

♦ acantholysis is focal and microscopic, unlike Hailey–Hailey disease

♦ level of epidermal involvement varies from suprabasilar to the entire squamous cell layer

♦ may show dyskeratotic cells similar to that of Darier's disease

♦ lymphocytic infiltration of the dermis and parakeratosis are often seen; eosinophils are usually sparse and there is no eosinophilic spongiosis

(continued next page)

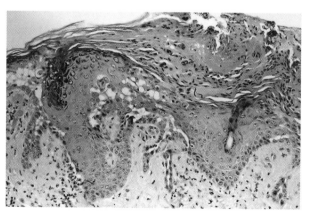

- multiple itchy papules and occasionally papulovesicles on the trunk and thighs in people >40 years of age
- clinical differential diagnosis: folliculitis; bites; and dermatitis
- diagnosis should be considered when lesions demonstrate mixed or variable acantholytic foci that mimic pemphigus, or Hailey–Hailey or Darier's disease
- note the microscopic and focal nature of the acantholysis
- microscopic focus of acantholysis associated with dyskeratosis resembles Darier's disease histologically, but the latter is usually not in the clinical differential diagnosis (scaly crusted papules in 'seborrheic areas', V-shaped nicking of the nails, punctate keratoses on the palms and soles are seen in Darier's disease)

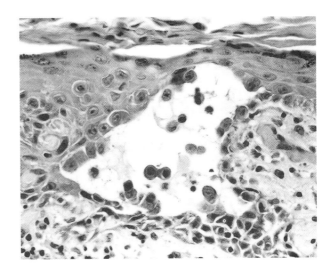

ACANTHOLYSIS CONFINED TO THE SUPERFICIAL EPIDERMIS

4.4 Pemphigus foliaceus
- acantholysis involves the superficial epidermis and may be confined to the subcorneal (granular) layer
- as a result, intact blisters are rarely seen clinically as the roof of the blister is fragile and readily denuded, and the superficial blisters are prone to erosion
- eosinophilic infiltration and spongiosis may be the only changes seen in biopsies of early lesions
- presence of acantholysis differentiates this from spongiotic dermatitis and should be looked for among the squamous cells forming the floor of the lesion
- secondary infection, inflammation, and epidermal hyperplasia may be seen
- direct immunofluorescence shows intercellular C3 and IgG autoantibodies
- recurrent crops of superficial erythematous crusted erosions are seen on the face, scalp, and trunk
- mucosal involvement is rare (unlike pemphigus vulgaris)
- endemic Brazilian variant (**fogo selvagem**)
- clinically may resemble impetigo (and pustular positive bacterial culture), seborrheic dermatitis (no acantholysis)

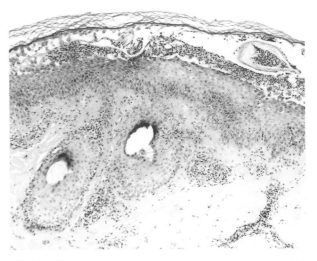

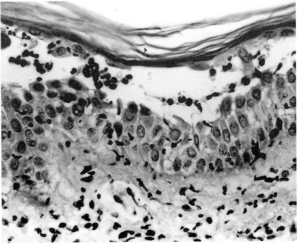

4.5 Subcorneal pustular dermatosis

♦ skin lesion of bullous impetigo (upper picture) shows a subcorneal collection of neutrophils

♦ acantholysis of the superficial epidermis is sometimes seen in subcorneal pustular lesions

♦ acantholytic squamous cell (lower picture, arrow) is seen among the polymorphonuclear leukocytes

♦ **bullous impetigo**, **staphylococcal scalded skin syndrome**, and **subcorneal pustular dermatosis (Sneddon–Wilkinson disease)** are subcorneal pustular skin lesions that may have identical histopathologic appearances; the occasional acantholytic cell is seen within the pustules

♦ neutrophilic nature of the infiltrate and clinical presentation help to differentiate this group of diseases from the true acantholytic skin lesions

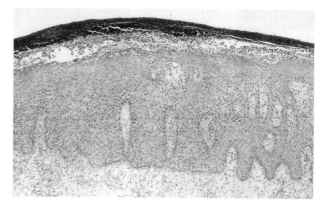

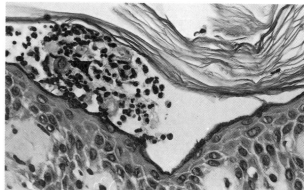

ACANTHOLYSIS CONFINED TO THE SUPRABASILAR LAYERS

4.6 Pemphigus vulgaris

♦ suprabasal cleft with basal cells adherent to the underlying basement membrane, but separate from one another, resembling a row of tombstones

♦ slight inflammation with occasional eosinophils in early lesions

♦ established lesions show considerable inflammation, eosinophils, and plasma cells

♦ intercellular IgG and C3 seen with direct immunofluorescence

♦ circulating IgG seen with indirect immunofluorescence

♦ mucosal involvement is common

♦ flaccid blisters on the skin break readily, leaving areas of denudation

♦ positive Nikolsky (separation of epidermis from dermis when lateral pressure is applied to normal-looking skin) and Asboe–Hansen (pressure applied directly over the surface of the intact blister produces lateral spread of the lesion) signs

♦ increased incidence in Jewish and Mediterranean populations

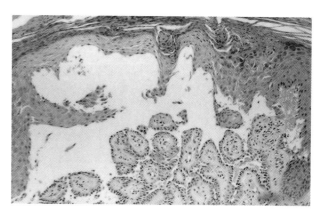

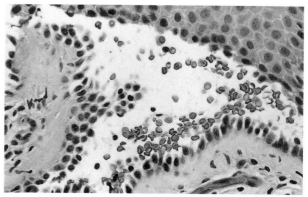

4.7 Pemphigus vegetans

♦ variant of pemphigus vulgaris sharing the common feature of suprabasilar acantholysis

♦ marked verrucous epidermal hyperplasia; the long-standing lesion shown here has an inflammatory exudate on the surface (upper picture, arrow)

♦ this section shows characteristic eosinophilic pustules within the epidermis

♦ eosinophilic spongiosis and eosinophilic intraepidermal abscesses are characteristic; a few nuclei of acantholytic cells (lower picture, arrows) are present among the eosinophils

♦ suprabasilar acantholysis may be focal and subtle

♦ involves intertriginous areas and oral mucosa

♦ may start as pemphigus vulgaris with flaccid weeping vesicles showing little epidermal change with healing; the lesions then become hyperkeratotic and papillomatous with pustules at the periphery

♦ intertriginous lesions resemble Hailey–Hailey disease clinically

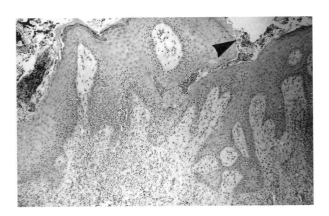

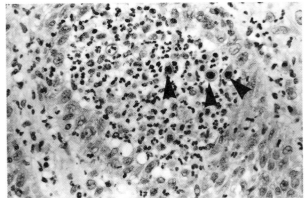

4.8 Darier's disease (keratosis follicularis)

♦ suprabasilar spaces or lacunae are the result of dyskeratosis and acantholysis

♦ no well-formed blisters with a defined 'roof' and 'floor'

♦ dyskeratosis results in corps ronds and grains

♦ grains (upper picture, large arrow) are dyskeratotic cells with shrunken nuclei and minimal cytoplasm, and may be seen within lacunae

♦ corps ronds (upper picture, small arrow) are basophilic round bodies in the superficial epidermis produced by abnormal keratinization

♦ numerous corps ronds possess condensed peripheral cytoplasm around a pyknotic nucleus imparting a halo-like appearance

♦ follicular plugging is characteristic

♦ autosomal-dominant disorder of keratinization

♦ scaly crusted papules seen in 'seborrheic areas'

♦ V-shaped nicking of nails, punctate keratoses on the palms and soles

♦ warty papules on the dorsum of the feet and hands

♦ white papules with central depression on oral mucosa

♦ clinical differential diagnosis: seborrheic dermatitis (no acantholysis); and Hailey–Hailey disease (dilapidated brick-wall appearance)

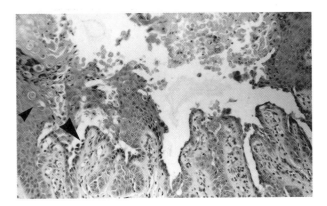

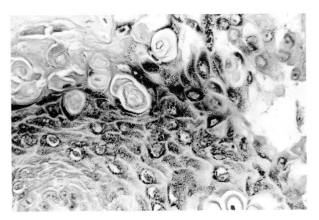

4.9 Warty dyskeratoma (isolated dyskeratosis follicularis)

♦ suprabasilar acantholysis and dyskeratosis form a central crater filled with keratinous debris and dyskeratotic cells

♦ hyperplasia of the epidermis and elongation of the rete ridges are more marked than in Darier's disease

♦ solitary papule or nodule with keratotic umbilicated center

♦ usually found on the head and neck

♦ small papule without the typical central crater of a warty dyskeratoma, but showing acantholytic dyskeratosis, has been called a **focal acantholytic dyskeratoma**

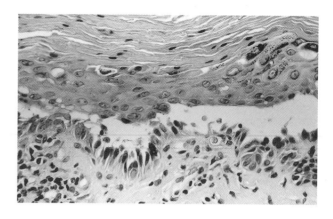

4.10 Actinic keratosis

♦ focal suprabasilar acantholysis is common

♦ nuclear pleomorphism and hyperchromasia in the acantholytic cells or adjacent squamous cells

♦ elastosis and lymphocytic infiltration of the dermis

♦ reddish-brown, rough, scaly macule on sun-exposed skin, especially the face and backs of the hands

♦ usually not difficult to identify clinically, but may mimic seborrheic keratosis, basal cell carcinoma, porokeratosis and squamous cell carcinoma

♦ does not clinically resemble other conditions with acantholysis

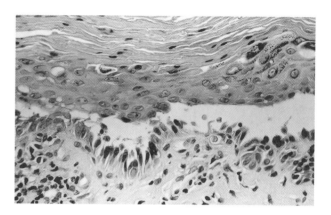

4.11 Adenoid (acantholytic) squamous cell carcinoma

♦ pseudoglandular, tubular, and alveolar structures formed from acantholytic neoplastic keratinocytes

♦ nuclear pleomorphism and hyperchromasia, and dyskeratosis are visible using higher magnifications

♦ usually no difficulty in recognizing the squamous origin of the tumor

♦ primary adenocarcinomas of the skin are rare; the majority are of adnexal gland origin

♦ adenoid squamous cell carcinoma does not have distinguishing clinical features; as with other squamous cell carcinomas, it is a reddish-brown scaly papule or nodule, with or without ulceration, usually on sun-exposed skin of elderly people

♦ most are well-differentiated carcinomas, which have a better prognosis

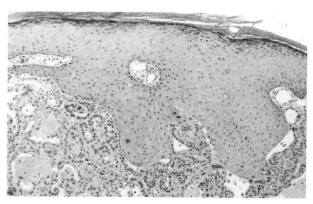

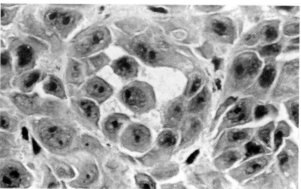

4.12 Incidental focal acantholytic dyskeratosis

♦ microscopic foci of suprabasal acantholysis with dyskeratosis may be seen in a variety of benign and malignant skin lesions, including **melanocytic nevi**, **basal cell carcinomas**, and **melanomas**

♦ shown here is a focal area of acantholysis lying adjacent to a benign nevus

♦ significance is unknown; occurrence is considered to be incidental

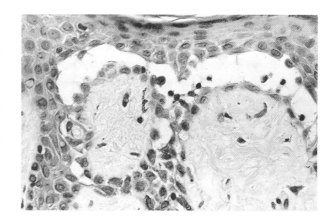

DYSKERATOSIS AND DYSPLASIA

Dyskeratosis refers to the faulty, premature keratinization of individual squamous cells. Two types are described:

Acantholytic dyskeratosis is dyskeratosis secondary to acantholysis. It does not imply malignancy. Characteristic cells include corps ronds and grains: corps ronds are present in Darier's disease and warty dyskeratoma, and have a large pyknotic nucleus surrounded by a clear halo and an outer rim of condensed basophilic cytoplasm; grains have a small pyknotic nucleus and a scant amount of cytoplasm, and are seen most commonly in the superficial layers of the epidermis. Except for these abnormal cells, nuclear pleomorphism and dysplastic features are absent in the surrounding epidermis in acantholytic dyskeratosis.

Neoplastic dyskeratosis is abnormal keratinization seen in precancerous and cancerous lesions such as actinic keratosis, Bowen's disease and squamous cell carcinoma. Some actinic keratoses and adenoid squamous cell carcinomas may also show acantho-

lytic dyskeratosis. Differentiating neoplastic from acantholytic dyskeratosis is seldom difficult as cytologic changes (nuclear pleomorphism and increased mitotic activity) are always seen diffusely in the former whereas individual dyskeratotic cells are usually outnumbered by normal epidermal cells in the latter.

Histopathologically, **dysplasia** describes a disorderly, yet non-invasive, proliferation of cells. It is usually encountered in descriptions of epithelial tissues, although the term has also been borrowed to describe atypical proliferations of melanocytes, such as dysplastic nevus.

Dysplasia is characterized by loss of uniformity of individual cells, pleomorphism, enlarged dark-staining nuclei, increased mitotic activity (especially above the basal layer), and loss of maturation (dyskeratosis). The process affects a large area of the epidermis (field change). Although dysplasia does not always progress to frankly invasive cancer, dysplastic squamous cells are hallmarks of a precancerous dermatosis that should be recognized and reported.

5.1 Acantholytic dyskeratosis
♦ **grains** (small arrow) are dyskeratotic cells with small
pyknotic nuclei and a scant amount of cytoplasm
seen mostly in the superficial layers of the epidermis
♦ **corps ronds** (large arrow) are dyskeratotic cells within the squamous cell layer with enlarged vesicular
nuclei surrounded by halos and an outer rim of condensed basophilic cytoplasm
♦ in this case of Darier's disease, note the relative lack
of nuclear pleomorphism and mitotic activity in the
surrounding epidermal cells

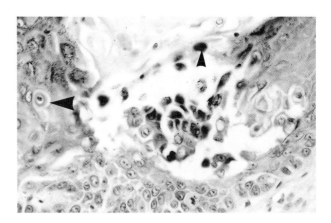

5.2 Neoplastic dyskeratosis and dysplasia
♦ dyskeratosis is often overshadowed by the increased
nuclear : cytoplasmic ratio of the epidermal cells and
the apparent cellularity of the entire epidermis as
seen here in this case of Bowen's disease
♦ there is a loss of cell uniformity, pleomorphism, and
increased mitotic activity
♦ corps ronds, when present, have atypical nuclei
♦ grains are not common in dysplastic dyskeratosis
because of nuclear enlargement

ACANTHOLYTIC DYSKERATOSIS

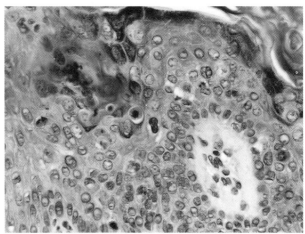

5.3 Darier's disease (keratosis follicularis)
♦ acantholytic dyskeratotic cells are characteristic
♦ multifocal change along the epidermis and prominence
of dyskeratosis help to distinguish Darier's disease
from warty dyskeratoma and Grover's disease; clinically, however, these conditions are rarely confused
♦ scaly crusted papules are seen in 'seborrheic areas',
punctate keratoses on the palms and soles, warty
papules on the dorsum of the feet and hands, V-
shaped nicking in the nails, and white papules with
central depression on the oral mucosa; inheritance
is autosomal-dominant
♦ clinical differential diagnosis: seborrheic dermatitis; and
Hailey–Hailey disease

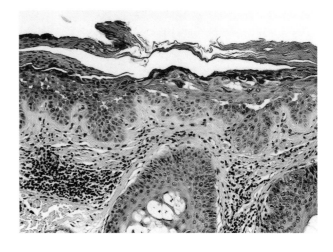

5.4 Warty dyskeratoma

♦ solitary, larger, crater-like lesion on the head and neck showing dyskeratotic cells and suprabasilar acantholysis

♦ hyperplasia of the rete ridges is usually marked (arrow)

♦ clinical differentiation from Darier's disease and Grover's disease is not a problem

♦ solitary warty papulonodule with a keratotic umbilicated center, typically on the head and neck

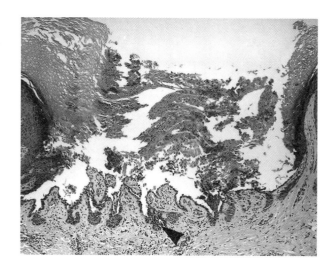

5.5 Grover's disease
(transient acantholytic dermatosis)

♦ although the histologic appearance may be identical to Darier's disease, the resemblance is only on microscopy; the clinical presentations are different

♦ Grover's disease is manifested by multiple itchy papules and, occasionally, papulovesicles on the trunk and thighs in people > 40 years of age whereas greasy crusted papules in the 'seborrheic' areas are seen in Darier's disease

♦ variable degrees of spongiosis, dyskeratosis, and extent and level of acantholysis and focal changes favor Grover's disease

♦ clinical differential diagnosis: folliculitis; bites; and dermatitis; however, on histology, these conditions are clearly distinct from each other

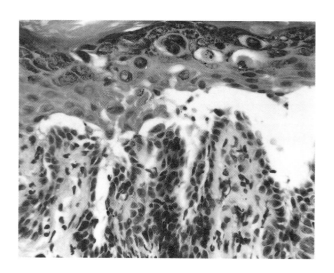

NEOPLASTIC DYSKERATOSIS AND DYSPLASIA

5.6 Bowen's disease
(squamous cell carcinoma in situ)

♦ corps ronds-like dyskeratotic cells are present, but grains are infrequent

♦ dysplastic cellular changes involving the entire thickness of the epidermis are typical

♦ as shown here, clusters of larger dysplastic cells are easily discernible as they are morphologically very different from the surrounding epidermal cells

♦ this 'clonal phenomenon of Jadassohn' may also be observed in seborrheic keratosis, Paget's disease, melanoma, and hidroacanthoma simplex

(continued next page)

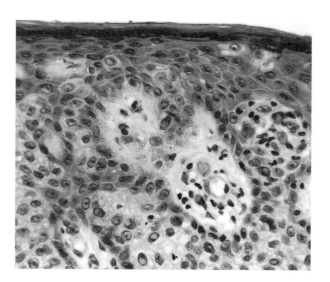

♦ single, dysplastic, squamous cells scattered throughout the thickness of the epidermis may be confused with superficial spreading melanoma or Paget's disease

♦ increased mitotic activity and abnormal mitotic figures are common

♦ parakeratosis and thickening of the epidermis are secondary to the neoplastic cell proliferation

♦ biopsy should include the dermis so that invasive carcinoma can be excluded

♦ clinically presents as a slowly enlarging, erythematous, sharply demarcated patch, commonly on the trunk and extremities

♦ clinical differential diagnosis: dermatophytosis; psoriasis; nummular dermatitis; and discoid LE

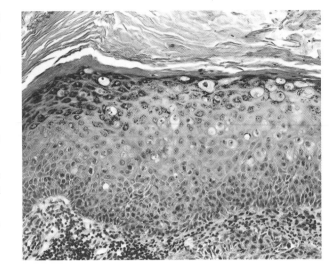

5.7 Bowenoid papulosis

♦ microscopic features are similar to those of Bowen's disease

♦ associated with the human papillomavirus

♦ multiple, small, red- to tan-colored papules on the penis and the vulva give a cobblestone appearance

♦ bowenoid papulosis may spontaneously regress

♦ bowenoid papulosis is distinguished from Bowen's disease on the basis of the clinical appearance and the younger age group affected

♦ be cautious of diagnosing Bowen's disease of the genitalia in the absence of a persistent erythematous or brown scaly patch; vulvar Bowen's disease may be multifocal, but does not usually present as multiple small papules

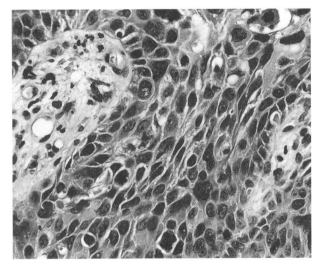

5.8 Actinic (solar) keratosis

♦ suprabasilar acantholysis with dyskeratotic cells may occasionally be seen in actinic keratosis

♦ look for dysplasia and nuclear pleomorphism

♦ parakeratosis is usually present

♦ dermis should be included in the biopsy to rule out malignant degeneration and invasion

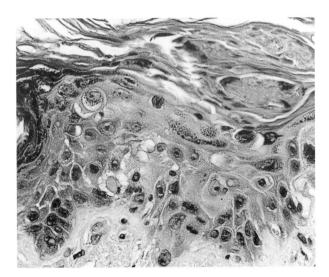

SQUAMOUS CELL DEGENERATION

An injured squamous cell often shows characteristic 'degenerative' cellular changes that suggest a cause of injury. Ballooning and reticular degeneration, koilocytosis, and formation of colloid bodies are characteristic changes of damaged keratinocytes. The first three are typically seen in viral infections.

Ballooning degeneration is an injurious change of squamous cells as a result of cytoplasmic swelling and acantholysis. It is commonly seen with herpes simplex and varicella–zoster viral infections, but may be observed in other forms of severe squamous cell injury, such as in erythema multiforme. The cell bodies become rounded and a peripheral rim of condensed cytoplasm marks the cell boundary.

Reticular degeneration, like ballooning degeneration, is common in certain viral infections, but may be also be encountered in other diseases with severe epidermal damage, such as erythema multiforme, fixed drug eruption, pityriasis lichenoides et varioliformis acuta, and acute contact dermatitis. Reticular degeneration affects a large area of the epidermis, unlike balloon cell degeneration which involves cells individually. Severe intracellular edema and cellular necrosis leave behind ghostly outlines of cell walls. These outlines form a faint eosinophilic lacy network of septa. Eventual coalescence of the smaller locules in reticulation results in intraepidermal vesicles. Clinically, these superficial vesicles rupture easily and quickly become eroded.

Koilocytosis is associated with human papillomavirus infection. The nucleus is hyperchromatic and enlarged – up to twice the size of a normal nucleus. There is vacuolation and cavitation of the cytoplasm. The cytoplasmic clearing has sharp and angulated margins.

Colloid bodies are eosinophilic degenerated keratinocytes which result from immune-mediated damage or apoptosis. When seen in lichen planus, these cells are called **Civatte bodies** whereas, in phototoxic reactions, they are termed **sunburn cells**. They are referred to as **Kamino bodies** when they occur within the junctional nests of a Spitz nevus.

Ballooning degeneration	6.1
Reticular degeneration	6.2
Koilocytosis	6.3
Colloid bodies	6.4

Differential diagnoses

Ballooning degeneration

Herpes simplex virus and varicella–zoster virus infections	6.5

Reticular degeneration

Fixed drug eruption	6.6
Hand-foot-and-mouth disease	6.7

Koilocytosis

Verruca plana	6.8
Deep palmoplantar wart	6.9

Colloid bodies

6.1 Ballooning degeneration
♦ injurious change in squamous cells as a result of cytoplasmic swelling and acantholysis
♦ commonly seen with herpes simplex and varicella–zoster virus infections, but may be observed in other forms of severe squamous cell injury, such as erythema multiforme
♦ cell bodies become rounded and a peripheral rim of condensed cytoplasm marks the cell boundary
♦ in the cytoplasm, there is a central zone of clearing, probably hydropic degeneration, creating a halo around a rounded central nucleus

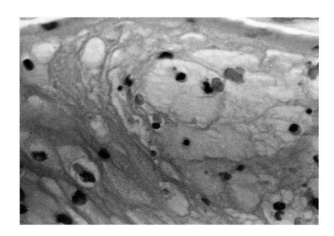

6.2 Reticular degeneration
♦ unlike balloon cell degeneration, which involves cells individually, reticular degeneration affects a large area of the epidermis
♦ severe intracellular edema and cellular necrosis leave behind ghostly outlines of cell walls, forming a faint, lacy, eosinophilic network of septa
♦ eventual coalescence of the smaller locules results in intraepidermal vesicles

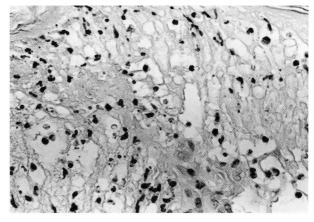

6.3 Koilocytosis
♦ koilocytosis is characteristic of human papillomavirus infection
♦ hyperchromatic and enlarged nuclei – up to twice the size of a normal nucleus
♦ vacuolation and cavitation of the cytoplasm
♦ cytoplasmic clearing shows sharp angulated margins

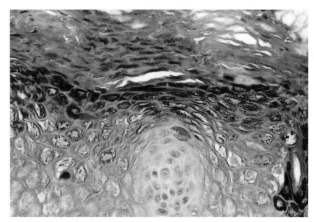

6.4 Colloid bodies

♦ eosinophilic degenerated keratinocytes are the result of immune-mediated damage or apoptosis

♦ shown here are lymphocytic exocytosis and colloid bodies at various stages of development

♦ a keratinocyte in contact with a lymphocyte in the parabasal cell layer is damaged and shows karyorrhexis and eosinophilic shrinkage of the cytoplasm

♦ fully formed colloid body (arrow) is a round hyaline mass with or without a remnant of the nucleus at the periphery

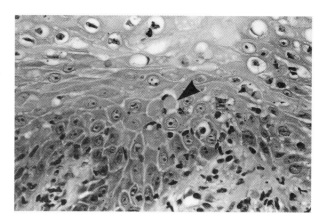

BALLOONING DEGENERATION

6.5 Herpes simplex virus infection

♦ in addition to balloon cell change, many keratinocytes have swollen 'washed-out' nuclei with an empty steel-gray center and thickened nuclear membrane

♦ multinucleated keratinocytes with prominent nuclear molding are typical of herpetic infections and may be seen on the Tzanck smear

♦ **herpes simplex** and **varicella–zoster virus** infections cannot be differentiated either histologically or by Tzanck smear; they need to be differentiated clinically by monoclonal-antibody testing and with viral culture

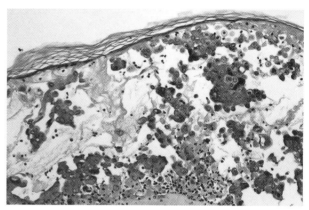

RETICULAR DEGENERATION

6.6 Fixed drug eruption

♦ massive superficial dermal edema lifts the epidermis

♦ epidermal necrosis is a frequent finding

♦ lacy eosinophilic fibers called 'gossamer fibers', typical of reticular degeneration, are observed

♦ fixed drug eruptions are characterized by one or a few, well-demarcated, erythematous to violaceous plaques or bullae, which often heal with postinflammatory hyperpigmentation

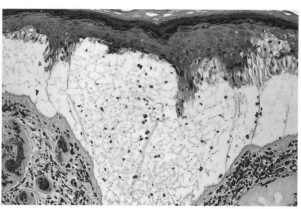

6.7 Hand-foot-and-mouth disease

♦ severe reticular degeneration

♦ lymphocytic exocytosis

♦ squamous cells have no specific viral inclusions

♦ caused by coxsackievirus

♦ seen primarily in children

♦ small vesicles, which may ulcerate, are seen in the mouth, and on the palms and soles

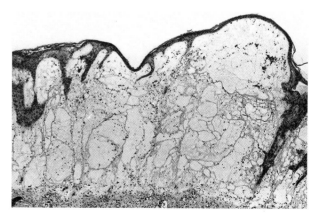

KOILOCYTOSIS

6.8 Verruca plana

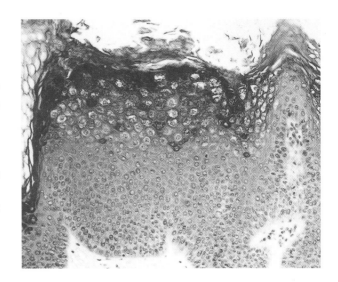

♦ koilocytotic cells are easily discernible in the superficial layers; in lesions of the uterine cervix, they tend to be subtle in genital and cutaneous warts, and in other human papillomavirus infections

♦ nuclear hyperchromasia and enlargement shown here

♦ cytoplasmic clearing shows sharp angulated margins

♦ parakeratosis is subtle or absent compared with verruca vulgaris

♦ flesh- or tan-colored, barely elevated, papules that are often grouped or linear

♦ common on the face, neck, and legs

♦ clinical differential diagnosis: seborrheic keratosis

6.9 Deep palmoplantar wart

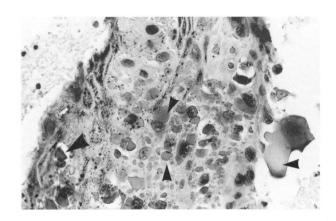

♦ koilocytosis (large arrow) is less conspicuous than in flat warts

♦ prominent large eosinophilic keratohyaline granules of varying sizes (small arrows)

♦ eosinophilic inclusions mimic molluscum bodies; molluscum contagiosum (pearly dome-shaped papules with central umbilication) is usually easily differentiated clinically from warts

♦ keratinocyte nuclei in warts are not displaced to the periphery

♦ plantar warts are keratotic papules with 'black dots' secondary to thrombosed capillaries

♦ clinical differential diagnosis: callus; corn; and verrucous squamous cell carcinoma

COLLOID BODIES

6.10 Erythema multiforme (EM)

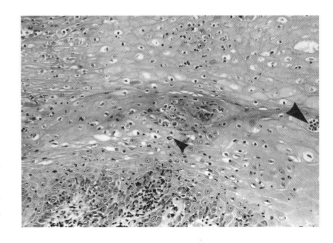

♦ varying degrees of squamous cell necrosis, from single colloid bodies (small arrow) to confluent necrosis

♦ colloid bodies may be scattered throughout the layers of the epidermis

♦ colloid bodies surrounded by lymphocytes and neutrophils are referred to as 'satellite cell necrosis' (large arrow)

♦ lymphocytic infiltration of the epidermis

♦ extensive basal cell necrosis may cause bullous EM, a subepidermal blistering lesion

♦ lymphocyte-mediated hypersensitivity reaction of the skin and/or mucosa; often secondary to drugs or infections

♦ 'iris' and 'target' lesions seen clinically, but widespread blisters may occur with severe disease

6.11 Acute graft versus host (GVH) reaction

♦ lymphocytic infiltration is slight and focal, and not band-like

♦ colloid bodies are usually sparse and seen in the basal cell layer

♦ severe forms may resemble erythema multiforme on microscopy, making differentiation from a possible drug reaction difficult

♦ GVH is seen as a sequela of bone marrow transplantation where immunocompetent donor lymphocytes mount an inflammatory reaction to host tissue; it has also developed after blood transfusion in immuno-suppressed patients, and after transfer of maternal leukocytes to the immunodeficient fetus

♦ erythematous macules, subtle papules and, sometimes, vesicles arise 10–40 days after transplantation or blood transfusion

♦ history of bone marrow transplantation or a transfusion is essential for the diagnosis

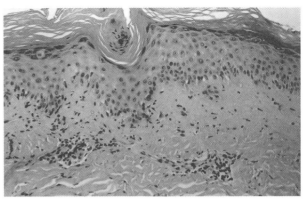

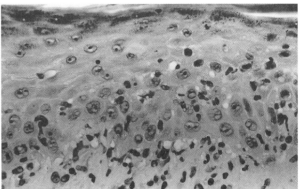

6.12 Lichen planus

♦ colloid bodies due to confluent basal cell degeneration are confined to the basal cell layer

♦ confluence of the necrotic basal cells may result in a subepidermal cleft (Max–Joseph spaces)

♦ band-like lymphocytic infiltration

♦ other changes of lichen planus include compact hyperkeratosis, wedge-shaped hypergranulotic beading, 'saw-tooth' epidermal hyperplasia, and dermal melanophages

♦ pruritic, polygonal, purple, planar papules with lacy, reticulated, Wickham's striae on the lower extremities, and flexor aspects of the wrists and forearms; may be generalized; oral and genital involvement common; may show nail changes

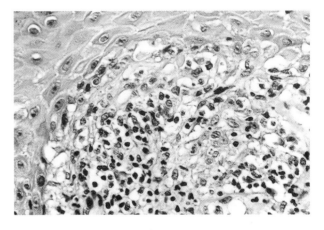

6.13 Pityriasis lichenoides

♦ colloid bodies are numerous in the acute form (pityriasis lichenoides et varioliformis acuta), but much less noticeable in the chronic form (pityriasis lichenoides chronica)

♦ parakeratosis, basal cell degeneration, and neutrophilic exocytosis are other epidermal changes

♦ epidermal necrosis and ulceration may occur in acute lesions

♦ lymphocytic vasculitis in the dermis and extravasation of red cells are seen

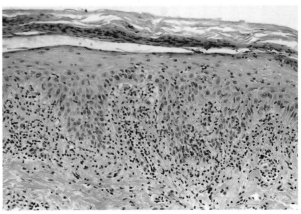

6.14 Spitz nevus

♦ colloid (Kamino) bodies are common in the basal cell layer; in the vicinity of junctional cell nests, they may be present in the papillary dermis (arrows)

♦ colloid bodies may also be found in melanomas; thus, their presence should not be taken as conclusive evidence of a benign nevus

♦ a Spitz nevus is usually a solitary red to brown telangiectatic papule or nodule, most commonly seen in children and young adults

♦ clinical differential diagnosis: pyogenic granuloma; hemangioma; juvenile xanthogranuloma; mastocytoma; arthropod bites; dermatofibroma; leiomyoma; melanocytic nevi; and sarcoid. However, these conditions may all be differentiated histologically

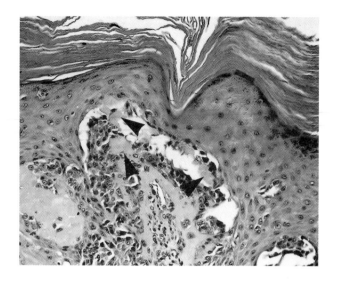

BASAL CELL DEGENERATION

Basal cell degeneration refers to necrosis of the basal keratinocytes. It is often described as vacuolar degeneration because dying basal cells exhibit cytoplasmic vacuoles that are large enough to be observed in tissue sections. The nucleus is lost in the degenerated basal cell (karyolysis) and cytoplasmic remnants form colloid bodies. Individual basal cells are involved initially, but loss of many contiguous basal cells in an area may lead to the production of clefts along the epidermodermal junction and, occasionally, true vesicles. Significant basal cell damage is often associated with the liberation of melanin pigment into the dermis (pigmentary incontinence). In addition, melanophages are often seen in the papillary dermis.

T lymphocyte-mediated cytotoxic damage is the usual cause of basal cell degeneration and, not surprisingly, lymphocytes are often seen in close proximity to the degenerated basal keratinocytes.

Basal cell degeneration	7.1

Differential diagnoses

Basal cell degeneration with band-like lymphocytic infiltrate

Lichen planus	7.2
Benign lichenoid keratosis	7.3
Lichenoid dermatitis	7.4

Basal cell degeneration with perivascular infiltrate

Lupus erythematosus	7.5
Dermatomyositis	7.6
Erythema multiforme	7.7
Toxic epidermal necrolysis	7.8
Graft versus host (GVH) reaction	7.9
Pityriasis lichenoides et varioliformis acuta (Mucha–Habermann disease)	7.10
Lichen sclerosus et atrophicus	7.11

7.1 Basal cell degeneration

♦ swarms of lymphocytes are seen in the basal cells

♦ vacuolar change of the basal cells

♦ colloid bodies (arrows) within the epidermis or dermis

♦ pigmentary incontinence

♦ marked spongiosis of the basal cell layer and edema of the papillary dermis in dermatitis may mimic cytoplasmic vacuoles of degenerated basal cells

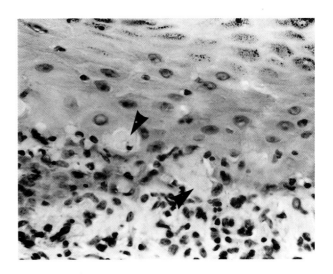

BASAL CELL DEGENERATION WITH BAND-LIKE LYMPHOCYTIC INFILTRATE

7.2 Lichen planus

♦ compact hyperkeratosis and wedge-shaped hypergranulosis

♦ basal cell degeneration with a band-like lymphocytic infiltrate remains the hallmark of lichen planus

♦ subepidermal cleft due to confluent basal cell degeneration is called a Max–Joseph space (upper picture, arrow)

♦ colloid (Civatte) bodies are easy to identify (lower picture, arrow)

♦ resolving lesions have an increased number of dermal melanophages with less intense inflammation

♦ a common cause of postinflammatory pigmentary incontinence

♦ clinically characterized by pruritic, polygonal, purple, planar papules with lacy, reticulated, Wickham's striae

♦ affects the lower extremities, and flexor aspects of the wrists and forearms

♦ may be generalized

♦ oral and genital involvement is common

♦ may show nail changes

♦ hypertrophic lesions may clinically mimic psoriasis and lichen simplex chronicus

♦ lichen amyloidosus, with discrete, small, itchy papules which coalesce to form hyperkeratotic plaques typically on the shins, may be clinically mistaken for this, but is readily differentiated histologically by Congo red staining

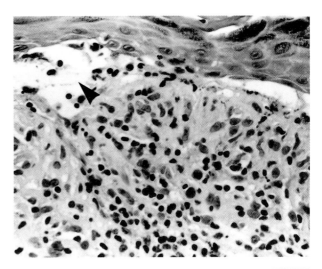

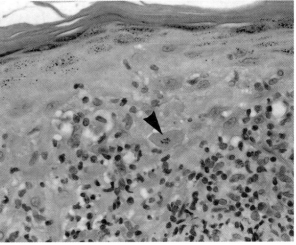

7.3 Benign lichenoid keratosis

- marked focal hyperkeratosis and parakeratosis
- plasma cells and eosinophils may be components of the lichenoid infiltrate
- basal cell degeneration, colloid bodies, and pigmentary incontinence
- solitary, red, violaceous, or brown, scaly papule on the upper chest or trunk
- represents a benign keratosis or hyperkeratotic squamous papilloma with lichenoid inflammation
- clinical differential diagnosis: actinic keratosis; and basal cell carcinoma
- clinical correlation helps to differentiate from lichen planus (solitary *vs* multiple lesions and different clinical appearance)

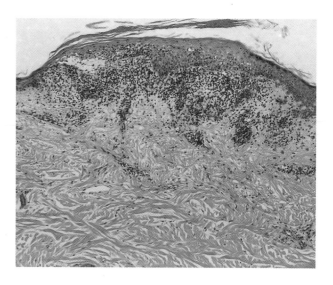

7.4 Lichenoid dermatitis

- resembles lichen planus in both gross and microscopic appearances
- presence of parakeratotic foci and eosinophils and/ or plasma cells may be the only clues to differentiate from lichen planus
- may be seen with reactions to certain drugs (thiazides and antimalarials) and to gold
- seen in some forms of neurodermatitis
- clinical correlation required for histologic diagnosis

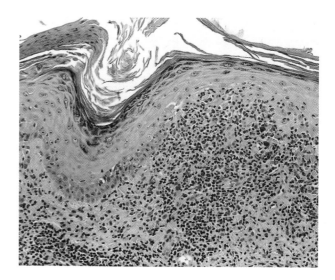

BASAL CELL DEGENERATION WITH PERIVASCULAR INFILTRATE

7.5 Lupus erythematosus (LE)

- hyperkeratosis, hypergranulosis, epidermal atrophy
- vacuolar change of basal cells is usually focal
- confluent basal cell degeneration may rarely lead to a bullous form, which needs to be distinguished from other subepidermal blistering diseases
- irregular hyaline thickening of the basement membrane
- lymphocytic infiltrate is perivascular and periadnexal, and may extend into the subcutaneum
- focal lichenoid infiltrate may be superimposed
- dermal mucin accumulation and destruction of elastic fibers
- discoid lesions are usually seen on the face and scalp, appearing as well-demarcated, erythematous, or violaceous, scaly plaques which may develop central atrophy and hyperpigmentation

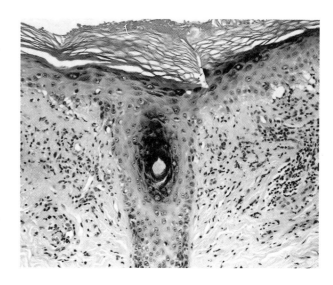

7.6 Dermatomyositis

♦ histologic changes in the skin lesions may be indistinguishable from those of systemic lupus erythematosus (SLE)
♦ vacuolar degeneration of the basal cells is focal and often associated with epidermal atrophy, except in the lesions over the knuckles (Gottron's papules)
♦ a slight perivascular lymphocytic infiltrate is usually present, and may involve the deep dermis and subcutaneous vessels
♦ periorbital heliotrope eruption and edema, poikoloderma, photosensitivity, periungual telangiectasia, Gottron's papules

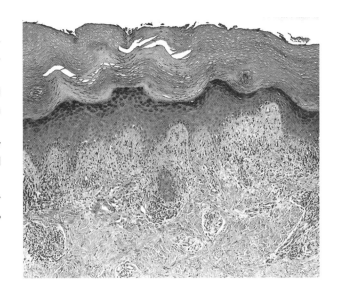

7.7 Erythema multiforme (EM)

♦ basal cell degeneration is almost always present; it is usually focal, but may be confluent in severe cases (Stevens–Johnson syndrome) and result in a subepidermal blister
♦ lymphocytic infiltrate is variable and primarily involves the superficial dermis
♦ eosinophils may be present, especially when secondary to a drug reaction
♦ EM is a hypersensitivity reaction triggered by various insults, particularly drugs and infections
♦ characteristic clinical lesions are the iris and target lesions
♦ widespread blisters may occur with severe disease

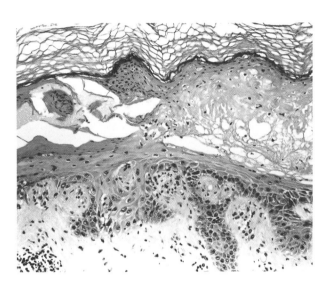

7.8 Toxic epidermal necrolysis (TEN)

♦ extensive epidermal necrosis and basal cell degeneration resulting in a subepidermal blister
♦ epidermal changes are identical to those of EM
♦ patients are acutely ill, with tender generalized morbilliform eruptions which quickly blister, then exfoliate in sheets, leaving raw denuded areas similar to those seen in victims with severe burns
♦ extensive mucous membrane involvement with oral ulcerations
♦ usually secondary to drugs

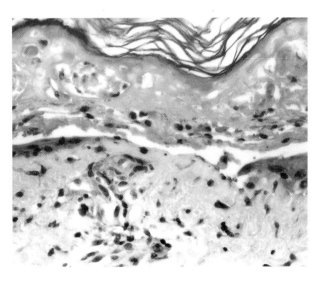

7.9 Graft versus host (GVH) reaction

♦ acute lesions display basal cell degeneration that is usually subtle and focal

♦ necrotic keratinocytes are not confined to the basal epidermis

♦ slight spongiosis may be present

♦ lymphocytic infiltration is mild, but diffuse

♦ there is sometimes dermal extravasation of red cells

♦ chronic lesions may show lichenoid inflammation with a few necrotic keratinocytes

♦ GVH is a sequela of bone marrow transplantation in which immunocompetent donor lymphocytes mount an inflammatory reaction to host tissue

♦ GVH may occur after blood transfusion in immuno-suppressed patients, and after transfer of maternal leukocytes to the immunodeficient fetus

♦ acute GVH is characterized by a generalized, erythematous, violaceous, maculopapular or vesicular eruption

♦ acute GVH may resemble an acute drug eruption clinically; biopsy may help to distinguish between these two entities

♦ chronic lesions may resemble lichen planus or scleroderma clinically, or may be poikilodermatous

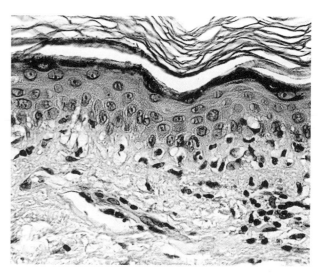

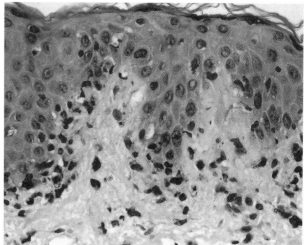

7.10 Pityriasis lichenoides et varioliformis acuta (PLEVA; Mucha–Habermann disease)

♦ microscopic appearance is dominated by extravasation of red cells and lymphocytic vasculitis

♦ focal basal cell degeneration is often a minor feature, but necrotic keratinocytes may be numerous in the superficial epidermis

♦ confluence of necrotic keratinocytes causes ulceration and a neutrophilic exudate

♦ parakeratosis and hyperkeratosis are present

♦ histologic changes are diagnostic, as seen on biopsy of fully developed lesions (shown here)

♦ generalized eruption with abrupt onset of crops of reddish-brown scaly papules, which may become vesicular and necrotic, and eventually ulcerate

♦ clinical differential diagnosis: varicella; leukocytoclastic vasculitis; and insect bites

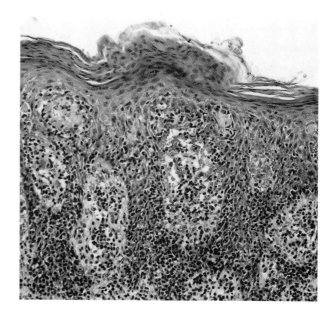

7.11 Lichen sclerosus et atrophicus

♦ basal cell degeneration is focal (shown here; arrow), but may lead to 'subepidermal' clefts and separation of epidermis from dermis
♦ epidermis is atrophic with compact hyperkeratosis
♦ eosinophilic change of the papillary dermal collagen (shown here) may occur
♦ a band of lymphocytes is seen in the middermis separating the edematous and / or hyalinized superficial dermis from the normal lower dermis
♦ lesions are genital and extragenital
♦ flat-topped white papules with follicular plugging

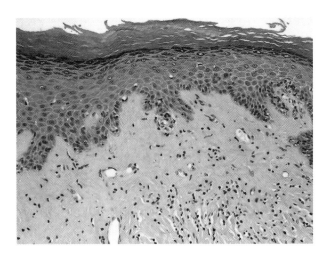

LYMPHOCYTIC EXOCYTOSIS

Exocytosis describes transmigration and infiltration of the epidermal cell layers by inflammatory cells. With the inflammation and inflammatory cellular infiltration, there is usually intercellular edema (spongiosis).

Spongiosis is a term indicating intercellular edema in the spinous layer. The intercellular space is widened and the intercellular bridges accentuated. On low-power microscopy, the appearance of the epidermis has been likened to that of a sponge. With massive edema, the bridges become overstretched and rupture, resulting in vesicle formation. These vesicles are frequently intensely pruritic. In dyshidrotic dermatitis, vesicles resembling tapioca are seen in clusters on the sides of the fingers and toes, and on the palms and soles. Occasionally, the

vesicles may coalesce to form bullae but, usually, the tapioca-like appearance is maintained. In acute contact dermatitis, such as poison ivy dermatitis, intercellular edema frequently results in vesicles that ooze. In poison ivy dermatitis, the vesicles are characteristically linear. Recognizing spongiosis is useful because it implies that the process is, at least in part, inflammatory.

Lymphocytes are commonly seen with marked spongiosis in all benign inflammatory dermatoses. When lymphocytic infiltration of the epidermis is not associated with a significant degree of spongiosis, the term **epidermotropism** is used. An affinity for the epidermal cells is implied by this name and the presence of epidermotropism suggests a non-inflammatory or neoplastic infiltrative process such as mycosis fungoides.

8.1 Lymphocytic exocytosis

♦ in contrast to the epidermotropism seen in mycosis fungoides, an inflammatory lymphocytic infiltration of the epidermis is always associated with an appreciable degree of spongiosis

♦ edema fluid between the squamous cells forces the cells apart, thus rendering the intercellular bridges prominent

♦ intercellular bridges may become overstretched and rupture, forming a vesicle (shown here)

♦ lymphocytes are seen in all levels of the epidermis and do not aggregate along the basal cell layer

♦ lymphocytes do not exhibit nuclear atypia

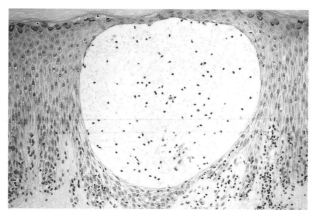

8.2 Epidermotropic lymphocytes in mycosis fungoides

♦ the number of lymphocytes infiltrating the epidermis is disproportionate to the degree of spongiosis, which is minimal (as seen here)

♦ neoplastic lymphocytes may have slightly enlarged nuclei (arrow) and vacuolated cytoplasm

♦ lymphocytes with discernible convoluted nuclei are difficult to find in most lesions

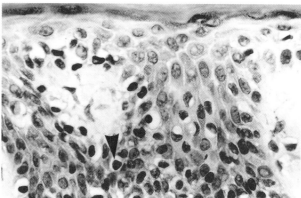

8.3 Dermatitis

♦ varying degrees of hyperkeratosis, parakeratosis, lymphocytic exocytosis, and spongiosis

♦ slight perivascular lymphocytic infiltrate in the superficial dermis

♦ normal epidermis with more than a slight degree of dermal inflammatory infiltrate and/or inflammatory involvement of the deep dermis should suggest a diagnosis other than dermatitis (such as mycosis fungoides)

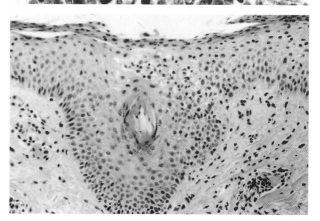

8.4 Hand dermatitis

♦ note the thick stratum corneum typical for this anatomical location

♦ check keratin layer for dermatophytes (should not be present)

♦ etiology of dermatitis cannot be made on the basis of pathological examination

♦ skin biopsy is used to exclude specific papulosquamous eruptions such as psoriasis, lichen planus, secondary syphilis, dermatophytosis, LE and mycosis fungoides

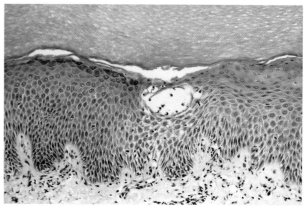

8.5 Pityriasis rosea

♦ regular parakeratotic cell mounds with spongiosis that is most marked under the parakeratotic foci

♦ extravasation of red cells in the papillary dermis

♦ lymphocytic infiltration of the superficial dermal vessels is variable; marked inflammation and involvement of deep dermal vessels, especially in the herald patch

♦ clinical correlation is usually required for a histopathologic diagnosis as the histologic features are non-specific

♦ in ≈25% of patients, the large herald patch is followed by a Christmas tree-like arrangement of smaller macules and papules with a collarette of fine scale, attached at the periphery and free at the center, primarily on the trunk

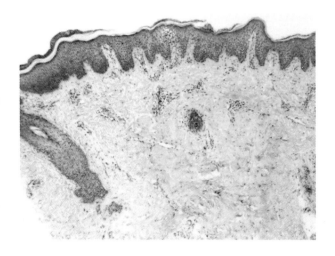

8.6 Dermatophytosis

♦ exocytosis and spongiosis may be slight; here, dermatophytosis with an almost normal-looking biopsy on low-power examination (upper picture) shows sligh pallor (small arrow) of the epidermis, suggesting spongiosis, and a slight degree of lymphocytic infiltration of the vessels in the superficial dermis (large arrow)

♦ dermatophytes are usually visible by routine H & E staining if examined on high magnification (lower picture, × 400, arrow)

♦ the species of dermatophyte cannot be identified on histology; fungal culture is necessary (results are available within ≈ 3–4 weeks)

♦ PAS staining after diastase digestion (to remove glycogen) highlights the organisms

♦ consider staining multiple sections in suspected cases

♦ diagnosis is usually made clinically and after potassium hydroxide (KOH) examination of skin scrapings for hyphae

♦ biopsies of dermatophytosis are usually performed if KOH examination and fungal cultures are negative and the patient fails to respond to treatment

♦ in dermatophyte fungal infections, scale is often seen at the periphery of the lesion and central clearing is common

♦ skin scrapings and biopsy should be taken from the edge of the lesion

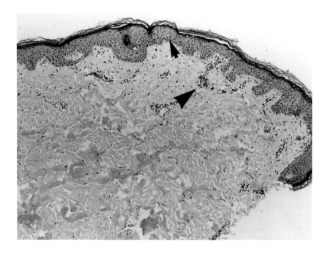

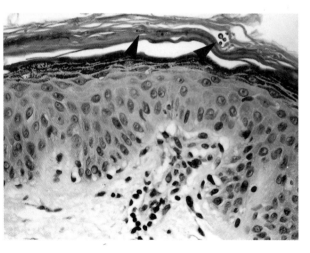

8.7 Photodermatitis

♦ patient's history is essential for making this diagnosis

♦ nevertheless, dermatitis with a disproportionate degree of dermal edema and/or lymphocytic infiltration around the deep dermal vessels should raise the possibility of photoeruptions

♦ **photodermatoses** occur in sun-exposed areas such as the face, the 'V' of the neck, dorsum of the hands, and extensor aspects of the arms

♦ **polymorphous light eruption** usually onsets in the spring with pruritic erythematous papules which may be eczematous

♦ **actinic reticuloid** is manifested as chronic, pruritic, lichenified, red, scaly plaques in older men; the face may have a leonine appearance; a biopsy is often carried out to rule out lymphoma

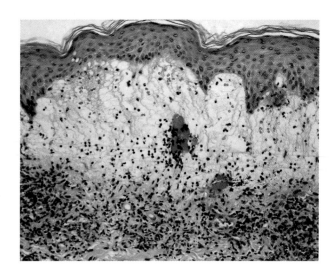

8.8 Mycosis fungoides

♦ in contrast to dermatitis, spongiosis is minimal and lymphocytes are often seen along the basal cell layer (epidermotropism)

♦ lymphocytes may have hyperchromatic and slightly enlarged nuclei with perinuclear halos

♦ actual convoluted nuclei are usually difficult to visualize; they are better seen in thin 3–4-μ sections or on electron microscopy

♦ mitoses are rare

♦ dermal lymphocytic infiltration is slight and tends to be band-like

♦ cases of persistent refractory dermatitis should be biopsied to rule out mycosis fungoides; two biopsies should be taken – one for routine histopathology and the other for electron microscopy

♦ upper picture shows heavy lymphocytic infiltration of the epidermis and papillary dermis, but with minimal spongiosis

♦ lower picture shows higher magnification of the epidermotropic lymphocytes with central slightly enlarged dark nuclei and clear cytoplasm

♦ there is an aggregate of atypical lymphocytes forming the so-called Pautrier's microabscess (arrow)

♦ Lutzner cells (lymphocytes with convoluted nuclei) are not usually observed, but some degree of nuclear pleomorphism and hyperchromasia are often apparent (lower)

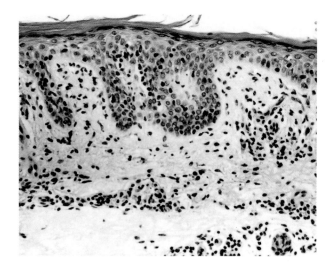

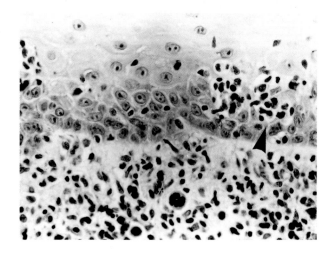

NEUTROPHILIC EXOCYTOSIS

Neutrophils are the effector cells in the acute inflammatory response of most tissues except the skin. Many of the acute inflammatory lesions of the skin are not associated with a neutrophilic response. Neutrophils, for example, are not normally present in acute dermatitis, a T lymphocyte-mediated reaction. The presence of neutrophilic exocytosis should raise the possibility of ulceration, excoriation and / or superimposed bacterial infection in a dermatitis or other differential diagnoses.

Large accumulations of neutrophils within the superficial epidermal layers may result in the formation of a clinically apparent pustule. **Pustules** may be sterile (pustular psoriasis, Reiter's disease, subcorneal pustular dermatosis, acropustulosis of infancy, acne vulgaris, rosacea) or contain bacteria (bullous impetigo, bacterial folliculitis). The vesicles in some viral diseases may become pustular (herpes simplex, varicella–zoster) and inflammatory dermatophyte skin infections may have pustules at the periphery. Follicular pustules are seen in folliculitis, acne vulgaris, and rosacea. A central hair is usually seen in folliculitis. Folliculitis may be missed on biopsy if follicles are not present in the sections examined. When crusts and pus are seen, additional sections should be taken so that at least one follicle is examined. Pustules develop in acne vulgaris after the follicular wall has ruptured and the comedonal contents have extruded into the dermis. In contrast to acne vulgaris, comedones are not a feature of rosacea.

Differential diagnoses

Non-pustular

Excoriated and impetiginized dermatitis	9.1
Psoriasis	9.2
Pale cell (clear cell) acanthoma (Degos' tumor)	9.3
Seborrheic dermatitis	9.4
Dermatophytosis	9.5
Necrolytic migratory erythema	9.6
Pityriasis lichenoides et varioliformis acuta	9.7
Epidermal necrosis	9.8

Vesicular / pustular

Miliaria crystallina	9.9
Herpes simplex / orf / zoster	9.10
Dermatitis herpetiformis	9.11
Pustular psoriasis	9.12
Keratoderma blennorrhagica / Reiter's syndrome	9.13
Folliculitis / acne vulgaris / acne rosacea	9.14
Subcorneal pustular dermatosis (Sneddon–Wilkinson disease) / impetigo / staphylococcal scalded skin syndrome / acropustulosis of infancy	9.15
Erythema elevatum diutinum	9.16

NON-PUSTULAR

9.1 Excoriated and impetiginized dermatitis

♦ epidermal atrophy and eosinophilic change of the superficial epidermal cell layers (large arrow) are the results of excoriation

♦ neutrophils with their multilobated nuclei are easily recognizable within the superficial squamous cell layers and fibrinous exudate; their presence does not imply an acute dermatitis

♦ neutrophils are also seen around congested dermal vessels (small arrow)

♦ clumps of bacteria are seen within the fibrous exudate if there is secondary infection

♦ differentiated from psoriasis by the absence of confluent parakeratosis and presence of spongiosis

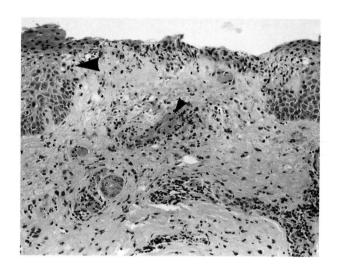

9.2 Psoriasis

♦ neutrophils are seen in all levels of the epidermis, but the greatest concentration is observed in the parakeratotic layer and superficial epidermis where there is hypogranulosis (arrow)

♦ collections of neutrophils in the parakeratotic layer and superficial epidermis are known as microabscesses of Munro and Kogoj, respectively

♦ in pustular psoriasis, epidermal cells in the center of the microabscess of Kogoj undergo cytolysis to form a unilocular pustule

♦ neutrophilic exocytosis in psoriasis is usually seen with only minimal spongiosis; vesicles are rare unless there is a superimposed dermatitis

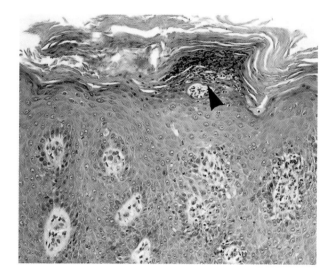

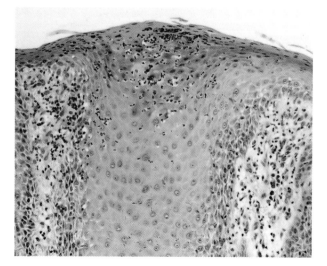

9.3 Pale cell (clear cell) acanthoma (Degos' tumor)

♦ neutrophilic exocytosis is often seen in this benign tumor (arrow)

♦ pallor of the epidermal cell cytoplasm is due to accumulation of glycogen secondary to deficient glycogen phosphorylase

♦ epidermal cells are PAS-positive and diastase-sensitive due to their abnormal glycogen content

♦ clinically, typically presents as a solitary, red to brown nodule or plaque, 1–2 cm in diameter, with wafer-like peripheral scale on the lower legs which often bleeds when the scale is removed

♦ diagnosis is rarely made clinically; often mistaken for a pyogenic granuloma, dermatofibroma, or amelanotic melanoma, but all are histopathologically distinct

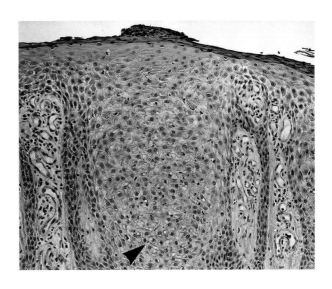

9.4 Seborrheic dermatitis

♦ focal parakeratosis, sometimes with trapped neutrophils, resembling Munro's microabscesses of psoriasis

♦ usually an appreciable degree of spongiosis accompanies the neutrophilic exocytosis

♦ epidermal acanthosis is mild and without the regular rete ridge hyperplasia seen in psoriasis

♦ lesions typically located near follicular ostia

♦ clinically seen as erythematous patches with greasy yellowish scales on the scalp, eyebrows, mustache area, paranasal area, central chest and, occasionally, axillae and groin

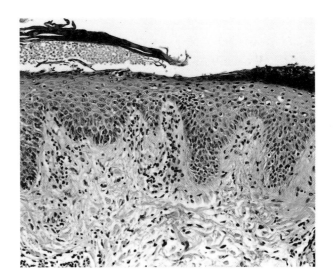

9.5 Dermatophytosis

♦ degree of epidermal spongiosis and exocytosis of neutrophils may be slight

♦ neutrophilic exudate in the keratin layer; the histologic appearance resembles that of an excoriated dermatitis

♦ neutrophilic infiltrate is seldom marked

♦ high index of suspicion required

♦ always examine the keratin layer for fungal spores and hyphae in histologic cases of apparent dermatitis

♦ hyphae may be accentuated with PAS staining

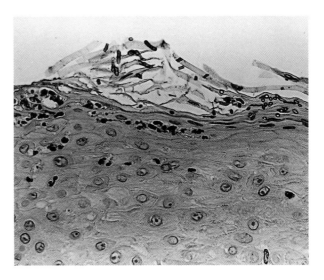

9.6 Necrolytic migratory erythema

♦ focal parakeratosis and sometimes pallor of the superficial epidermal cells with slight neutrophilic exocytosis (arrow)

♦ necrolysis of the superficial epidermal cells is seen as pale epidermal cells with pyknotic nuclei

♦ cleft formation secondary to necrolysis may result in blisters seen clinically

♦ biopsies should be taken from the edge of early lesions to see the characteristic epidermal changes

♦ recurrent episodes of annular and serpiginous erythematous scaly patches with crusting and sometimes blister formation on the extremities and trunk, and perioral and genital skin

♦ oral erosions are common and may mimic candidiasis

♦ most commonly associated with pancreatic glucagonoma

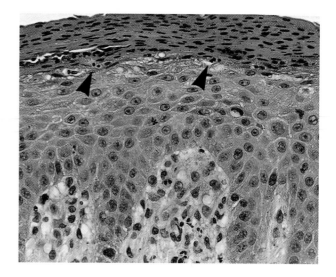

9.7 Pityriasis lichenoides et varioliformis acuta (PLEVA)

♦ neutrophilic exocytosis is often seen where there are many colloid bodies and extensive epidermal necrosis (small arrow)

♦ some lesions of PLEVA are ulcerated

♦ there is a lymphocytic vasculitis involving the superficial and deep dermal vessels

♦ marked extravasation of red cells in papillary dermis (large arrow)

♦ histopathologic changes may resemble EM, but are clinically different (generalized eruption with abrupt onset of crops of reddish-brown scaly papules which may become vesicular and necrotic, and ulcerate in PLEVA in contrast to the iris and target lesions and bullae seen in EM)

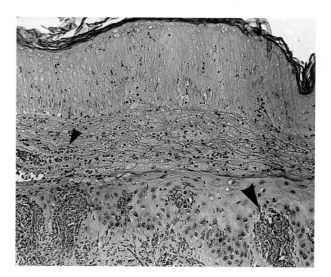

9.8 Epidermal necrosis

♦ neutrophilic infiltration of the epidermis is frequently seen in areas of necrosis, irrespective of the cause

♦ epidermal roof of any blister duration may become necrotic with time

♦ extensive epidermal necrosis associated with neutrophilic exocytosis in **erythema multiforme** is seen in this picture

(continued next page)

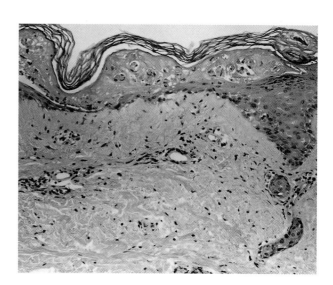

♦ neutrophilic infiltration of an area of epidermal necrosis due to **ischemia** in arteriosclerosis is seen in this picture

♦ neutrophilic infiltration of the epidermis may also be seen in a **traumatized skin tag** and **inflamed seborrheic keratosis**

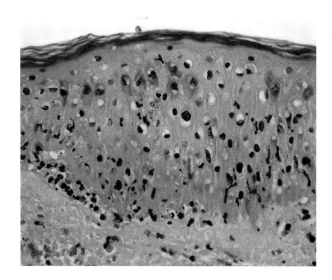

VESICULAR / PUSTULAR

9.9 Miliaria crystallina

♦ forms as a consequence of intracorneal or superficial intraepidermal obstruction of the eccrine sweat duct

♦ observe the subcorneal pustule; neutrophils are present in the lumen of the sweat duct

♦ vesicles are in direct communication with an underlying sweat duct

♦ superficial clear, non-inflammatory, small asymptomatic vesicles resembling dewdrops are seen clinically

♦ stratum corneum overlying the vesicles is easily rubbed off

♦ usually develops in sunburned areas after exercise or after sudden vigorous sweating associated with a high fever

♦ diagnosis is usually made clinically; a biopsy is rarely necessary

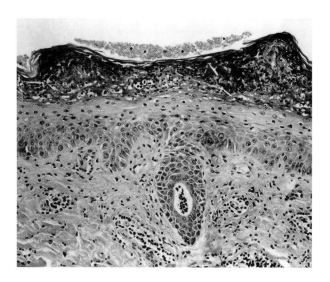

9.10 Herpes simplex

♦ ballooning degeneration and necrosis of infected keratinocytes are often associated with heavy neutrophilic exocytosis and sometimes grossly pustular lesions

♦ similar epidermal necrosis with intraepidermal vesicles and pustules may be seen in lesions of **orf** (a poxvirus infection endemic in sheep)

♦ **herpes simplex** and **herpes zoster** cannot be distinguished histologically; monoclonal antibody testing of smears taken from the base of fresh vesicles and viral culture are required

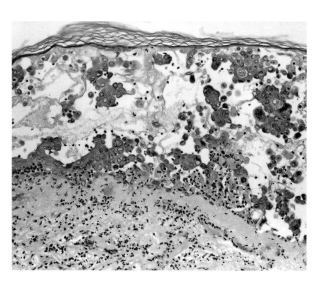

9.11 Dermatitis herpetiformis

♦ epidermal layers forming the roof of vesicles and blisters, irrespective of whether they are sub- or intraepidermal, usually degenerate eventually and become chemotactic factors for neutrophils

♦ despite the presence of neutrophils, lesions are sterile

♦ as shown here, neutrophils may also come from ruptured neutrophilic vesicles, as also seen in **linear IgA dermatosis** and **acropustulosis of infancy**

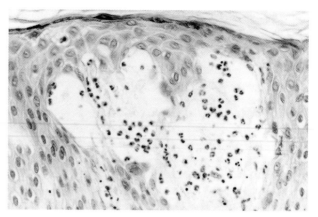

9.12 Pustular psoriasis

♦ psoriasis with markedly exaggerated neutrophilic exocytosis forming macroabscesses and pustular lesions

♦ may have pustules, erythema, and scaling on the palms and soles particularly in middle-aged women, around the fingers associated with nail changes (acropustulosis), and locally within plaques or generalized pustules (von Zumbusch)

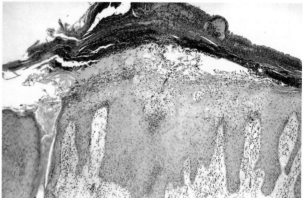

9.13 Keratoderma blennorrhagica

♦ indistinguishable histologically from pustular psoriasis, although a thickened, parakeratotic, horny layer is more suggestive of keratosis blennorrhagica

♦ clinically, thick, hyperkeratotic, crusted, pustules with a mollusk-like appearance are seen on the palms and soles

♦ associated with **Reiter's syndrome**

♦ urethritis, arthritis, and conjunctivitis are other features of Reiter's syndrome

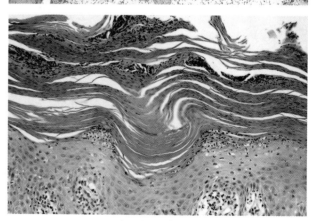

9.14 Folliculitis

♦ follicle is infiltrated and distended by neutrophils

♦ ulceration of follicular epithelium leading to dermal abscess, perifollicular granulomatous inflammation, and vascular reaction

♦ histopathologic changes are basically the same for acne vulgaris and acne rosacea

♦ **folliculitis**: tender follicular pustules on an erythematous base; bacterial culture usually positive for *Staphylococcus aureus*

♦ **acne vulgaris**: papules; pustules; comedones; cysts on face, chest, shoulders, back and upper arms; primarily in teenagers

♦ **acne rosacea**: facial erythema; papules; pustules; telangiectasia; flushing; occasionally, small cysts; no comedones

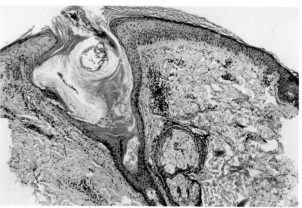

9.15 Subcorneal pustular dermatosis (Sneddon–Wilkinson disease)

♦ neutrophils are located primarily within a subcorneal blister; there is usually spongiosis and a slight degree of acantholysis in the underlying epidermis layers forming the floor of the blister

♦ identical histologic features are seen in **bullous impetigo** (shown here), **staphylococcal scalded skin syndrome**, and **acropustulosis of infancy**

♦ **bullous impetigo** is usually caused by *Staphylococcus aureus* or, less commonly, β-hemolytic streptococci which may be cultured; the face, hands, and genitalia are frequently affected

♦ **staphylococcal scalded skin syndrome** generally affects children age <5 years and is caused by an exotoxin from *S. aureus*; tenderness, erythema, superficial blistering, and desquamation are seen most commonly on the face, neck, axillae, and groin

♦ **acropustulosis of infancy** onsets at birth or during infancy with recurrent crops of pruritic 1–2-mm vesiculopustules on the palms, soles, and distal extremities; blacks are primarily affected; spontaneous clearing occurs at age 2–3 years

♦ **subcorneal pustular dermatosis** is seen primarily in women age >40 years as symmetric, discrete, flaccid pustules on normal or slightly erythematous skin in intertriginous areas; there is no involvement of the face, scalp, or mucous membranes

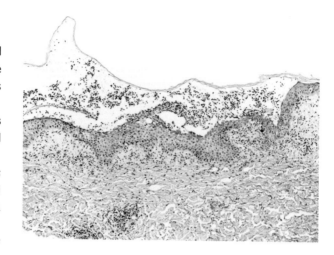

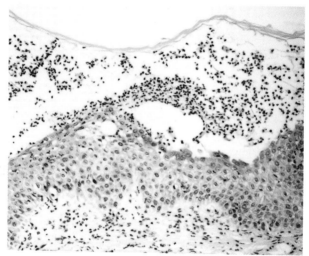

9.16 Erythema elevatum diutinum

♦ heavy infiltration of the dermis by neutrophils in this chronic vasculitic skin condition may lead to marked spongiosis and neutrophilic exocytosis (shown here)

♦ symmetric, persistent, violaceous to brown papules, nodules, and plaques on the extensor surfaces of the extremities, typically over joints and, occasionally, on the buttocks, face, and torso

♦ may be associated with monoclonal gammopathy (usually IgA), multiple myeloma, myelodysplasia, and chronic or recurrent infections

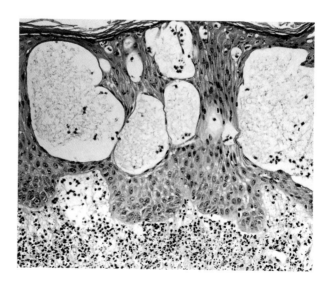

EOSINOPHILIC EXOCYTOSIS

Traditionally, eosinophils are the cells associated with type I allergic reactions which are initiated by specific binding of antigens to IgE-class antibodies on the surface of mast cells. In allergic rhinitis, for example, activation of intraepithelial mast cells, through the release of eosinophil chemotactic factor of anaphylaxis (ECF-A), eventuates in eosinophilic infiltration of the nasal mucosa. Eosinophils may also phagocytose antigen–antibody complexes and mast cell granules. In its role as a modulator of inflammation, eosinophils are often present in significant numbers in various immune-complex-mediated diseases such as leukocytoclastic vasculitis, pemphigus, and pemphigoid.

A few eosinophils are sometimes found with lymphocytes in non-specific dermatitis, but marked eosinophilia or the presence of eosinophilic spongiosis should raise the possibility of diagnoses other than banal dermatitis.

Eosinophilic exocytosis / bullous pemphigoid	10.1

Differential diagnoses

Erythema toxicum neonatorum	10.2
Incontinentia pigmenti	10.3
Scabies / tick bites	10.4
Bullous pemphigoid / herpes gestationis	10.5
Pemphigus vegetans / foliaceus	10.6
Pruritic urticarial papules and plaques of pregnancy	10.7

10.1 Eosinophilic exocytosis
- microabscess composed primarily of eosinophils is seen here at the tip of the dermal papilla in a case of **bullous pemphigoid**
- refractile eosinophilic cytoplasmic granules (arrows) from degranulated eosinophils

10.2 Erythema toxicum neonatorum
- erythematous macules with a pinpoint central vesicle or perifollicular pustule filled with eosinophils and some neutrophils
- surrounding skin and macular area show dermal edema and eosinophilic infiltrate
- occurs in up to 50% of newborns; rarely biopsied
- lesions often present birth or develop within the first 1–2 days and fade within a few days
- clinically, may be mistaken for transient neonatal pustular melanosis; however, neutrophils rather than eosinophils predominate in the latter, which is seen primarily in blacks

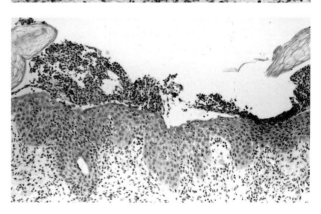

10.3 Incontinentia pigmenti

♦ eosinophilic spongiosis is characteristic of the vesicular (first) stage of the disease, presenting at birth or in the early neonatal period with linear vesicles over the trunk and extremities ± peripheral eosinophilia

♦ mimics childhood pemphigoid histologically, but direct immunofluorescence shows linear IgG deposition along the epidermal basement membrane in pemphigoid only

♦ epidermolysis bullosa presenting during infancy may show eosinophilic exocytosis, but distinguishing the two diseases is seldom clinically difficult

♦ X-linked dominant condition lethal to males; four stages of evolution: vesiculobullous; verrucous; swirled hyperpigmentation; and linear hypopigmentation

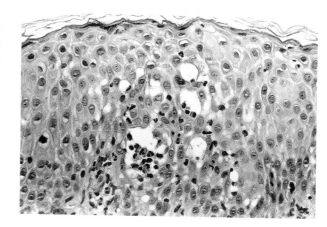

10.4 Scabies

♦ this biopsy of the epidermal furrow in scabies reveals numerous mites in cross-section

♦ marked eosinophilic exocytosis and spongiosis; an eosinophilic microabscess is present in the epidermis (arrow)

♦ eosinophilic exocytosis is especially common at or around the site of an arthropod bite, but the offending arthropod is not commonly seen in the tissue section; fragments of the mouthpiece may be embedded in the tissue (as seen in **tick bites**)

♦ infiltrate tends to be polymorphous: lymphocytes, plasma cells, and histiocytes are seen in varying numbers

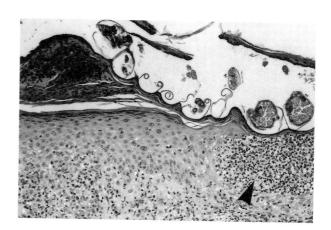

10.5 Bullous pemphigoid

♦ eosinophilic spongiosis is the earliest histologic change and precedes the subepidermal blister

♦ degree of eosinophilic infiltration is variable, and biopsy of non-inflamed skin shows few eosinophils

♦ direct immunofluorescence demonstrates a linear band of IgG and / or C3 at the basement membrane zone

♦ circulating IgG antibasement membrane antibodies may be demonstrated with indirect immunofluorescence

♦ large tense bullae seen on normal or erythematous skin

♦ **herpes gestationis** has identical histologic and clinical features, but occurs during pregnancy whereas bullous pemphigoid occurs primarily in the elderly

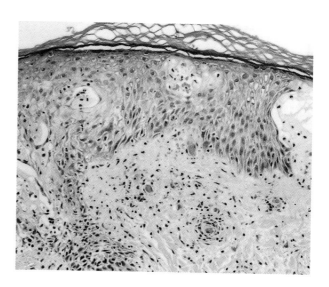

10.6 Pemphigus vegetans
♦ although often described as the typical inflammatory cell in all types of pemphigus, eosinophils are seldom the exclusive inflammatory cells
♦ eosinophilic pustules are characteristic of **pemphigus vegetans** whereas neutrophils are often seen in **pemphigus foliaceus**, a condition in which blisters are usually eroded
♦ acantholysis may be present within or next to areas of eosinophilic spongiosis; suprabasilar acantholysis differentiates pemphigus vulgaris and vegetans from pemphigus foliaceus and erythematosus, which both show acantholysis of the superficial epidermis
♦ flaccid vesicles which rupture easily
♦ mucosal involvement is common

10.7 Pruritic urticarial papules and plaques of pregnancy (PUPPP)
♦ histologic changes are identical to those of dermatitis, but with an increased number of eosinophils in the dermis and slight eosinophilic spongiosis (arrow)
♦ clinical history and presentation of the rash are essential for a definitive diagnosis
♦ predilection for primigravidas in the third trimester of pregnancy
♦ intensely pruritic urticarial papules and plaques that start in the abdominal striae, but may become generalized
♦ regresses spontaneously after delivery

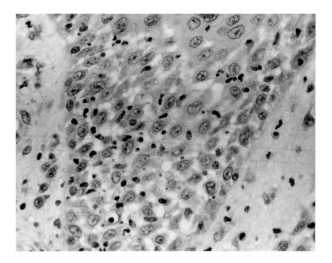

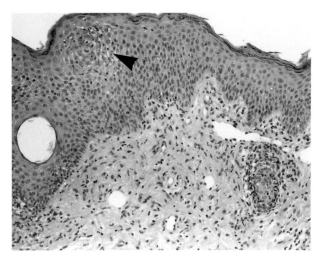

MELANOCYTES, AND EPITHELIOID AND LANGERHANS CELLS

Keratinocytes are not the only cells that proliferate within the epidermis. Melanocytes, Langerhans cells, and glandular cells of adnexal origin may do so as well. The normal density of melanocytes varies, but is approximately 1 in 10 basal cells. Langerhans cells account for up to 4% of all the cells in the epidermis.

Melanocytic proliferation

Intraepidermal melanocytic proliferation is a common occurrence. These cells may retain dendritic processes, vacuolated cytoplasm and eccentric nuclei typical of normal basal melanocytes in so-called **lentiginous hyperplasia**. Alternatively, cells may become **epithelioid** with rounded cell bodies, pale-staining cytoplasm, and central nuclei (as seen in junctional nevus, melanoma in situ).

Intraepidermal melanocytic proliferation is usually seen clinically as a flat hyperpigmented macule. Raised papular lesions usually involve cellular growth into the dermis.

Lentiginous hyperplasia is seen in simple lentigo, solar lentigo, lentigo maligna, and nevus spilus. All of these lesions are flat and not raised above the skin surface. A simple lentigo is a commonly seen brown or brownish-black macule 1–5 mm in diameter. It appears in childhood, but may arise at any time throughout life. It cannot be distinguished from junctional nevus clinically, although the latter shows epithelioid, rather than lentiginous, hyperplasia on histology.

A simple lentigo is darker than a freckle (ephelis) and, unlike a freckle, does not darken or increase in number with exposure to sunlight. Freckles are brown macules which do not result from melanocytic proliferation. The number of melanocytes is not increased, but the melanocytes produce more pigment.

A solar lentigo appears as a uniformly brown macule in areas of chronic sun-exposure, usually on the backs of the hands, face, and extensor aspects of the forearms after age 40 years. It is larger than a simple lentigo and has less regular borders. Multiple solar lentigines on the upper back are usually indicative of previous blistering sunburn and may be seen in younger persons.

A lentigo maligna is a variously colored patch on sun-exposed skin, usually the face, in elderly people.

A nevus spilus is a solitary, brown patch, 1–20 cm in diameter, containing several smaller, dark-brown, freckle-like macules. It is clinically similar to a café au lait patch except that the latter does not contain multiple freckle-like macules or papules. Café au lait patches show an increase of pigment in the basal cell layer of the epidermis with giant pigment granules in the keratinocytes and melanocytes. Dark-brown café au lait patches have an increased number of melanocytes.

Becker's nevus may also present as a solitary large brown patch. It is most commonly seen on the shoulders; coarse terminal hair may grow within the lesion. In contrast to nevus spilus, there is no increase in the number of melanocytes. In Becker's nevus, the epidermis is thickened and the basal layer hyperpigmented.

Epithelioid cell hyperplasia

The epithelioid melanocytes seen in intraepidermal epithelioid melanocytic hyperplasia, especially in atypical hyperplasia, need to be distinguished from the dysplastic squamous cells of Bowen's disease, epithelioid tumor cells of Paget's disease, and malignant Langerhans cells in histiocytosis X. The lymphocytes in spongiotic dermatitis may also, on occasion, assume an epithelioid appearance. These conditions can usually be distinguished clinically.

Langerhans cell proliferation

Langerhans cells are antigen-presenting cells which may be increased in contact dermatitis, seborrheic keratosis, verrucous epidermal nevus, Bowen's disease, and inflamed keratoacanthoma. However, their number remains relatively small in comparison to other epidermal cells; indeed, it is often difficult to appreciate the increased number of Langerhans cells by routine staining.

Self-healing reticulohistiocytosis and solitary Langerhans cell histiocytoma (solitary Hashimoto–Pritzker disease) are rare conditions that involute spontaneously. Congenital or perinatal, the rapidly growing ulcerating papulonodules resolve spontaneously within 1–3 months. These conditions may be indistinguishable clinically and histologically from histiocytosis X. However, the former have a benign course and lack systemic involvement.

Histiocytosis X is a malignant proliferation of the Langerhans cells with three clinical expressions: Letterer–Siwe disease (an acute disseminated form); Hand–Schüller–Christian disease (a chronic progressive form); and eosinophilic granuloma (a localized form). Onset of Letterer–Siwe disease is usually in the first 2 years of life as an eruption resembling seborrheic dermatitis. Purpura may be seen in Letterer–Siwe disease, but is not a feature of seborrheic dermatitis. Cutaneous lesions are only seen in approximately 30% of patients with Hand–Schüller–Christian disease, a disorder characterized by bony lesions, diabetes insipidus, and exophthalmos. Eosinophilic granuloma typically affects the bones, and cutaneous lesions are rare.

Differential diagnoses

11.1 Lentiginous hyperplasia with dendritic melanocytes
♦ arrows indicate some of the melanocytes
♦ located in the basal epidermis
♦ vacuolated cytoplasm
♦ dark, eccentric, crescent-shaped nucleus
♦ dendritic cell processes not visible by H & E staining

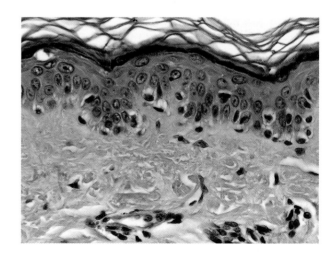

11.2 Epithelioid melanocytes
♦ rounded cell body with pale-staining amphophilic cytoplasm (arrow)
♦ may have intracytoplasmic melanin granules
♦ central vesicular nucleus
♦ no cell junctions, but typically seen in clusters
♦ more than three cells constitute a junctional nest

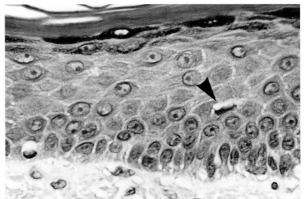

11.3 Normal Langerhans cells
♦ a small cell with a round nucleus and clear cytoplasm found between keratinocytes of the squamous cell layer (arrow)
♦ dendritic cell bodies are not appreciable on routine H & E staining
♦ weakly S100 protein-positive and OKT6-positive
♦ Birbeck granules are characteristic cytoplasmic structures seen ultrastructurally

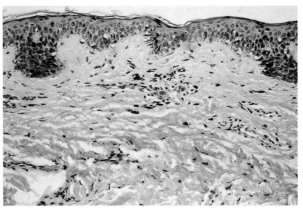

LENTIGINOUS HYPERPLASIA

11.4 Simple lentigo (lentigo simplex)
♦ regular rete ridge elongation
♦ basal epidermal hyperpigmentation
♦ increase in the number of basal melanocytes
♦ basal melanocytes are cytologically uniform; their usual dendritic cell bodies, vacuolated cytoplasm, and eccentrically located nuclei are retained
♦ nesting of melanocytes and epithelioid cell change may be seen in the occasional simple lentigo
♦ common, brown to brownish-black, sharply demarcated macule 1–5 mm in diameter, seen anywhere on the skin

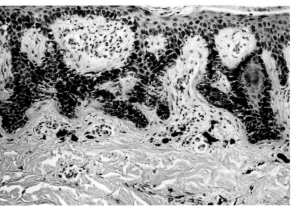

11.5 Solar lentigo (lentigo senilis)
♦ elongation of rete ridges; basal epidermal hyperpigmentation
♦ melanocytic hyperplasia
♦ epidermis between the rete ridges may be atrophic
♦ no nesting of melanocytes
♦ very common, uniformly brown, macule with an irregular border seen in the elderly on sun-exposed areas, particularly on the backs of the hands

11.6 Lentigo maligna (Hutchinson's freckle)

♦ epidermis is usually atrophic
♦ no rete ridge hyperplasia
♦ epidermal hyperpigmentation, especially in the basal cell layer
♦ melanocytic hyperplasia with atypical melanocytes
♦ enlarged hyperchromatic pleomorphic nuclei
♦ cytoplasm may appear vacuolated
♦ proliferation of melanocytes seen along adnexal structures
♦ dermal elastosis always present
♦ large, irregularly pigmented, and contoured patch on sun-damaged skin, particularly the face
♦ usually in the elderly and almost always in whites
♦ precursor of lentigo maligna melanoma
♦ intraepidermal growth phase is prolonged and 10–30 years may pass before malignant transformation

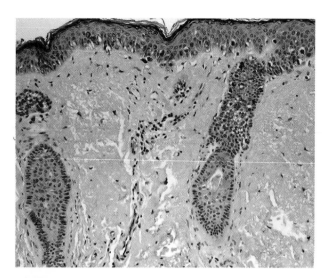

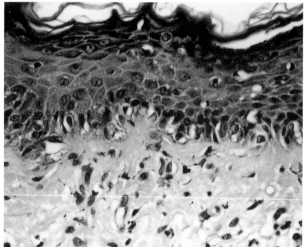

11.7 Speckled lentiginous nevus (nevus spilus)

♦ lentiginous melanocytic hyperplasia seen in the light brown patch
♦ nevic cell nests are found along the basal epidermis and in the speckled darker areas of the dermis, as seen here
♦ no cytologic atypia
♦ no dermal architectural alterations of dysplastic nevus
♦ solitary brown patch 1–20 cm in diameter showing multiple darker flat or raised 'freckles' within it
♦ usually appears in childhood on the trunk and extremities
♦ diagnosis usually made clinically; a biopsy is usually not necessary, but may be performed to rule out malignant transformation if part of the lesion changes

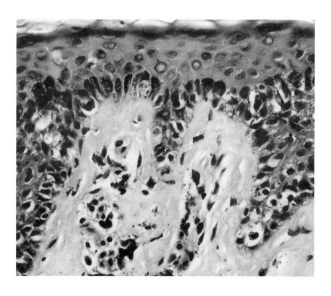

EPITHELIOID CELL HYPERPLASIA

11.8 Junctional nevus

- ♦ melanocytes become epithelioid nevic cells and cluster to form nests at the epidermodermal junction
- ♦ junctional nevi on the extremities, and in children especially, may show concomitant lentiginous hyperplasia with single melanocytes scattered along the basal epidermis
- ♦ no nuclear atypia
- ♦ brown to brownish-black macule 1–5 mm in diameter and seen anywhere on the skin
- ♦ nevi of the palms and soles are usually junctional
- ♦ junctional nevi which are almost black in color and variable in shape should be biopsied to rule out melanoma

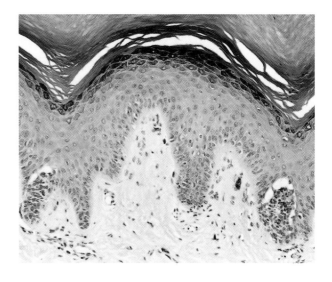

11.9 Regenerating nevus

- ♦ dermal scar (large arrow); residual dermal nevic cells are present on the right side of the scar
- ♦ when partially excised nevi regrow, the proliferating nevic cells are most commonly seen within the epidermal cell layers
- ♦ regenerating nevic cells are often atypical with enlarged nuclei and nucleoli
- ♦ single cells may be seen in the squamous cell layer of the regenerating epidermis, simulating Pagetoid spread (small arrows)
- ♦ clinical history, histologic presence of a dermal scar or residual dermal nevic cells that are benign should suggest this diagnosis

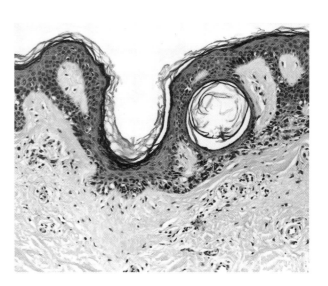

11.10 Atypical (dysplastic) nevus with slight dysplasia

- ♦ histologic diagnosis based on cytologic atypia, architectural atypia, and host response
- ♦ cytologic atypia is most demonstrable in junctional cells
- ♦ grading of atypia is subjective and not reproducible
- ♦ low-grade dysplasia is characterized by slight nuclear enlargement and cytologic atypia, absence of nucleoli, and the very occasional single epithelioid nevic cell
- ♦ architectural atypia manifested by asymmetry, eosinophilic and/or lamellar fibroplasia, lentiginous melanocytic hyperplasia with spindle or epithelioid melanocytes in nests of variable size, bridging adjacent rete ridges

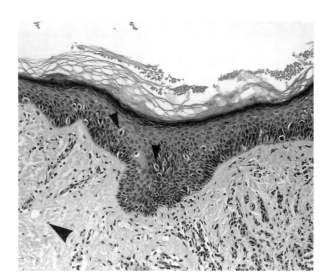

(continued next page)

- host response, seen as dermal infiltration of lymphocytes, is variable in degree, but usually present
- clinically, atypical nevi are often large (> 8 mm) and of variable color, with a slightly elevated center and a border that fades into the surrounding skin
- may be difficult to distinguish clinically from melanoma
- patients with multiple atypical nevi, especially if there is a family history of melanoma, are at an increased risk for melanoma
- any atypical nevus with clinical evidence of change should be biopsied to rule out malignant degeneration

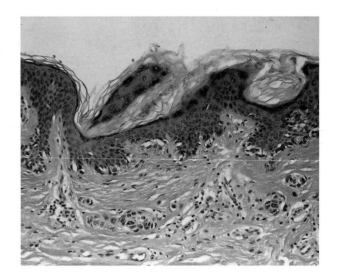

11.11 Atypical (dysplastic) nevus with severe dysplasia

- high-grade dysplasia is akin to melanoma in situ with Pagetoid cells invading the epidermis and marked cytologic atypia
- individual atypical melanocytes are located not only in the basal layer, but also within the superficial epidermal cell layers
- 'shoulder' phenomenon, with intraepidermal melanocytes extending beyond the main dermal component
- dermal nevic cells, if present in a compound lesion, are small and often distributed in a plate-like arrangement, as seen in an acquired nevus
- multiple sections of a severely dysplastic nevus should be examined to exclude early invasion and transformation into invasive melanoma
- pleomorphic dermal nevic cells in a dysplastic nevus raise the concern of invasive malignant melanoma

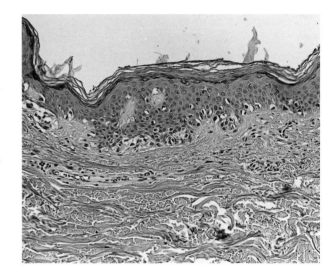

11.12 Malignant melanoma in situ

- intraepidermal proliferation of atypical melanocytes and Pagetoid spread of neoplastic nevic cells are similar to those seen in a severely dysplastic atypical nevus
- multiple levels of the biopsy should be examined to exclude early microscopic invasion or focal regression
- missing a focus of invasion or regression may explain cases of 'thin' melanomas giving rise to metastases

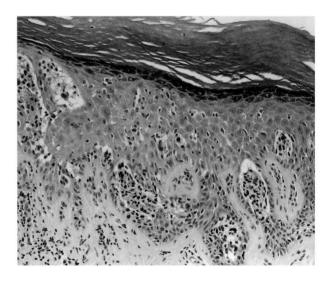

11.13 Superficial spreading invasive malignant melanoma

♦ atypical epithelioid melanocytes infiltrate the entire thickness of the hyperplastic epidermis (as here)

♦ epidermis may atrophy or even ulcerate

♦ in the squamous cell layers, tumor cells are scattered singly or in small clusters

♦ with their enlarged nuclei and abundant, faintly eosinophilic, cytoplasm, they resemble the tumor cells of Paget's disease (Pagetoid invasion)

♦ presence of atypical nevic cells in the dermis distinguishes invasive melanoma from an in situ lesion and severe dysplasia

♦ melanoma should be suspected when a pigmented lesion is asymmetric and >6 mm, with irregular borders and a variegated color

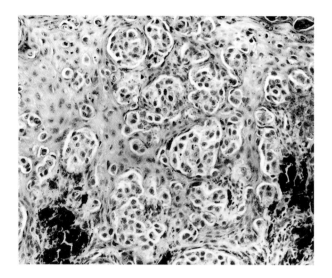

11.14 Acral lentiginous melanoma

♦ the name refers to melanomas of the nail bed and extremities

♦ atypical lentiginous melanocytic proliferation is common in this form of melanoma, although Pagetoid cells, such as those in superficial spreading melanoma, are also seen in around one-third of cases

♦ histologic appearance is similar to mucosal melanomas

♦ more common in blacks and Asians

♦ poorer prognosis than melanomas at other sites

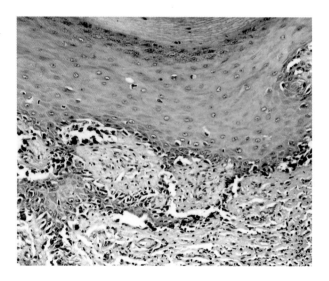

11.15 Paget's disease

♦ malignant glandular cells of lactiferous duct or sweat gland origin proliferate in epidermal cell layers

♦ Paget cells are large and round with a pale-staining cytoplasm surrounding a central, rounded, vesicular nucleus (arrows)

♦ Paget cells are easily discernible from the surrounding keratinocytes

♦ there are no intercellular bridges

♦ luminal differentiation is sometimes observed

♦ cytoplasmic mucin is demonstrable by immunohistochemistry (PAS with diastase) in most cases of extramammary Paget's disease, but the result is inconsistent in mammary Paget's disease

♦ the occasional cell may show intracytoplasmic melanin pigmentation

♦ Paget cells are carcinoembryonic antigen (CEA)-positive

(continued next page)

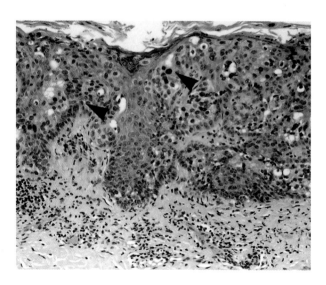

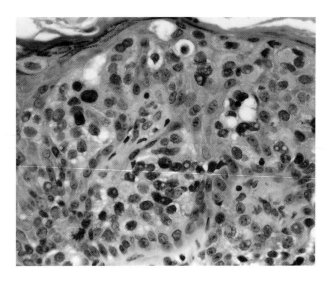

♦ Paget cells are not positive for S100 protein and cytokeratin

♦ S100 protein, CEA, and cytokeratin stains are most reliable in differentiating melanoma (S100-positive, CEA- and cytokeratin-negative) and Bowen's disease (cytokeratin-positive, CEA- and S100-negative) from Paget's disease

♦ **Paget's disease of the breast** presents as a red scaly patch on the nipple and is invariably associated with an underlying intraductal or invasive ductal carcinoma

♦ **extramammary Paget's disease** may occur on anogenital skin or, less frequently, in the axillae or eyelids where, in most patients, it is associated with an underlying malignancy, usually adenocarcinoma

♦ all patients with extramammary Paget's disease should be investigated for underlying malignancy

♦ any persistent eczematous eruption of the nipple or anogenital area should be biopsied to rule out Paget's disease

11.16 Bowen's disease

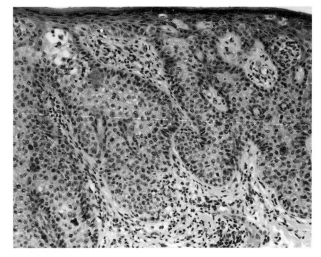

♦ squamous cell carcinoma in situ

♦ atypical and dysplastic keratinocytes are present in all layers of the epidermis

♦ frequent mitotic figures, including abnormal forms

♦ although resembling Paget cells, Bowen cells are squamous cells with intercellular bridges and eosinophilic keratinizing cytoplasm

♦ as in normal squamous cells, intracytoplasmic melanin pigment may be present

♦ cytokeratin-positive, S100- and CEA-negative

♦ scaly eczematous patch with notched, serrated, irregular margins

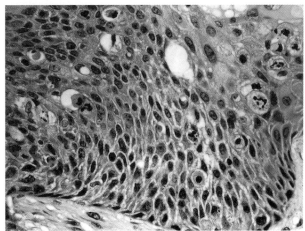

11.17 Gianotti–Crosti syndrome

♦ lymphoid cells may occasionally appear to be epithelioid and present as Pagetoid cells within the epidermal cell layers (arrows)

♦ **dermatitis** usually shows spongiosis, exocytosis of lymphocytes, and a slight superficial perivascular lymphocytic infiltrate

♦ suspect **Gianotti–Crosti syndrome** and **mycosis fungoides**, although spongiosis is usually minimal in the latter

♦ diagnosis of Gianotti–Crosti requires clinicopathologic correlation (seen primarily in children as an eruption of asymptomatic erythematous papules on the extremities, face, and buttocks, which lasts for a few weeks; associated with anicteric hepatitis due to hepatitis B and Epstein–Barr virus)

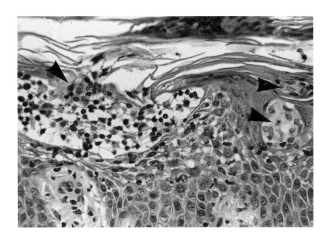

LANGERHANS CELL PROLIFERATION

11.18 Histiocytosis X

♦ malignant Langerhans cells with an epithelioid appearance infiltrate the epidermis and dermis

♦ Birbeck granules may be seen on electron microscopy

♦ should be suspected in children < 2 years of age who have a persistent eruption similar to seborrheic dermatitis with brown scaly papules on the scalp or groin, especially if some are ulcerated or purpuric

♦ may have lymphadenopathy, hepatosplenomegaly, chronic or recurrent osteomyelitis, or other infections such as pneumonia

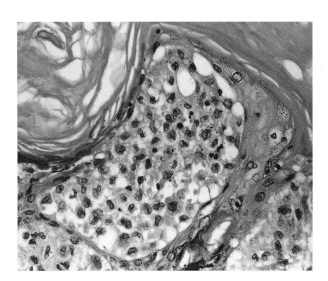

SUBCORNEAL VESICLES, BULLAE, AND PUSTULES

In any vesiculobullous eruption, intact vesicles should be biopsied if possible. If a punch biopsy is to be taken, it should be 1–2 mm larger than the vesicle so that the potential for vesicular rupture during the procedure is minimized. The superficial location and thin surfaces of subcorneal vesicles render them particularly vulnerable to rupture. Erosions and crusts are commonly seen in superficial subcorneal vesicular conditions; it is not uncommon for the microscopist to find no intact vesicles in this group of disorders.

Subcorneal blisters are seen in miliaria crystallina, erythema toxicum neonatorum, transient neonatal pustular melanosis, acropustulosis of infancy, staphylococcal scalded skin syndrome, bullous impetigo, subcorneal pustular dermatosis, pemphigus foliaceus and erythematosus, and friction blisters. Clinicopathologic correlation is important as the histologic appearance of skin biopsies from these conditions is very similar. The age and gender of the patient, and clinical appearance of the lesions aid in the diagnosis. In pemphigus foliaceus and erythematosus, the tissue changes are more distinctive because the blisters develop secondary to acantholysis of the superficial layers of the epidermis. Nevertheless, some degree of acantholysis may be present in subcorneal pustular dermatosis and bullous impetigo.

A **pustule** develops when there is a collection of neutrophils in a blister. The presence of neutrophils does not necessarily imply infection. Although, by routine H & E staining, clumps of bacteria may be seen among inflammatory exudates in impetiginized dermatitis, bacteria are seldom observed in staphylococcus scalded skin syndrome as it is caused by a toxin. Tissue Gram staining is of limited usefulness in the differential diagnosis of the pustular skin lesions.

Differential diagnoses

12.1 Miliaria crystallina

♦ obstructed sweat ducts at acrosyringium due to fever, sunburn, and exposure to hot humid environments
♦ obstruction at the stratum corneum is referred to as **miliaria crystallina**, manifested as small, superficial, clear, non-inflammatory, asymptomatic vesicles
♦ obstruction within the spinous layer is referred to as **miliaria rubra** (prickly heat) because of its erythematous prickly papulovesicles
♦ miliaria crystallina resolves more quickly because it is more superficial
♦ serial sectioning may be required to demonstrate contiguity with sweat ducts in both types of miliaria

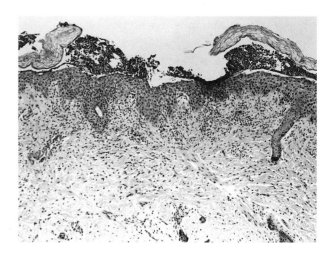

12.2 Erythema toxicum neonatorum

♦ very common eruption occurring in up to 50% of newborns
♦ in its most vivid form, it is characterized by a perifollicular subcorneal pustule filled with eosinophils and occasional neutrophils
♦ often prominent papillary dermal edema
♦ asymptomatic erythematous macules, papules, and pustules appearing anywhere on the body except the palms and soles
♦ usually appears during the first 3–4 days of life and lasts for 2 days
♦ rarely present at birth

12.3 Subcorneal pustular skin lesions of infancy

♦ this includes two histologically similar diseases: **acro-pustulosis of infancy** and **transient neonatal pustular melanosis** (shown here)

♦ both diseases show intra- or subcorneal accumulation of neutrophils and are more common in black infants

♦ **transient neonatal pustular melanosis** presents at birth as superficial vesiculopustules that easily rupture within 1–2 days, leaving a collarette of fine white scales around an area of hyperpigmentation that usually fades within weeks to months

♦ focal basilar hyperpigmentation is seen in the areas of hyperpigmentation

♦ in contrast to erythema toxicum neonatorum, palms and soles may be involved

♦ **acropustulosis of infancy** onsets during infancy with recurrent crops of itchy vesiculopustules 1–2 mm in diameter on the palms, soles, and distal extremities; clears by age 2–3 years

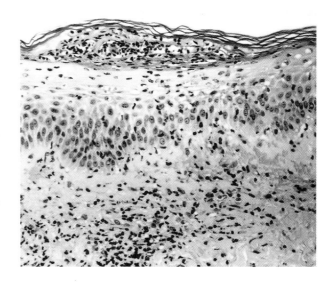

12.4 Staphylococcal scalded skin syndrome (SSSS)

♦ bullae form in subgranular zone or within stratum granulosum

♦ acantholytic cells may be seen

♦ neutrophils are present in the epidermis and blister

♦ **SSSS** is due to a bacterial exotoxin produced by an infection at a different site; fever, malaise, skin tenderness, erythema, superficial blistering and desquamation typically on the face, neck, axillae, and groin are seen, usually in children <5 years of age

♦ **bullous impetigo** has a similar histologic appearance, but a different clinical appearance (large flaccid pustules and crusts which are not usually accompanied by fever or skin tenderness)

♦ both are caused by *Staphylococcus aureus*, although β-hemolytic streptococci may also cause impetigo

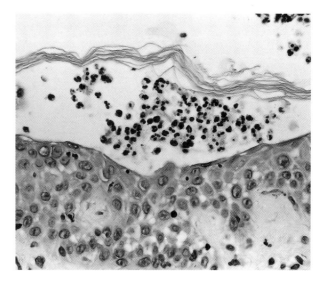

12.5 Subcorneal pustular dermatosis (Sneddon–Wilkinson disease)

- characterized by sterile pustules located deep to the stratum corneum
- neutrophils and infrequent eosinophils are found within the pustules
- intracelluar edema and spongiosis are usually present in the vicinity of the pustule
- condition primarily of women > 40 years of age
- symmetric, discrete, flaccid pustules on normal or slightly erythematous skin in intertriginous areas
- no facial, scalp, or mucous membrane involvement

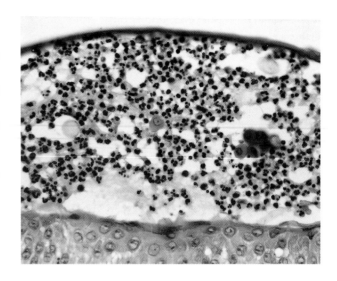

12.6 Pemphigus foliaceus

- acantholysis in upper spinous and granular layers
- eosinophilic spongiosis (small arrows point to eosinophils)
- some neutrophils with their multisegmented nuclei are also present
- subcorneal blister with acantholytic keratinocytes (large arrow)
- intercellular IgG autoantibodies seen with direct and indirect immunofluorescence, and C3 with direct immunofluorescence
- **fogo selvagem** is a variant endemic in Brazil
- crusted erosions seen on the face, scalp, and trunk
- intact blisters are rare
- mucosal involvement is rare
- clinically may mimic non-bullous impetigo

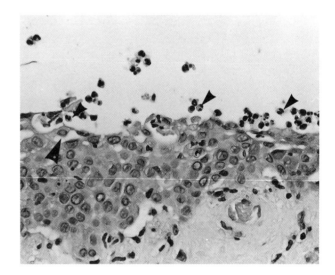

12.7 Friction blister

- blister roof contains the stratum corneum and stratum granulosum
- degenerated keratinocytes are seen on the floor of the blister
- rest of epidermis appears normal
- minimal inflammatory cellular infiltrate
- caused by shearing forces within the epidermis
- occurs primarily on the feet after prolonged walking, or on the palms or palmar aspects of the fingers after certain activities (such as shovelling) or sports

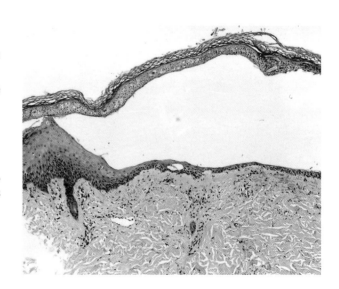

12.8 Pustular psoriasis

♦ expansion of Munro and Kogoj microabscesses forms the pustules of pustular psoriasis (arrow)

♦ in contrast to impetiginized dermatitis, spongiosis is slight and disproportionate to the severe neutrophilic infiltration

♦ regular papillated epidermal hyperplasia is evident

♦ diagnosis is usually made clinically and histologic confirmation is usually not indicated

♦ clinical differential diagnosis: bacterial or viral infection; acute exanthematous pustulosis; pustular drug eruptions; subcorneal pustulosis dermatosis; and miliaria with secondary infection

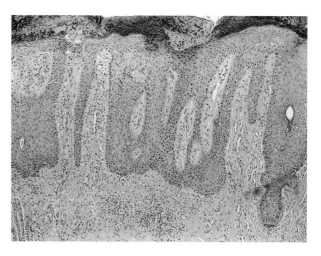

INTRAEPIDERMAL VESICLES AND BULLAE

Intraepidermal vesicles of the squamous cell layer may form as a result of forced separation of the epidermal cells (spongiosis), loss of cell adhesion (acantholysis), or keratinocyte necrosis (herpetic viral infections). Identification of stretched spinous cell processes in spongiosis, rounded acantholytic cells, and degenerative squamous cell changes is therefore of key importance to the histologic differential diagnosis of vesiculobullous lesions of the squamous cell layer.

Contact allergic dermatitis, such as poison ivy dermatitis and dyshidrotic eczema, often leads to the formation of spongiotic vesicles. These diagnoses are usually easily made clinically and a biopsy is rarely necessary. Incontinentia pigmenti usually presents at birth or shortly thereafter with linear vesiculobullae, and is often biopsied to rule out herpetic infections and to confirm the clinical diagnosis. It has an X-linked dominant inheritance that is lethal in males. Confirmation may be required if there are other associated congenital abnormalities or if the parents wish to have more children in the future. Hailey–Hailey disease may be diagnosed clinically, especially if there is a family history (autosomal-dominant inheritance), but a biopsy is usually taken for histologic confirmation. Hailey–Hailey disease may be clinically mistaken for impetigo, pemphigus vulgaris, pemphigus vegetans, and Darier's disease.

13.1 Intraepidermal vesicle

♦ intraepidermal location of the vesicle is seen in this case of eczema on the hand
♦ vesicle roof is formed by the granular and cornified cell layers
♦ floor of the vesicle is formed by layers of epidermal basal cells
♦ spongiosis is almost always associated with exocytosis of lymphocytes

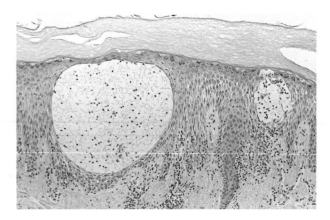

SPONGIOTIC

13.2 Spongiotic dermatitis

♦ spongiosis and exocytosis of inflammatory cells
♦ vesicle is formed by exudate forcing keratinocytes apart
♦ desmosomal cell junctions are stretched and become easily visible in early lesions
♦ with profound edema, epidermal cells lose their cell connections and may undergo reticular degeneration

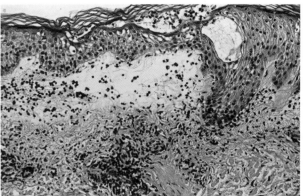

13.3 Incontinentia pigmenti

♦ eosinophilic spongiosis with intraepidermal vesicles filled with eosinophils is seen in the first stage, which occurs at birth or infancy with crops of linear vesicles or bullae over the trunk and extremities; this first stage lasts for weeks to months
♦ flaking, dyskeratotic, squamous cells
♦ X-linked dominant disease which is lethal to males
♦ Four stages: vesiculobullous; verrucous; swirled hyperpigmentation; and linear hypopigmentation
♦ may have peripheral eosinophilia, alopecia, ocular, dental, bony, and neurological abnormalities

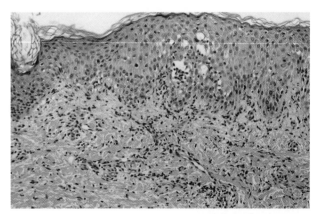

ACANTHOLYTIC

13.4 Hailey–Hailey disease
(benign familial pemphigus)

♦ acantholysis may involve the full thickness of the stratum malpighii (dilapidated brick-wall appearance)
♦ unusual to see dyskeratotic cells (corps ronds and grains)
♦ remember: Grover's disease may mimic Hailey–Hailey on microscopy, but acantholysis is seldom extensive in Grover's disease
♦ autosomal-dominant disease with flaccid blisters and crusts in intertriginous areas and on the neck

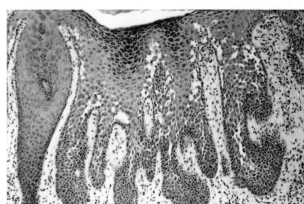

NECROTIC

13.5 Herpes simplex / varicella–zoster / orf

♦ **herpes simplex**, **varicella** and **zoster** lesions are histologically identical; immunofluorescent assays with monoclonal antibodies or viral culture are required to differentiate the viruses

♦ intraepidermal vesicles develop as a result of reticular and ballooning degeneration of the keratinocytes

♦ multinucleated keratinocytes are common

♦ **orf** (a poxvirus infection in sheep) may show similar intraepidermal necrotic vesicles that progress to pustules, but the characteristic herpetic keratinocyte nuclear changes (enlarged 'washed-out' and multiple nuclei) are absent

♦ widespread vesicles and pustules at various stages of development in chickenpox; dermatomal painful vesicles in herpes zoster and simplex; recurrent oral and genital lesions with herpes simplex *vs* solitary infection in older or immunocompromised patients with herpes zoster

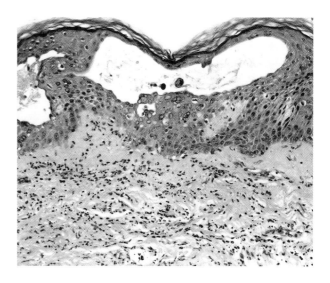

13.6 Bullous erythema multiforme

♦ keratinocyte necrosis is usually spotty; however, confluence of the necrotic cells in severe cases may result in intraepidermal or subepidermal blisters

♦ note the perivascular lymphocytic infiltration in the dermis and lack of viral changes in the keratinocytes

♦ bullae and erythematous urticarial targetoid lesions in an acutely ill patient

♦ mucosal lesions are common

♦ hypersensitivity reaction often secondary to drugs, or herpes or *Mycoplasma* infections

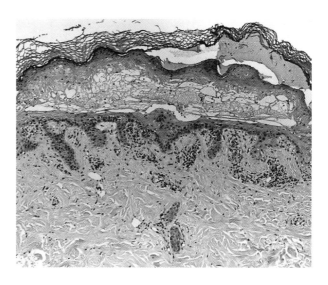

SUPRABASAL VESICLES AND BULLAE

In contrast to the vesiculobullous lesions of the squamous cell layer in which several different mechanisms may result in blistering, acantholysis is the only pathogenic mechanism in suprabasal vesicles. In pemphigus vulgaris and vegetans, intercellular autoantibodies may be demonstrated whereas Darier's disease is a genodermatosis with defective cell adhesion and dyskeratosis. Other lesions, such as actinic keratosis, Grover's disease (transient acantholytic dermatosis) and warty dyskeratoma, may show suprabasal clefts or lacunae which are microscopic intraepidermal slit-like spaces.

Intact blisters are commonly seen in pemphigus vulgaris in contrast to pemphigus foliaceus, in which the split is more superficial and the vesicles are more prone to rupture. Mucosal involvement is common in pemphigus vulgaris, but uncommon in pemphigus foliaceus. Several drugs (such as penicillamine, piroxicam, penicillin, captopril, enalapril, thiopronine, alpha-mercaptopropionylglycine, and phenobarbital) may cause a pemphigus-like eruption. Approximately 7% of patients treated with penicillamine for at least 6 months develop pemphigus. The eruption most usually resembles pemphigus foliaceus, but may also suggest pemphigus vulgaris. The eruption usually clears once the drug is discontinued, but some patients require systemic corticosteroids and / or immunosuppressive agents to achieve control.

Warty papules are seen in Darier's disease whereas, in Grover's disease, itchy papules and, occasionally, papulovesicles occur. Vesicles are never seen clinically in actinic keratosis or warty dyskeratoma.

Suprabasal cleft and acantholysis	14.1

Differential diagnoses

Suprabasal vesicles

Pemphigus vulgaris	14.2
Darier's disease (keratosis follicularis)	14.3
Grover's disease (transient acantholytic dermatosis)	14.4
Actinic keratosis	14.5
Warty dyskeratoma	14.6

14.1 Suprabasal cleft and acantholysis
♦ cleft or lacuna due to suprabasal acantholysis is seen here in this case of Darier's disease
♦ dyskeratotic cells (large arrow shows a corps ronds and small arrow shows a grain) and downward proliferation of the basal cells are common to both warty dyskeratoma and Darier's disease

SUPRABASAL VESICLES

14.2 Pemphigus vulgaris
♦ acantholytic cells in blister, but no dyskeratosis
♦ row of dyscohesive basal cells, resembling tombstones, forms the floor of the blister (arrow)
♦ a few eosinophils are present in the papillary dermis
♦ direct and indirect immunofluorescence show IgG antibody staining between epidermal cells
♦ mucosal involvement common
♦ flaccid blisters on the skin break readily, leaving areas of denudation
♦ positive Nikolsky (separation of epidermis from dermis when lateral pressure is applied to normal-looking skin) and positive Asboe–Hansen (pressure applied directly over the surface of the intact blister produces lateral spread of the lesion) signs
♦ increased incidence in Jewish and Mediterranean populations

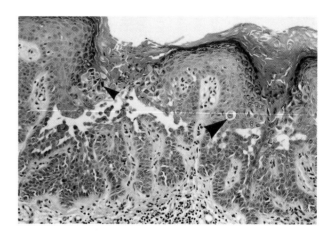

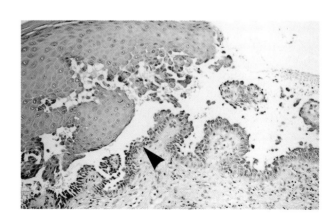

14.3 Darier's disease (keratosis follicularis)
♦ suprabasal clefts without well-formed blisters
♦ lacunae containing corps ronds and grains
♦ autosomal-dominant disorder of keratinization
♦ scaly crusted papules in seborrheic areas
♦ V-shaped nicking of nails, and punctate keratoses of the palms and soles
♦ warty papules on dorsum of feet and hands
♦ white papules with central depression on oral mucosa
♦ does not resemble pemphigus clinically
♦ clinical differential diagnosis: seborrheic dermatitis (no acantholysis); and Hailey–Hailey disease (dilapidated brick-wall appearance)

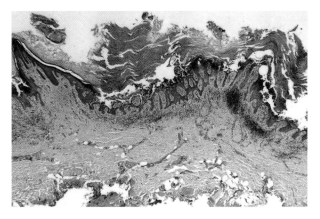

14.4 Grover's disease (transient acantholytic dermatosis)
♦ acantholytic focus is microscopic and acantholysis may not be confined to suprabasal layer
♦ may have dyskeratotic cells, as seen in Darier's disease
♦ multiple itchy papules and, occasionally, papulovesicles on the trunk and thighs in those > 40 years of age
♦ not clinically similar to Darier's disease
♦ clinical differential diagnosis: folliculitis; bites; and dermatitis; however, these conditions are all histologically distinctive

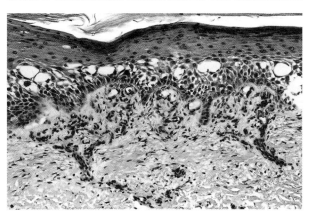

14.5 Actinic keratosis
♦ suprabasal acantholysis is not an uncommon histopathologic change, and has no apparent prognostic significance
♦ vesicles are not seen clinically; may be easily differentiated clinically from any of the other conditions showing suprabasal acantholysis
♦ look for dysplastic squamous cell changes and irregular hyperplastic rete ridges
♦ reddish-brown, rough, raised, scaly lesions with the texture of fine sandpaper seen on sun-exposed skin, especially the face and backs of the hands

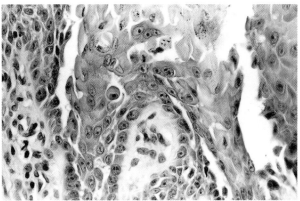

14.6 Warty dyskeratoma
♦ suprabasal acantholysis and dyskeratosis forming an obvious central crater
♦ epidermal hyperplasia and elongation of the rete ridges
♦ solitary papule or nodule with a keratotic umbilicated center usually found on the head and neck
♦ not clinically similar to pemphigus, Darier's disease or Grover's disease

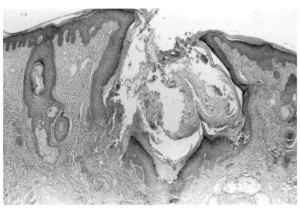

SUBEPIDERMAL VESICLES AND BULLAE

As the name implies, a subepidermal blister is located below the epidermis. The epidermis forms the roof and the underlying dermis is the floor. These blisters are often large and tense, and rupture less easily than more superficial blisters.

Formation of a subepidermal blister may involve defective attachment or structural integrity of the basal cells, epidermal basement membrane, or anchoring fibrils in the papillary dermis. Blistering conditions due to tissue separation above the lamina densa of the basement membrane (bullous pemphigoid) usually do not heal with scarring whereas those below it (dermal epidermolysis bullosa) do.

Although indistinguishable in appearance by routine H & E staining on light microscopy, the plane of separation and pathogenesis of the various subepidermal blistering diseases is different. Immune deposits, for example, are seen in the papillary dermis rather than in the lamina lucida in epidermolysis bullosa acquisita (EBA) on immunoelectron microscopy although, on light and immunofluorescence microscopy, EBA and bullous pemphigoid are morphologically identical.

Ancillary techniques such as PAS staining to show the location of the basement membrane, immunohistochemical staining of type IV collagen, electron microscopy to demonstrate the lamina densa, and direct and indirect immunofluorescence salt-split skin techniques, and clinical findings may aid in the classification of difficult cases.

The individual blisters seen in bullous pemphigoid, acquired epidermolysis bullosa and porphyria cutanea tarda (PCT) are clinically similar, but often appear with different patterns of distribution. In bullous pemphigoid, a disease primarily of the elderly, blisters may develop on normal or erythematous skin, and usually on the medial thighs, flexor aspects of the forearms, axillae, groin, and abdomen. Mucosal involvement, especially oral, is common. Because the split is above the basement membrane, blisters usually heal without scarring.

In EBA, the blisters occur in areas of trauma. Blisters in PCT are usually seen on the hands and are often associated with skin fragility, milia, hyperpigmentation, hypertrichosis, and sclerodermoid changes.

Linear IgA dermatosis and dermatitis herpetiformis may be histologically identical and occasionally clinically indistinguishable, but they differ in their direct immunofluorescence appearances. Linear IgA dermatosis has linear, rather than granular, IgA deposition and a much lower association with gluten-sensitive enteropathy. In-linear IgA dermatosis, IgA antibodies are deposited in the lamina lucida and / or sublamina densa; circulating IgA antibasement membrane antibodies are common.

Basal cell degeneration

Extensive basal cell degeneration and loss of the lowermost layer of the epidermis may result in blister formation that appears to be subepidermal on light microscopy. Such confluent basal cell necrosis may be seen in erythema multiforme, toxic epidermal necrolysis, graft versus host reaction, pityriasis lichenoides et varioliformis acuta, bullous lupus erythematosus, bullous lichen planus, and bullous lichen sclerosus et atrophicus. Bullous variants of most of these conditions are rare; the typical histologic changes are discussed in Chapter 7. Epidermolytic epidermolysis bullosa is also due to cytolysis of basal cells, but develops secondary to trauma and, unlike the other conditions, has an autosomal-dominant inheritance.

Massive dermal edema

The epidermis may be lifted by massive amounts of edema fluid in the papillary dermis so that a histologic appearance mimicking a subepidermal vesicle may be encountered in skin lesions with a marked degree of dermal edema. Conditions where severe dermal edema is often encountered include acute phototoxic reaction, polymorphous light eruption, acute fixed drug eruption, and erythema multiforme. The presence of epidermal rete ridges, vessels, and dermal collagen fibers in the subepidermal space favors edema. However, bullous pemphigoid may present as an urticarial lesion so that an edematous dermis without subepidermal vesiculation does not necessarily exclude the diagnosis of pemphigoid.

15.1 Subepidermal blister

♦ a subepidermal blister in a case of bullous pemphigoid is seen here
♦ the roof is formed by the basal cell layer and the full thickness of the epidermis
♦ location of the PAS-positive epidermal basement membrane is variable and disease-dependent
♦ be aware of regenerating epidermis, which may give a false impression of an intraepidermal blister

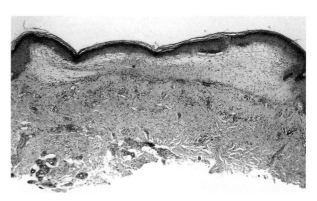

15.2 Basal cell degeneration resulting in a basal cleft

♦ coalescence of degenerating basal cells (the holes along the basal epidermis) forms an incipient basal cleft in erythema multiforme
♦ colloid bodies and lymphocytes are present
♦ progressive vacuolar degeneration of the basal cells may result in a subepidermal bulla

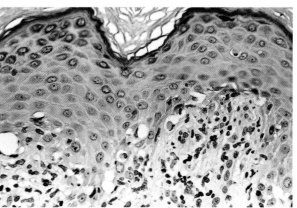

15.3 Dermal edema in polymorphous light eruption

♦ pallor and widening of the papillary dermis are due to edema and fluid accumulation
♦ the epidermis appears to be lifted, suggesting a sub-epidermal blister
♦ distinct from a subepidermal blister, although dermal fibers and epidermal rete ridges (arrow) are seen with an inflammatory infiltrate (lymphocytes) and fibrin strands in massive dermal edema

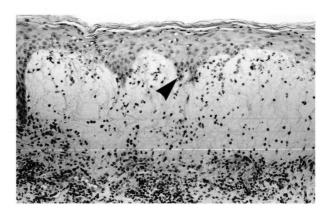

15.4 Bullous pemphigoid

♦ early lesions of bullous pemphigoid (BP) may be urti-carial or dermatitic (upper picture)
♦ bullae in BP are subepidermal (through lamina lucida) and all cell layers of the epidermis form the roof of the blister
♦ the blister floor is formed by the flattened dermis
♦ dermal papillae are not preserved
♦ varying degrees of superficial, dermal, perivascular, in-flammatory infiltration and eosinophils are usually in abundance as well as neutrophils and lymphocytes
♦ urticarial lesions may show eosinophilic spongiosis
♦ regenerating epidermis (arrows; lower picture) along the floor of the blister is indicative of a chronic lesion and should not be taken as evidence of an intraepidermal blister
♦ it is important to be able to recognize epithelial regen-eration along the blister floor (lower picture) as it may be mistaken for an intraepidermal blister

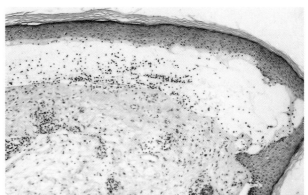

♦ direct immunofluorescence shows linear IgG and C3 along the epidermal basement membrane zone (BMZ); anti-BMZ antibodies in the patient's serum bind to the epithelial side of salt-split normal skin
♦ an eruption of large, tense, subepidermal blisters com-monly seen in the elderly
♦ blisters may develop on normal or erythematous skin

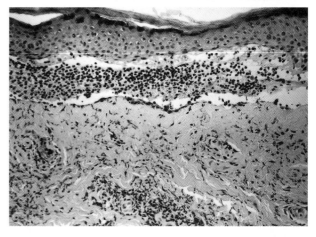

15.5 Herpes gestationis (HG)

♦ HG and **cicatricial pemphigoid** (CP) are histologi-cally identical to bullous pemphigoid
♦ HG occurs in pregnant women and is clinically similar to BP
♦ CP primarily involves the mucosa, and head and neck (where BP is uncommon)
♦ in contrast to BP, few blisters are seen in CP and the lesions heal with scarring

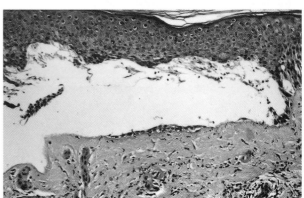

15.6 Junctional epidermolysis bullosa (EB)
♦ separation occurs in the lamina lucida
♦ appears as a subepidermal blister by light microscopy
♦ inflammation is slight except with secondary infection
♦ PAS-positive basement membrane material is seen along the floor (arrow)
♦ electron microscopy may show a reduced number of and/or abnormal hemidesmosomes of the basal cells and/or subbasal dense plate
♦ includes generalized gravis, generalized mitis, inversa, minimus, progressiva, and cicatricial variants
♦ all have autosomal-recessive inheritance
♦ blisters present at birth (onset at ages 5–8 years in progressiva variant)

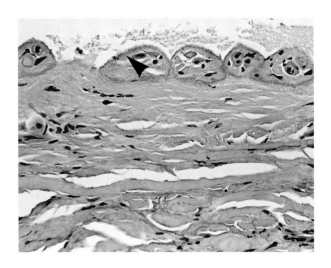

15.7 Dystrophic epidermolysis bullosa (EB)
♦ absent or reduced type VII anchoring fibrils in papillary dermis results in sublamina densa cleavage
♦ PAS-positive basement membrane material along roof of the blister (arrow), or slit between the epidermal roof and dermal floor
♦ dystrophic types may be either autosomal-dominant or -recessive
♦ skin fragility, generalized blisters at birth and in areas of trauma, scarring, milia, oral erosions, dystrophic or absent nails
♦ **EB acquisita** is an autoimmune disorder characterized by subepidermal deposition of IgG antibodies to type VII collagen (primary component of anchoring fibrils) and C3 on direct immunofluorescence; it has similar light microscopic features, skin fragility, blisters in areas of trauma, and scarring

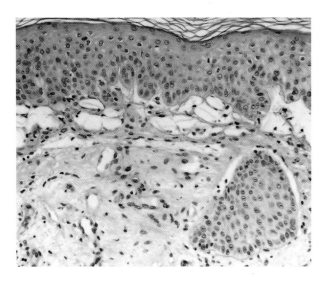

15.8 Porphyria cutanea tarda
♦ subepidermal bulla without inflammatory cell infiltrate
♦ prominent 'rigid' dermal papillae which extend upward into cavity (so-called festooning)
♦ dermal papillae and the walls of the dermal papillary capillaries are filled with a PAS-positive diastase-resistant material (small arrow)
♦ 'caterpillar bodies' are PAS-positive, diastase-resistant, elongated, and segmented structures that may be seen in the epidermal roof
♦ basement membrane (large arrow) is seen along the floor of the blister
♦ blisters primarily on the hands are associated with skin fragility, milia, hyperpigmentation, sclerodermoid changes, and hypertrichosis

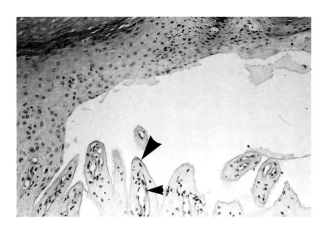

15.9 Dermatitis herpetiformis (DH)

♦ neutrophilic microabscesses in the tips of the dermal papilla

♦ leukocytoclasis may be present; presence of degenerated neutrophils and nuclear dust may be mistaken for leukocytoclastic vasculitis

♦ carefully examine the vessels of the papillary dermis to confirm that the neutrophilic infiltration is not angiocentric

♦ granular IgA in papillary tips on direct immunofluorescence of involved and uninvolved skin

♦ intensely pruritic papules and vesicles appear typically on the elbows, knees, buttocks, and scalp

♦ with gluten-sensitive enteropathy, usually not clinically evident and only identifiable with small bowel biopsy

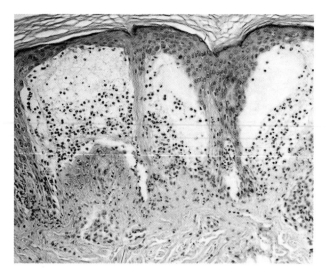

15.10 Linear IgA dermatosis

♦ accumulations of neutrophils and fibrin at dermal papillae (papillary microabscesses) and in bullae identical to those of dermatitis herpetiformis

♦ linear IgA deposition at the dermoepidermal junction (within the lamina lucida and / or below the lamina densa)

♦ autoantibodies to a 97-kD antigen anchoring filament antigen, a 230-kD hemidesmosome antigen, or 290-kD type VII collagen

♦ may develop in adults or in children (**chronic bullous disease of childhood**), or be drug-induced (for example, vancomycin)

♦ unlike DH, rarely associated with gluten-sensitive enteropathy

♦ large bullae with annular and / or polycyclic shapes, forming a 'cluster of jewels', are seen on normal or erythematous skin of the trunk, buttocks, thighs, groin, or around the mouth

♦ clinical differential diagnosis: varicella; herpes simplex; and bullous impetigo; however, these entities are all easily distinguished on histology or bacterial culture (impetigo)

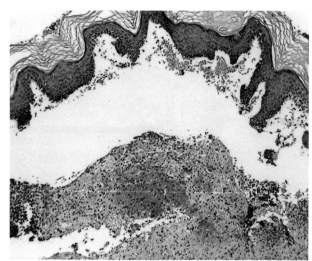

15.11 Epidermolytic epidermolysis bullosa

♦ histologic appearance mimics a subepidermal blister with minimal inflammation

♦ cleavage along the basal cell layer and epidermal separation is due to degeneration of basal cells

♦ PAS staining shows basement membrane (arrow) lining the floor of the blister

♦ blisters are formed as a consequence of trauma

♦ clinical variants include Koebner, Weber–Cockayne, Dowling–Meara, Ogna, and Kallin

♦ all have autosomal-dominant inheritance

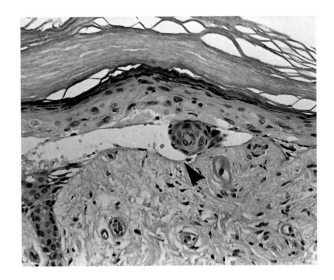

15.12 Bullous lichen sclerosus et atrophicus (LSA)

♦ in this bullous lesion of LSA, the subepidermal blister involves the right-hand side of the section

♦ formation of the blister is the result of extensive and confluent basal cell degeneration and necrosis

♦ as already mentioned (see page 93), so-called interface dermatitis may present as a subepidermal vesicular lesion if the basal cell degeneration is extensive

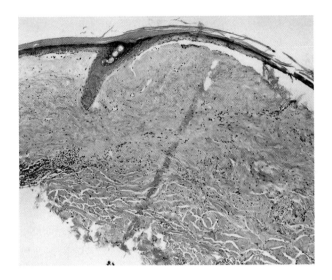

15.13 Fixed drug eruption

♦ severe papillary dermal edema in such conditions as **fixed drug eruption** and **polymorphous light eruption** give rise to histologic appearances that may be mistaken for a subepidermal blister

♦ the dermis shown here is heavily infiltrated by lymphocytes and eosinophils

♦ massive papillary dermal edema is present and strands of vertically oriented fibers span the subepidermal space

♦ rete ridges are stretched, but maintain contact with the dermis

♦ a dermal capillary (arrow) is an expected finding in dermal edema, but not in a subepidermal blister

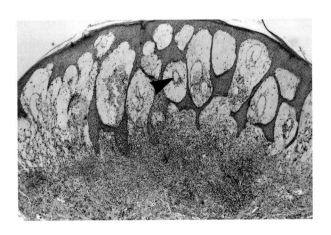

DERMIS

COLLAGEN AND ELASTIC FIBERS

Collagen

The term **sclerosis**, when used in histopathology, implies thickening, or an increased amount, of collagen within the dermis. In a sclerotic dermis, the collagen bundles are thickened and the spaces between the fibers diminished or lost. The histologic appearance contrasts with dermal mucinosis (see Chapter 17), in which the spaces between the fibers are increased. Sclerotic fibers are generally more eosinophilic, an appearance that may be referred to as hyalinization of the dermis. Variability of staining may, however, render this feature difficult to appreciate. Sclerosis is a characteristic feature of morphea.

An increased amount of newly formed fibrous tissue is also encountered in recent scars and tumors. Many tumors are characterized by a striking amount of fibrosis (the desmoplastic reaction). Even at low magnification, the malignant nature is easily recognized because of the increased cellularity and cellular pleomorphism of the tumor cells.

Atrophy of the dermis is a subtle histologic finding. It refers to thinning of the connective tissue layer which, in turn, brings the fat layer closer to the surface. The overlying epidermis often shows thinning. To ascertain atrophy, it may be necessary to take a biopsy from a normal uninvolved control site from the same part of the body (as dermal thickness varies with body location) for comparison. Dermal atrophy, if localized, is usually manifested clinically as a depressed area. If there is no epidermal atrophy, the skin is normal in color and the skin lines are retained. If epidermal atrophy is also present, the skin surface may be transparent, and the skin lines are lost. Dermal atrophy is usually secondary to inflammation or trauma.

Diseases of defective collagen production (such as Ehlers–Danlos syndrome) may show no histopathologic abnormalities unless the skin has been altered by trauma.

Hyaline is a descriptive term used in dermatopathology for a non-specific morphologic appearance which is often confined to extracellular dermal components. The hallmark feature of hyaline change is a homogeneous, pink, opaque appearance of the dermis on H & E-stained sections. It is important to appreciate that many different mechanisms involving many different extracellular proteins may produce this change. Hyaline change may be a result of altered collagen or elastin, or deposition of a protein not normally found in the dermis.

Hyaline change is a feature of lichen sclerosis, chronic radiation dermatitis, colloid milium, and amyloid. In lichen sclerosus, the collagen fibers become a pink amorphous mass (homogenization) whereas, in colloid milium, hyaline change represents degenerated elastic fibers. Amyloid is eosinophilic and homogeneous and, when present within the dermis, may mimic altered collagen. However, the collagen fibers are normal. Amyloid consists of deposits of rigid non-branching aggregated fibrillary proteins 7.5–10 nm in diameter and arranged in a β-pleated sheet configuration. Keratin is the protein precursor in lichen amyloidosus. Amyloid may be confirmed by Congo red staining.

Elastic fibers

Normal elastic fibers are difficult to evaluate in routine H & E-stained sections. When damaged, the elastic fibers become more visible and stain more strongly with hematoxylin. Elastic fibers are demonstrated with special stains such as Verhoeff–van Gieson and acid orcein. Abnormal proliferation of elastic fibers is referred to as **elastosis**, which is basophilic on H & E staining. Changes in elastic tissue may only be seen with microscopy, or may also be seen clinically as yellow papules and plaques (as in solar elastosis, pseudoxanthoma elasticum, or elastoma) or as erythematous keratotic papules in a serpiginous pattern (elastosis perforans serpiginosa). The eosinophilic deposits in colloid milium represent degenerated elastic fibers. These are pink-staining with H & E, but are stained blue in solar elastosis.

16.1 Collagen fibers in normal dermis
♦ collagen fibers in the papillary and periadnexal adventitial dermis are extremely fine with a diameter of 1–2 μ
♦ individual fibrils are difficult to appreciate on light microscopy, conferring an eosinophilic and amorphous appearance to the papillary dermis
♦ collagen fibers in the reticular dermis are organized into thick bundles, many of which lie parallel to the skin surface
♦ normal reticular dermis shows occasional fibroblasts and nuclei (arrow) between the collagen bundles

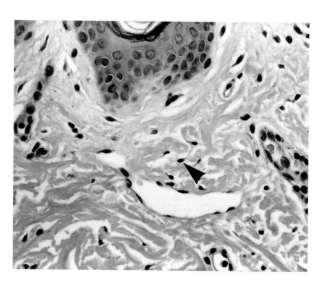

16.2 Verhoeff–van Gieson stain showing elastic fibers

♦ elastic fibers within the papillary dermis are fine and form a plexus (elaunin fibers) parallel to the epidermodermal junction

♦ the fine, vertical, elastic fibers in the papillary dermis are the oxytalan fibers

♦ elastic fibers in the reticular dermis are thicker and organized into coarser bundles

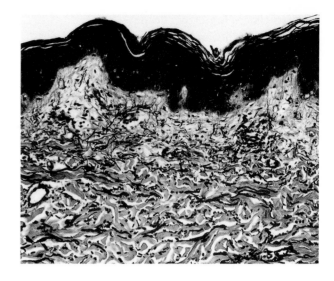

16.3 Dermal sclerosis

♦ note the thickened collagen fibers in the dermis and decreased spaces between the fibers in this case of morphea

♦ collagen fibers appear rigid; cleft-like artifacts are often observed

♦ paucity of cell nuclei in sclerotic collagen

♦ atrophic adnexal structures

♦ a small eccrine duct is shown here (upper center of this field)

SCLEROSIS

16.4 Hypertrophic scar

♦ the newly formed collagen in the superficial dermis is basophilic and cellular

♦ myofibroblasts, which have ovoid nuclei with indentations along the nuclear membrane, are present

♦ myofibroblasts share features of smooth muscle cells (actin filaments) and fibroblasts

♦ myofibroblasts provide the contractile force in wound closure and healing

♦ hypertrophic scars and keloids represent excessive proliferation of fibrous tissue during wound healing

♦ hypertrophic scars and keloids both appear red, raised, and firm with a smooth surface

♦ hypertrophic scars tend to flatten with time whereas keloids remain exuberant and may extend beyond the site of initial injury

♦ delayed development may clinically simulate sarcoid (granulomas)

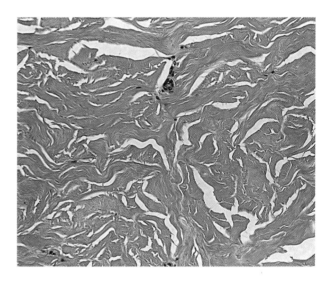

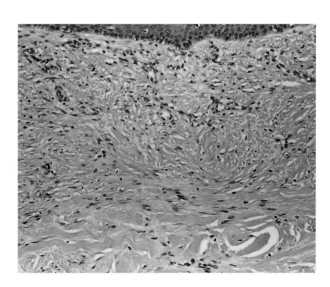

16.5 Keloid

♦ cellular dermal scar with proliferating myofibroblasts
♦ hyaline change of the collagen fibers is characteristic
♦ nodular formations of collagen fibers which are haphazardly arranged
♦ especially common in Orientals and blacks
♦ red, raised, firm, exuberant scar tissue which may extend beyond the site of initial injury

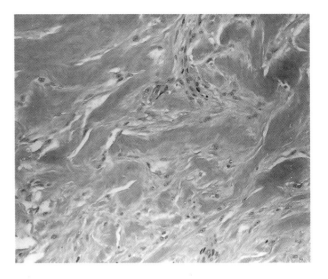

16.6 Collagenoma

♦ increased collagen fibers, but the increased thickness of the dermis may be difficult to visualize by microscopy unless there is homogenization of the collagen fibers or a concomitant increase in elastic fibers; biopsy from an uninvolved normal area may be helpful for comparison
♦ smooth, flesh-colored to yellow, oval, slightly raised papules which frequently coalesce to form a cobblestone pattern commonly over the trunk or thighs
♦ may be associated with tuberous sclerosis (**shagreen patch**) or osteopoikilosis (**Buschke–Ollendorff syndrome**)
♦ elastoma is clinically indistinguishable from collagenoma, but has an increase of elastic fibers rather than collagen fibers

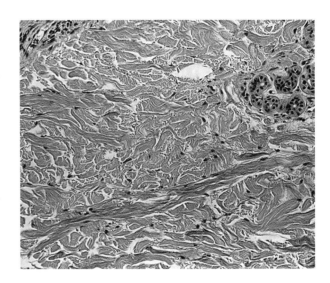

16.7 Morphea (localized scleroderma)

♦ histologic features are the same for all clinical types of morphea and systemic sclerosis
♦ a bulky dermis with straight edges and square corners at the deep margins of the biopsy (boxcar sign on skin punches)
♦ thickening of the dermal collagen and loss of spaces between the fibers, which stain strongly eosinophilic
♦ sclerotic fibrous tissue extends into subcutaneous fat
♦ lack of homogenization of the papillary dermal collagen may help to differentiate from lichen sclerosus
♦ epidermal atrophy and a few degenerated basal keratinocytes
♦ pigmentary incontinence with pigment-laden dermal melanophages
♦ early lesions of morphea are inflammatory with lymphocytes around dermal vessels
♦ only chronic lesions show characteristic eosinophilic sclerosis
♦ reduced number of adnexal structures, vessels, and fibroblasts

(continued next page)

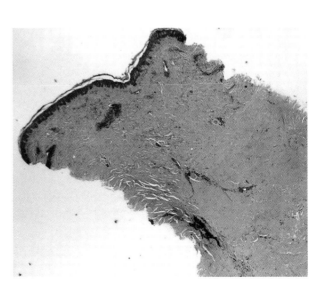

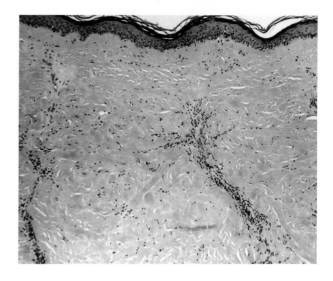

- characterized by indurated, ivory-white, round-to-oval, usually multiple, plaques with a violaceous border which may become atrophic and hyper- or hypopigmented with time
- linear morphea presents as linear, depressed, sclerotic bands and, in children, may be associated with lack of growth of the involved area
- clinically may be confused with lichen sclerosus; both conditions may also coexist
- an association with Lyme disease has been reported
- may resemble scleredema when acute
- may resemble atrophoderma of Pasini and Pierini when chronic

16.8 Desmoplastic tumor reaction

- describes the fibrous reaction to invasive malignancy
- fibrous tissue is cellular and disorganized, and accounts for the clinically firm consistency of tumors
- the fibrous reaction is marked in this case of sclerotic (morpheic) basal cell carcinoma
- tumor cells (arrow) may be so compressed that they are difficult to see
- desmoplastic melanoma is another example in which spindle-shaped melanomatous cells blend with, and are difficult to be distinguished from, the spindle fibrous tissue of desmoplastic fibrous stroma
- immunohistochemical stains such as cytokeratin and S100 protein may be used to highlight carcinomatous and melanomatous cells if necessary

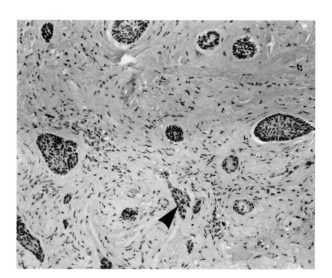

DERMAL ATROPHY

16.9 Atrophic dermal scar

- on microscopy, a well-healed dermal scar may be difficult to identify, but its presence may be of significance (evidence of a previous resection or biopsy in an atypical nevus)
- elastin staining is helpful to demonstrate focal absence of elastic fibers (shown here)
- histologic differential diagnosis: **striae distensae**, which show fragmentation, and focal fragmentation and loss of elastic fibers; wrinkling due to **middermal elastosis**, which shows focal loss of elastic fibers in the middermis; and **anetoderma**, which may show perivascular inflammation and eventual loss of elastic fibers
- clinical diagnosis is seldom a problem, especially if there is a history of trauma

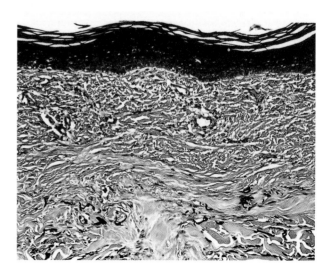

16.10 Atrophoderma of Pasini and Pierini

♦ histologic diagnosis usually requires a second biopsy of uninvolved skin from the same area of the body for comparison
♦ normal skin taken adjacent to the lesion (upper picture)
♦ biopsy of atrophoderma of Pasini and Pierini (lower picture) shows dermal thinning and atrophy
♦ hyaline thickening of collagen fibers and slight inflammation have been described, but these changes are not always present
♦ slate-colored, slightly depressed, patches primarily on the back which spread slowly over a number of years and then persist
♦ may be mistaken clinically for morphea, although the latter is usually indurated

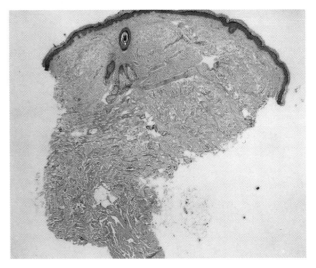

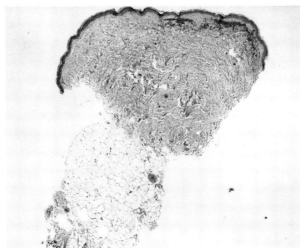

16.11 Anetoderma

♦ flattened epidermis, dermal edema, and a lymphocytic perivascular and periappendageal infiltrate early on
♦ fragmentation and loss of elastic fibers starting in the subpapillary zone and extending downward, resulting in a coin-shaped area without elastic fibers (as shown here)
♦ macules, which may initially be erythematous (**anetoderma of Jadassohn**), urticarial wheals (**anetoderma of Pellizari**), or flesh-colored papules (**anetoderma of Schweninger–Buzzi**), become wrinkled and atrophic, and may be indented by finger pressure through the rim of normal surrounding skin
♦ clinical differential diagnosis: atrophic scars; fat herniations in focal dermal hypoplasia; secondary macular atrophy in LE; syphilis; and acrodermatitis chronica atrophicans

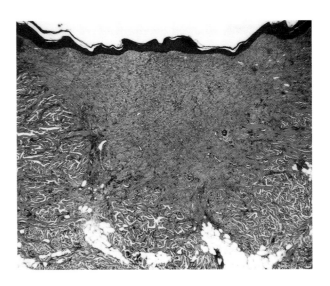

HYALINE CHANGE

16.12 Lichen sclerosus (et atrophicus)

- compact hyperkeratosis and epidermal atrophy
- eosinophilic change and homogenization of papillary dermal collagen
- fibrous arrangement of the collagen fibers is lost; the superficial dermis appears amorphous, although finer elastic fibers are still visible
- superficial dermis may be edematous and pale-staining, but deep dermal tissue is normal
- genital and extragenital lesions
- in women, genital involvement is typically seen as 'figure-of-eight' whiteness, hemorrhage, and itching
- extragenital lesions are flat-topped white papules with follicular plugs and dells which may coalesce to form plaques resembling morphea
- may coexist with morphea

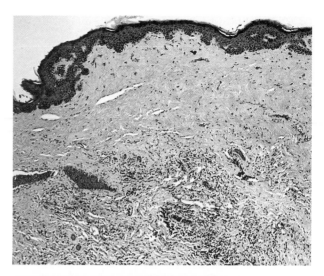

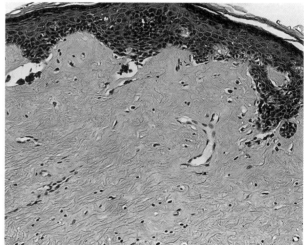

16.13 Chronic radiation dermatitis

- hyaline change of the dermal collagen, particularly in the superficial dermis
- dilated superficial vessels
- dermal edema in acute lesions and reactive stellate fibroblasts with pleomorphic nuclei in chronic lesions
- partial or complete loss of skin appendages
- epidermis has an irregular thickness with alternating areas of acanthosis, atrophy, hyperkeratosis, and patchy parakeratosis
- thin, dry, indurated hyper- or hypopigmented plaque with hyperkeratosis, telangiectasia and, sometimes, ulceration

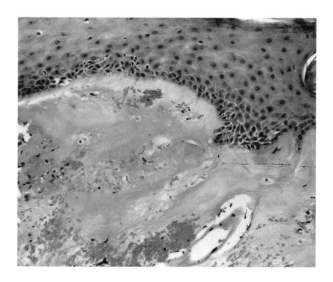

16.14 Lichen amyloidosus (LA)

♦ amount of amyloid is small and confined to the papillary dermis (arrows)
♦ amyloid material in LA is believed to originate from basal cells
♦ Congo red staining renders amyloid material red/orange in color which appears apple-green under polarized light
♦ amyloid also stains with crystal violet and thioflavine T
♦ more common in Orientals and South Americans
♦ brown/red/grey itchy lichenoid papules which may coalesce to form hyperkeratotic plaques clinically resembling lichen simplex chronicus or hyperkeratotic lichen planus, conditions which may be differentiated by histology

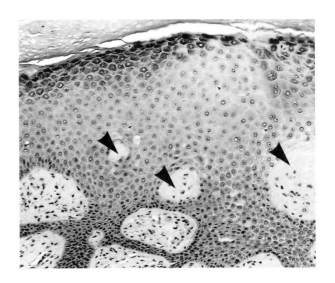

16.15 Colloid milium

♦ well-circumscribed dermal collections of eosinophilic homogeneous material with a striking resemblance to amyloidosis
♦ low magnification (upper picture) shows the papular nature of the lesion
♦ fractures consisting of hyaline material and clefts are typically seen (lower picture)
♦ in common with amyloid, stains with Congo red and exhibits apple-green birefringence
♦ electron microscopy reveals that, unlike amyloid, the filaments are degenerated elastic fibers
♦ 1–2-mm, yellow, translucent papules found in clusters on sun-exposed skin
♦ may release jelly-like material when punctured

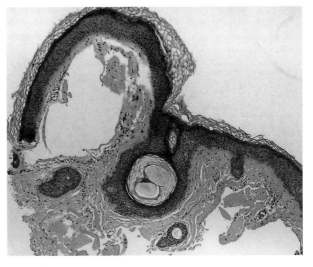

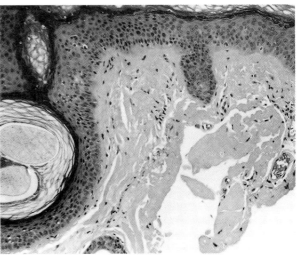

ABNORMAL ELASTIC TISSUE

16.16 Actinic elastosis

♦ although elastosis is recognizable with H & E (upper picture), abnormalities of the elastic fibers are best seen with an elastic fiber stain (lower picture)

♦ increased amount of thickened elastic fibers which eventually become curled and tangled, or amorphous in extreme cases

♦ amorphous aggregates of elastic fibers are basophilic and smudgy with H & E

♦ elastic-tissue changes confined to upper-third or -half of the dermis in less severe cases; tissue in the immediate subepidermal area is spared

♦ telangiectatic vessels

♦ often not visible clinically, but may present as yellow thickened wrinkled skin (Milian's citrine skin), yellow papules on the face associated with open comedones and cysts (Favre–Racouchot syndrome), yellow thickened skin with furrows on the nape of the neck (cutis rhomboidalis nuchae), or diffuse yellow plaques on the face or neck (Dubreuilh's elastoma)

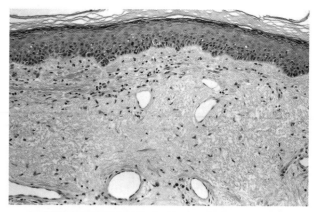

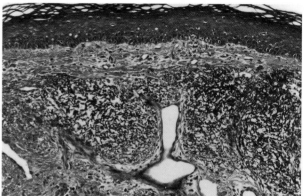

16.17 Pseudoxanthoma elasticum

♦ middermal elastic fibers appear coarsely granular and contain calcium hydroxyapatite

♦ abnormal fibers are more visible with elastic (lower picture) or von Kossa staining than with routine H & E staining (upper picture)

♦ massive calcification may occur, leading to foreign body granulomatous inflammation

♦ 1–3-mm yellow papules in a linear pattern forming plaques on the sides of the neck, axillae, abdomen, and groin

♦ may be associated with angioid streaks in the retina, hypertension, intermittent claudication, coronary artery disease, and cerebral or gastrointestinal hemorrhage

♦ autosomal-recessive or -dominant inheritance

♦ clinical appearance is usually diagnostic, especially if there is a positive family history

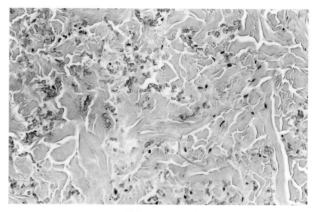

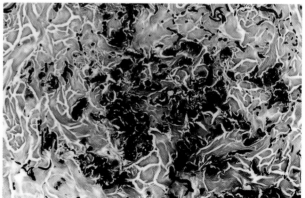

16.18 Elastosis perforans serpiginosa (EPS)

- ♦ two foci of transepidermal elimination of elastotic material can be seen (H & E; arrows)
- ♦ basophilic material in papillary dermis surrounded by inflammatory cells and foreign body granulomas
- ♦ claw-like epidermal downgrowth surrounds the lesion
- ♦ abnormal elastic fibers are eliminated with cellular debris and inflammatory cells through transepidermal defect, resembling Kyrle's disease and perforating folliculitis, although only EPS has an increased amount of elastic fibers in the dermis
- ♦ high-power view (lower picture) of an epidermal tunnel filled with curly elastic fibers and keratin highlighted by elastic staining
- ♦ serpiginous, pink, keratotic papules usually on the neck and arms
- ♦ may be associated with Down syndrome and penicillamine use
- ♦ clinical differential diagnosis: granuloma annulare (necrobiosis); porokeratosis of Mibelli (cornoid lamella); annular sarcoid (granulomas); and tinea corporis (hyphae in stratum corneum, no elastic tissue changes, positive KOH and fungal culture)

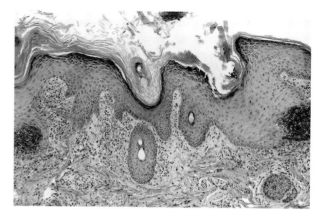

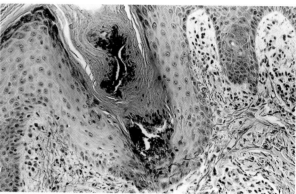

MUCIN DEPOSITION

Dermal mucin usually originates from fibroblasts in unusual inflammatory dermatoses or from glandular dermal neoplasms (benign or malignant). Mucin is composed of carbohydrate-rich glycoproteins (primarily hyaluronic acid and dermatan sulfate), which are also present in the ground substance of connective tissue. Excessive separation of collagen fibers suggests dermal mucinosis. Because mucin is largely water, it is easily removed by dehydration in processing. Thus, it often appears as a clear space or as basophilic shreds and granules in routine H & E-stained sections.

Fibroblast-derived acid mucin stains positively with alcian blue at pH 2.5 (but not at pH 0.5), toluidine blue, and colloidal iron, but negatively with PAS staining. As a large proportion of mucin is hyaluronic acid in cutaneous mucinoses (lichen myxedematosus, focal cutaneous mucinosis, myxedema, mucous cyst, and alopecia mucinosa), its presence may be further confirmed by pretreatment with hyaluronidase. Chondroitin sulfate is the predominant dermal mucin in Hurler and Hunter's syndromes. Unlike the acid mucin of the fibroblasts, epithelial mucin is neutral and positively stained by mucicarmine and PAS after diastase digestion.

Many unrelated conditions are characterized by dermal mucin deposition. Distinctive cutaneous mucinoses include lichen myxedematosus (papular mucinosis, scleromyxedema), myxedema, scleredema, storage diseases (mucopolysaccharidoses), reticular erythematous mucinosis (reticular erythematous infiltrated macules and papules on the upper torso which may be aggravated by sunlight), acral persistent papular mucinosis (papules on the backs of the hands and wrists), papular and nodular mucinosis associated with lupus erythematosus (LE; flesh-colored papules on the neck, trunk, and arms with papillary and middermal mucin deposits without the typical microscopic features of LE, although indirect immunofluorescence may show IgG, IgM, and / or C3 at the dermoepidermal junction), cutaneous focal mucinosis (a solitary lesion), self-healing juvenile cutaneous mucinosis (plaques and nodules with a predilection for the head and trunk in adolescents which spontaneously resolve within months), cutaneous mucinosis of infancy (discrete, pinpoint, grouped papules on the elbows and hands in infants), papular mucinosis of the toxic oil syndrome (reported in 1981 in Spain, with initial interstitial pneumonitis followed by white to yellow papules on the arms and legs, sclerodermoid changes, and neuromuscular disease), and mucous cyst (digital myxoid cyst and oral mucous cyst).

A number of diseases may also have dermal mucin deposition as an additional histopathologic feature, including collagen–vascular diseases (such as LE, dermatomyositis, scleroderma), Degos' disease, pachydermoperiostosis, hypertrophic scar, actinic elastosis, necrobiotic granulomatous reactions (for example, granuloma annulare, but usually less marked or absent in necrobiosis lipoidica and rheumatoid nodule), and hereditary progressive mucinous histiocytosis. Furthermore, many different cutaneous tumors, including basal cell carcinoma, various benign and malignant sweat gland tumors such as chondroid syringoma and colloid carcinoma of eccrine gland, and connective tissue tumors such as lipoma, liposarcoma, neurofibroma, neurilemmoma, and nerve sheath myxoma, may reveal demonstrable amounts of mucin on microscopy.

Although the various types of mucin are identical with H & E staining, the finding of epithelial cells within mucin pools strongly suggests a mucin-secreting neoplasm. Necrobiotic conditions may be identified by the presence of mucin in areas of necrobiosis surrounded by epithelioid histiocytes and giant cells.

Follicular mucin deposition may be seen as a distinctive feature of alopecia mucinosa, but may also be present in LE, lichen planus, lichen striatus, dermatitis, photodermatitis, angiolymphoid hyperplasia with eosinophilia, sarcoidosis, Hodgkin's and non-Hodgkin's lymphomas, and leukemia.

Differential diagnoses

Mucin deposition without epithelioid cells

Lichen myxedematosus / papular mucinosis	17.1
Lichen myxedematosus / scleromyxedema	17.2
Pretibial myxedema	17.3
Cutaneous myxoma (including Carney's complex)	17.4
Scleredema	17.5
Digital mucous (myxoid) cyst / mucocele	17.6
Lupus erythematosus	17.7

Mucin deposition with epithelioid cells

Primary mucinous (colloid) carcinoma	17.8
Myxoma of nerve sheath (neurothekeoma)	17.9

Necrobiotic granuloma with mucin

Granuloma annulare	17.10
Necrobiosis lipoidica	17.11
Rheumatoid nodule	17.12

Follicular mucin deposition

Alopecia mucinosa (follicular mucinosis)	17.13

MUCIN DEPOSITION WITHOUT EPITHELIOID CELLS

17.1 Lichen myxedematosus / papular mucinosis

♦ presence of mucin in the dermis is suggested by separation and spaces appearing between collagen fibers

♦ dermis is cellular because of an increased number of fibroblasts with slightly enlarged nuclei

♦ some degree of lymphocytic infiltration is common

♦ epidermis may be thinned due to pressure from the mucinous deposits beneath it

♦ extensive chronic eruption, typically on the hands, arms, and face, consisting of 2–3-mm waxy papules which are often linear

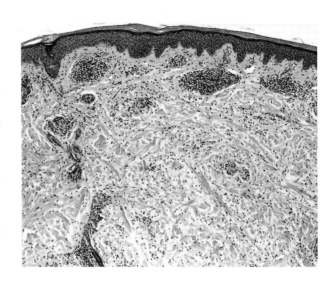

17.2 Lichen myxedematosus / scleromyxedema

♦ similar to papular mucinosis but, in addition, there is an increased irregular deposition of collagen

♦ there may be a proliferation of fibroblasts

♦ collagen fibers are split by increased tissue mucin

♦ clinically similar to papular mucinosis except that there is also a diffuse thickening of the skin

♦ strong association with monoclonal gammopathy, primarily IgG

♦ there may be mucin deposition in various organs

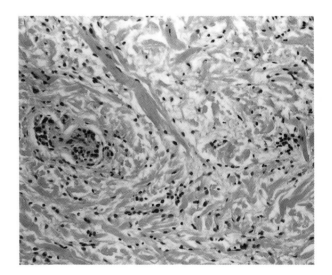

17.3 Pretibial myxedema

♦ epidermis and papillary dermis are normal, although hyperkeratosis may be present

♦ reticular dermis considerably thickened by voluminous mucin, which splits the collagen fibers

♦ stellate fibroblasts may be seen in mucin-rich areas

♦ flesh-colored to yellow / red / brown bilateral nodules and plaques with induration and prominent follicular orifices, giving a *peau d'orange* appearance primarily in the pretibial area

♦ usually associated with Graves' disease

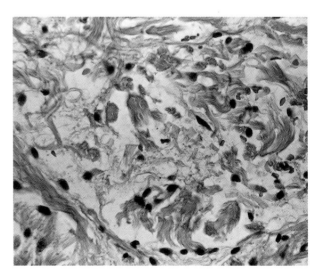

17.4 Cutaneous myxoma (including Carney's complex)

♦ freshly excised tumors exude a sticky mucoid fluid

♦ sharply circumscribed, rarely encapsulated, dermal and / or subcutaneous tumor

♦ within the myxoid stroma are stellate or spindle-shaped fibroblasts, branching capillaries, and scattered mast cells

♦ papule usually < 1 cm in diameter with a predilection for eyelids, ears, and nipples

♦ **Carney's complex** (also known as **LAMB** or **NAME**) refers to myxomas (cutaneous, cardiac, mammary), spotty pigmentation (lentigines and blue nevi on skin and mucous membranes), and endocrine overactivity (sexual precocity, large-cell calcifying Sertoli cell tumor of the testicle, acromegaly, Cushing's syndrome); may have autosomal-dominant inheritance; early detection of cutaneous myxoma may help detect cardiac myxoma

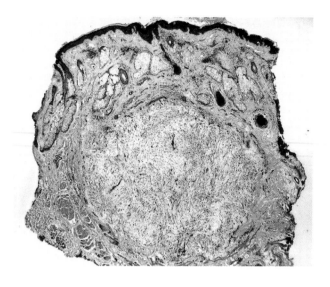

17.5 Scleredema

♦ normal epidermis

♦ dermis is thickened three- to fourfold due to infiltration of mucin between collagen fibers

♦ differs from lichen myxedematosus in that the number of fibroblast nuclei is not increased, although there is dermal thickening presumably due to excessive collagen production

♦ may have mild perivascular lymphocytic infiltrate in papillary dermis and an increased number of mast cells

♦ ill-defined woody induration of the upper back and neck which may extend to the face, trunk, and extremities

♦ often associated with a preceding viral or streptococcal infection or diabetes mellitus; may gradually involute (especially if postinfectious) or be relentless (especially if associated with diabetes mellitus)

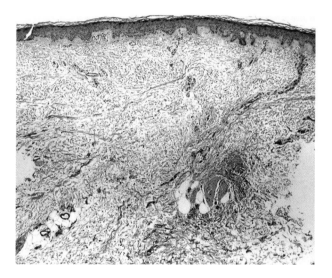

17.6 Digital mucous (myxoid) cyst

♦ poorly defined areas of dermal mucin initially but, with time, coalesces to form a well-demarcated lesion with cavity formation

♦ overlying epidermis may be thinned

♦ **digital mucous (myxoid) cyst** is a solitary nodule, located near the nail or distal interphalangeal joint, which exudes a clear, viscous, jelly-like material if incised; may be associated with osteoarthritis

♦ **mucocele** is an oral cyst, commonly found on the lower lip; it often develops after minor trauma, resulting in rupture of a mucous duct, mucous accumulation, and formation of a cyst with a histologic appearance similar to digital mucous cyst

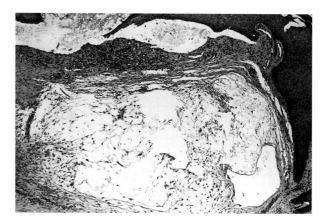

17.7 Lupus erythematosus (LE)

♦ often increased dermal mucin in typical LE lesions

♦ mucinous area is immediately below the epidermis, identifiable by the excessive amount of empty space present between collagen fibers

♦ acid mucin deposition may be confirmed by alcian blue staining

♦ other features of LE (epidermal atrophy, follicular plugging, vacuolar degeneration of basal cells) are seen

♦ discoid LE lesions are violaceous to reddish-brown plaques with hyperkeratosis and central atrophy, typically on the face and scalp

♦ subacute LE lesions are often annular with slight scale

♦ systemic LE lesions are usually erythematous plaques

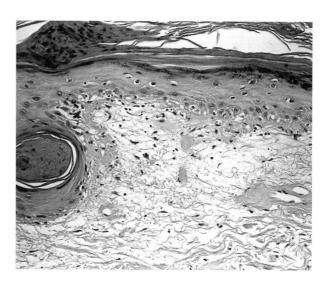

MUCIN DEPOSITION WITH EPITHELIOID CELLS

17.8 Primary mucinous (colloid) carcinoma

- mucin-producing adenocarcinoma of eccrine glandular origin
- mucin pools separated into compartments by thin fibrous strands
- small aggregates of well- to moderately differentiated tumor cells apparently floating in mucin (arrow)
- luminal and glandular differentiation may be seen
- histologically identical to metastatic colloid carcinoma of breast, stomach, colon, or ovary; diagnosis of a primary eccrine colloid carcinoma requires exclusion of a metastatic carcinoma
- slow-growing, small, flesh-colored, nodule ± telangiectasia and ulceration; metastases are uncommon
- clinical differential diagnosis: epidermoid cyst; basal cell carcinoma; squamous cell carcinoma; and pilomatricoma

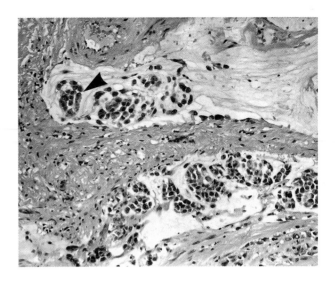

17.9 Myxoma of nerve sheath (neurothekeoma)

- mature lesions tend to be myxoid whereas immature nerve sheath myxomas are cellular and made up of epithelioid cells
- in the mature lesion shown here, lobules of mucinous tissue are surrounded by dense fibrous tissue (perineurium)
- spindle cells with fibrillary cell bodies and cytoplasmic processes are evident in the mucinous stroma
- in the immature type, margins are poorly defined and there is less mucin
- soft nodules on face and arms
- high magnification shows the mixed population of spindle and epithelioid cells, which may or may not be S100 protein-positive

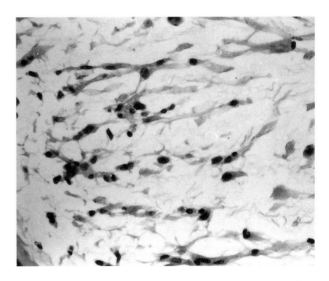

NECROBIOTIC GRANULOMA WITH MUCIN

17.10 Granuloma annulare (GA)

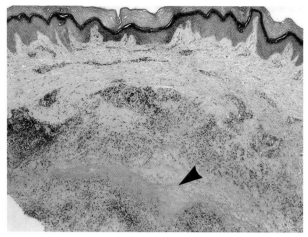

♦ necrobiotic type GA (upper picture) has a compact keratin layer on the skin surface, indicating a lesion of the extremities

♦ centrally, a cell-poor area with faintly basophilic mucin and necrobiotic degenerated collagen (arrow)

♦ multinucleated giant cells may be present in the surrounding layers of lymphohistiocytic cells

♦ histologically infiltrative type of GA (lower picture) shows minimal necrobiotic change of collagen fibers

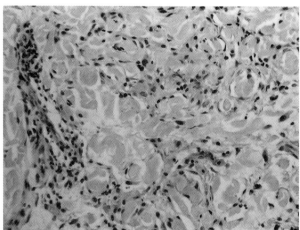

♦ only a slight amount of mucin deposition, but the collagen fibers are surrounded by histiocytic cells

♦ histologically infiltrative variant is an easy lesion to miss on microscopy

♦ firm, flesh-colored to pink papules in an annular arrangement on the extremities typically in children and young adults; approximately half are solitary

♦ subcutaneous GA is a disease of children with deep dermal or subcutaneous nodules on the lower legs, buttocks, hands, scalp, and periorbital area; often misdiagnosed as a rheumatoid nodule, causing unnecessary alarm and investigations; in contrast to rheumatoid nodule, mucin may be prominent

♦ generalized GA usually occurs in middle-aged adults as numerous papules particularly over the extremities; may be associated with diabetes mellitus

17.11 Necrobiosis lipoidica (NL)

♦ normal or atrophic epidermis

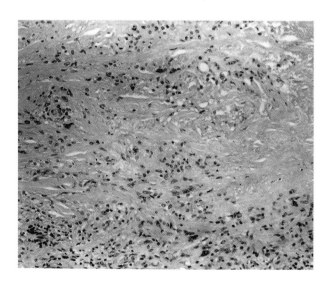

♦ unlike GA, minimal or no mucin; mucin staining may help to differentiate these two conditions with necrobiotic granulomatous inflammation

♦ more diffuse necrobiosis in NL compared with GA and the inflammation is usually granulomatous

♦ endothelial proliferation and blood vessel wall thickening with PAS-positive diastase-resistant material in NL

♦ no intracellular elastin (unlike GA, which may have this finding)

♦ typically, yellow plaques with telangiectasia and a violaceous to brown indurated border in the pretibial area; may be ulcerated; usually associated with diabetes mellitus

♦ usually a clinical diagnosis; if biopsy is necessary, the edge of the lesion should be biopsied and the patient warned that biopsy may cause ulceration

17.12 Rheumatoid nodule
- ◆ histologically similar to subcutaneous GA
- ◆ centrally, a characteristic cell-poor area of fibrinoid degeneration
- ◆ peripherally, surrounding lymphocytes and histiocytes, and the occasional multinucleated giant cell
- ◆ dermal mucin is minimal and may be absent; again, mucin staining is useful, although the clinical diagnosis is seldom difficult in a patient with rheumatoid arthritis
- ◆ outer zone of granulation tissue with a mononuclear and plasma cell infiltrate
- ◆ present in approximately 20% of adults with rheumatoid arthritis
- ◆ often associated with more severe disease
- ◆ firm, non-tender, flesh-colored nodules usually located on extensor surfaces of the extremities, particularly over the olecranon

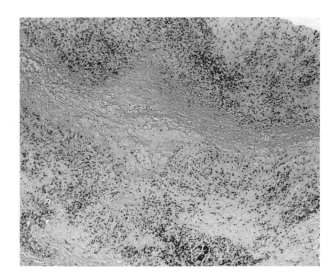

FOLLICULAR MUCIN DEPOSITION

17.13 Alopecia mucinosa (follicular mucinosis)
- ◆ mucinous degeneration of outer root sheath (large arrow) and sebaceous glands which may result in the formation of cystic spaces filled with mucin (small arrow)
- ◆ inflammation may be marked with lymphocytes, histiocytes, and eosinophils
- ◆ a few mutinucleated epithelioid histiocytic giant cells may be present, as seen here
- ◆ atypical lymphocytes and a band-like infiltrate suggest mycosis fungoides
- ◆ follicular papules or plaques which coalesce into one or more well-defined erythematous plaques on the head and neck; prominent follicular openings; alopecia is not prominent unless in a hairy area such as the beard or scalp
- ◆ may be benign and self-limiting (resolving within 2 months to 2 years), chronic and relapsing or persistent, and associated with cutaneous T-cell lymphoma

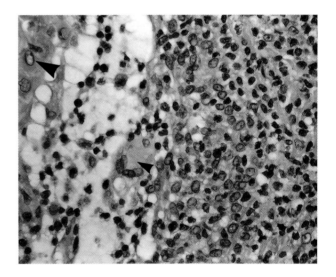

LYMPHOCYTIC INFILTRATION

Lymphocytic cellular infiltration of the dermal vessels is a basic histopathologic change common to all inflammatory skin diseases. Most papulosquamous eruptions and acute dermatitis show aggregation of lymphocytes around the superficial vessels. With increasing severity and / or chronicity, lymphocytes may be seen around the mid- and lower dermal vessels. However, heavy infiltration rather than a sprinkling of lymphocytes around deep dermal vessels should raise the suspicion of the conditions best remembered as the 'Five Ls': Jessner's benign Lymphocytic infiltration of the skin; the prototypical lesion Lupus erythematosus; Light eruptions; Lymphoma; and Lymphocytoma cutis. Insect bite reaction may also show a persistent, predominantly lymphocytic, response.

The importance of histologic examination of intra-dermal lymphocytic infiltration is to differentiate reactive (benign) dermatitides from malignancy. Typically, the cells in reactive conditions do not display cytologic atypia. The lymphocytic infiltrate may be diffuse (as in insect bite reactions) or well circumscribed (for example, in Jessner's benign lymphocytic infiltration). In cases of heavy reactive lymphocytic infiltrates, follicles with germinal centers are often seen.

Intradermal lymphoid malignancies may be primary or represent a cutaneous manifestation of leukemia or lymphoma elsewhere. In most leukemias and lymphomas, cytologic atypia is seen. Diffuse, nodular, and follicular patterns may be observed with malignant lymphomas. The 'follicles' of follicular lymphomas do not have tingible body macrophages or eccentrically shaped mantle caps. Distinguishing reactive lymphoid proliferations from cutaneous lymphoma / leukemia may be difficult and require immunohistochemical and / or gene rearrangement studies. Diagnosing cutaneous myelogenous leukemia requires a high degree of suspicion because the cytoplasmic granules, easily recognized with Wright–Giemsa staining (used with bone-marrow aspirates), are not conspicuous with routine H & E staining.

One feature that is helpful in distinguishing whether an infiltrate is reactive or neoplastic is its distribution within the dermis. If the bulk of the cells is deep ('bottom-heavy'), then the infiltrate is more likely to be neoplastic. Reactive infiltrates tend to be 'top-heavy'. However, malignant cutaneous lymphomatous infiltrates may not necessarily present as large nodular dermal cell aggregates. The patch stage of mycosis fungoides is a good example. Lymphoid tumors of the skin are further described in Chapter 31.

Clinically, lesions with a perivascular, lichenoid, or nodular lymphocytic infiltrate often present as erythematous papules or plaques. Jessner's benign lymphocytic infiltrate, lymphocytoma cutis, lupus erythematosus (LE), plaque-type polymorphous light eruption, plaque-stage mycosis fungoides, and other cutaneous lymphomas are often difficult to distinguish clinically, especially if there are only a few lesions; a biopsy is often required. Unfortunately, the histology is not always distinctive. Polymorphous light eruption (PMLE) may not only simulate LE clinically, but also histologically. Additional tests may be required. Serology [such as antinuclear antibodies (ANA), anti-Ro, and anti-La antibodies] and direct immunofluorescence are often positive in LE and not in PMLE.

Lymphocytic vasculitis implies primary lymphocyte-mediated endothelial cell damage rather than secondary vascular injury, which occurs in dermatitis. Perivascular lymphocytes are, however, present in both conditions. Extravasation of red cells and enlargement of endothelial cell nuclei are helpful in distinguishing the histologic features of lymphocytic vasculitis. Diseases thought to represent a lymphocytic vasculitis include progressive pigmented purpuric dermatosis and pityriasis lichenoides. Clinically, they are different from most dermatitides and do not resemble each other. The clinical appearance may be helpful if the histologic appearance is not typical.

18.1 Perivascular lymphocytic infiltration
- ♦ there is slight to moderate perivascular lymphocytic infiltration in this case of Jessner's benign lymphocytic infiltration
- ♦ small lymphocytes with rounded uniform nuclei and scant cytoplasm
- ♦ normal epidermis differentiates Jessner's from LE; furthermore, in lymphocytoma cutis, the infiltrate is nodular and dense

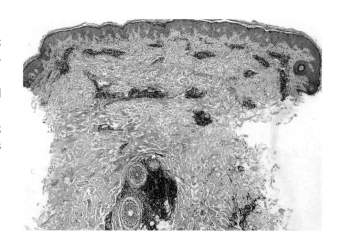

18.2 Nodular lymphocytic infiltration

♦ in contrast to 18.1, cutaneous malignant lymphomas are large tumor nodules, as seen here

♦ lymphomatous infiltrate is dense and replaces adnexal structures

♦ it is often bottom-heavy, with invasion of the subcutaneous tissue

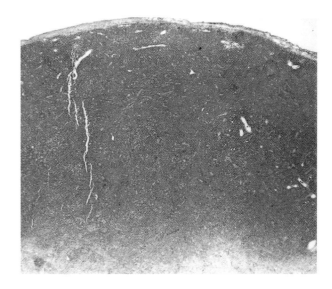

18.3 Lymphocytic vasculitis

♦ hallmark of a lymphocytic vasculitis is the finding of extravasation of red cells (large arrow) associated with lymphocytic infiltration of the dermal vessels, as in this case of Schamberg's progressive pigmented purpuric dermatitis

♦ swelling of the endothelial cell nucleus is often difficult to appreciate

♦ unlike leukocytoclastic vasculitis, thrombi are not usually seen

♦ the tiny granules seen here are hemosiderin pigment (small arrows), which stains brown with H & E

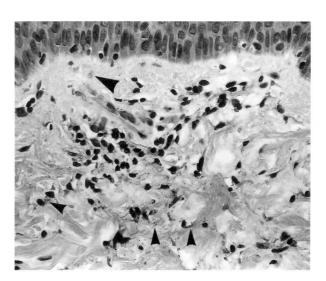

PERIVASCULAR LYMPHOCYTIC INFILTRATE WITH EPIDERMAL CHANGE

18.4 Dermatitis

♦ lymphocytic infiltration may vary from slight to moderate, but is never nodular; lymphocytes are perivascular, but only around the superficial dermal vessels

♦ lymphocytic exocytosis may be seen; epidermal hyperkeratosis, parakeratosis, and spongiosis are always present

♦ deviation from this histopathologic pattern, particularly if the inflammation involves the deep dermis, should cast doubt on the diagnosis

♦ red, scaly, itchy patches and plaques with or without papulovesicles

♦ small-plaque parapsoriasis may have similar histologic features; clinically, persistent, slightly scaly, erythematous, yellow-brown macules or thin plaques are seen on the trunk and proximal extremities

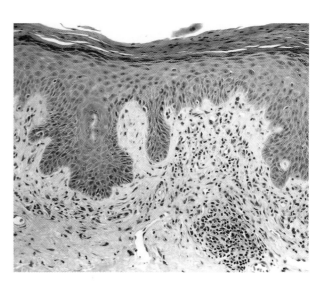

18.5 Lupus erythematosus (LE)

♦ lymphocytic infiltration involves superficial and deep vascular plexuses, is often periadnexal, and may be lichenoid

♦ usually moderately dense, as seen here, but may be slight in systemic LE and subacute LE

♦ occasional plasma cells, but no eosinophils

♦ compact hyperkeratosis and keratin plugging of hair follicles

♦ hyaline thickening of epidermal basement membrane in chronic lesions

♦ presence of basal cell degeneration helps to confirm the diagnosis

♦ discoid lesions occur most commonly on the face and scalp as erythematous to violaceous hyperkeratotic plaques with central atrophy

♦ lesions of systemic LE are often erythematous plaques

♦ subacute cutaneous LE lesions are erythematous and often annular with or without slight scale; they may be clinically mistaken for benign lymphocytic infiltration (no basal cell degeneration), psoriasis (epidermal microabscesses and no basal cell degeneration), seborrheic dermatitis (spongiosis and no basal cell degeneration), photodermatoses, dermatophyte fungal infections (positive fungal culture and PAS staining), and sarcoidosis (granulomas)

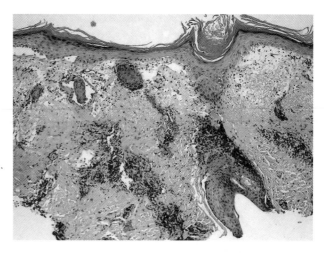

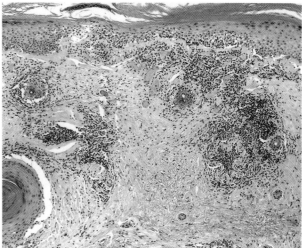

18.6 Gyrate erythema

♦ focal parakeratosis, slight spongiosis, and slight to moderate perivascular lymphocytic infiltration of dermal vessels

♦ as such a histologic appearance is common to dermatitis and many of the papulosquamous eruptions, clinical correlation is usually necessary for a histologic diagnosis

♦ pink papules enlarge to form large rings with central clearing

♦ edges may be flat, elevated, smooth, or slightly scaly

♦ lesions may last a few days or months and new lesions may develop over many years

♦ biopsy of the advancing edge only may reveal focal parakeratosis

♦ clinical differential diagnosis: dermatophytosis; LE; and sarcoidosis

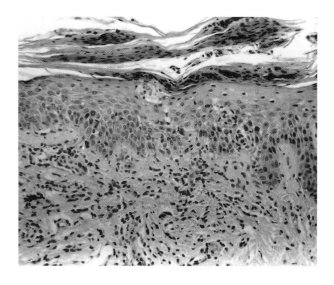

18.7 Erythema multiforme (EM)

♦ epidermal change consisting of spotty basal cell necrosis is usually prominent and overshadows the dermal inflammation (arrow)

♦ perivascular lymphocytic infiltration is slight, but may be variable

♦ primarily involves the superficial dermal vessels, but a heavy dermal infiltrate with minimal epidermal change resembling a photoreaction is sometimes observed (dermal-type EM)

♦ eosinophils may be present in the dermis in drug-induced EM

♦ drugs and infections, particularly with herpes simplex and *Mycoplasma*, are the most common causes

♦ characteristic clinical lesions are the iris and target lesions, but widespread blisters and mucosal involvement may occur

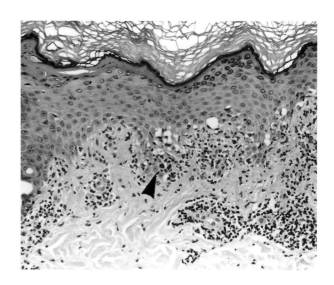

18.8 Polymorphous light eruption (PMLE)

♦ slight to moderate perivascular lymphocytic infiltration in superficial and deep dermis with a varying degree of edema, epidermal spongiosis, and hyperkeratosis

♦ histopathologic differential diagnosis includes LE, although true periappendageal lymphocytic infiltration and liquefaction degeneration are infrequent in PMLE, Jessner's, and dermatitis

♦ clinical history is required to diagnose photodermatitis

♦ **actinic prurigo** is a chronic photodermatitis, seen predominantly in North American Indians and often with a familial tendency, cheilitis, and an early age of onset, that may show similar histologic features

♦ **PMLE** is a pruritic papular, vesicular, plaque-type, or eczematous eruption on sun-exposed areas, but often spares the face (unlike LE), appearing within minutes to days after exposure, primarily in the spring or early summer, and persisting for hours to days; the eruption is monomorphous in the same individual

♦ clinical differential diagnosis: LE [direct immunofluorescence and serology (ANA, anti-Ro, and anti-La antibodies) may help differentiation if the histologic picture is ambiguous]; Jessner's; lymphocytoma cutis; dermatitis; and sarcoidosis

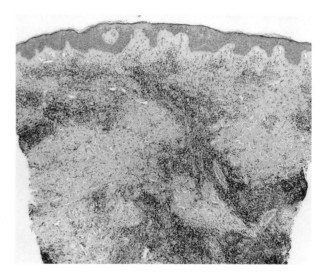

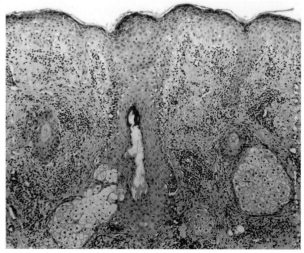

PERIVASCULAR LYMPHOCYTIC INFILTRATE WITHOUT EPIDERMAL CHANGE

18.9 Jessner's benign lymphocytic infiltration of the skin

♦ well-demarcated, densely cellular, dermal nodules composed almost entirely of lymphocytes

♦ lymphocytes form tight cuffs or sleeves around vessels and appendages

♦ no cellular atypia, exocytosis, or epidermotropism

♦ presence of a normal epidermis is the key to differentiation from LE

♦ well-demarcated, erythematous, non-scaly, solitary plaques, a few or many without follicular plugging (unlike LE) but, occasionally, with central clearing, most often located on the face; they heal spontaneously without scarring, but often recur

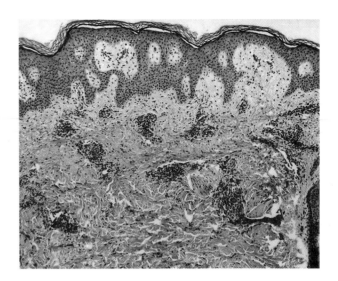

18.10 Arthropod bite reaction

♦ moderately dense, mixed inflammatory infiltrate consisting of many lymphocytes, eosinophils, and occasional plasma cells

♦ neutrophils and tissue necrosis may be seen with certain arthropods, such as spiders

♦ reactive lymphoid follicles may be present in chronic lesions

♦ histologic differential diagnosis: lymphomatoid papulomatosis (pleomorphic lymphoid cells); Hodgkin's lymphoma (Reed–Sternberg cells); and mycosis fungoides (atypical T lymphocytes with epidermotropism)

♦ itchy, erythematous, clustered papules often with a central punctum

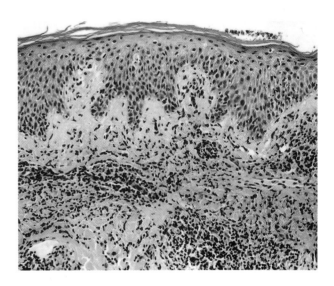

LICHENOID LYMPHOCYTIC INFILTRATE

18.11 Lichenoid dermatitis

♦ lymphocytic infiltration is band-like and obscures the dermoepidermal junction

♦ degenerated basal cells, colloid bodies, and pigment-laden dermal melanophages similar to lichen planus

♦ in contrast, parakeratosis and perivascular lymphocytic infiltration (arrow) are usual in lichenoid dermatitis

♦ **lichenoid keratosis** is a benign keratosis with a lichenoid inflammatory reaction which clinically mimics actinic keratosis, seborrheic keratosis, and basal cell carcinoma

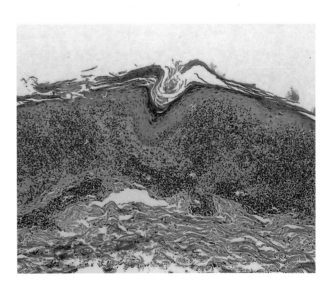

18.12 Mycosis fungoides
(patch and plaque stages)

♦ in addition to epidermotropic lymphocytes, the lymphocytic infiltrate is often band-like

♦ differentiate from lichenoid dermatitis by noting the absence of basal cell degeneration and colloid bodies

♦ epidermotropic lymphocytes have small dark nuclei and nuclear irregularities, and are difficult to visualize on histology

♦ look for a halo around the epidermotropic lymphocytes

♦ spongiosis is disproportionately slight in relation to the number of lymphocytes in the epidermis (unlike dermatitis)

♦ an aggregate of more than three lymphocytes along the basal epidermis is characteristic of a Pautrier's microabscess

♦ mycosis fungoides is a cutaneous T-cell lymphoma which may clinically mimic dermatitis

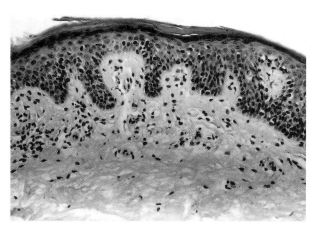

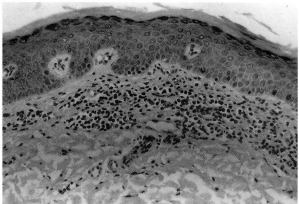

NODULAR LYMPHOCYTIC INFILTRATION

18.13 Lymphocytoma cutis
(benign cutaneous lymphoid hyperplasia)

♦ typically, there is a top-heavy dermal infiltrate composed of small and large lymphocytes as well as plasma cells and eosinophils

♦ small lymphocytes have round, uniformly basophilic nuclei and scant cytoplasm whereas larger lymphocytes have folded, vesicular, pale-staining nuclei and a voluminous cytoplasm

♦ follicles with reactive germinal centers (with tingible-body macrophages) are seen in fully developed cases

♦ in contrast to lymphoma, there is no cytologic atypia or a lack of monoclonal pattern with immunohistochemical staining

♦ single or multiple papules and nodules, usually on the face or ears, spontaneously resolve without scarring, but tend to recur

♦ clinical diagnosis requires histologic confirmation

♦ clinical differential diagnosis: Jessner's; LE; sarcoidosis; rhinophyma; lymphoma; granuloma faciale; and PMLE

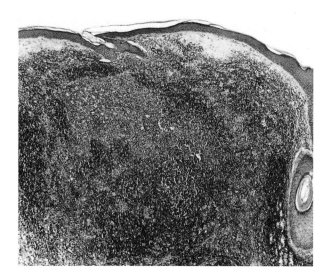

18.14 Halo nevus

♦ regressing compound nevi may show heavy lymphocytic cellular infiltration, but the nodule is solitary

♦ lymphocytes surround regressing nevic cells which often have pyknotic nuclei and indistinct cell bodies

♦ pigment-laden melanophages are usually present

♦ clinically, a white halo forms around an established nevus

LYMPHOCYTIC VASCULITIS

18.15 Schamberg's progressive pigmented purpuric dermatosis

♦ extravasation of red cells with lymphocytic infiltration of the superficial dermal vessels (large arrow)

♦ fine dust-like particles (small arrow) are hemosiderin pigment that stains yellow-brown with H & E

♦ hemosiderin may be intra- or extracellular and reacts positively with iron staining

♦ epidermal changes, (such as spongiosis, acanthosis, and parakeratosis) are common

♦ asymptomatic or, occasionally, slightly itchy chronic eruption composed of irregular, brown, macular, eczematous or lichenoid lesions with petechiae on the legs and, on occasions, elsewhere

♦ clinical diagnosis is usually not difficult and a biopsy is often not necessary

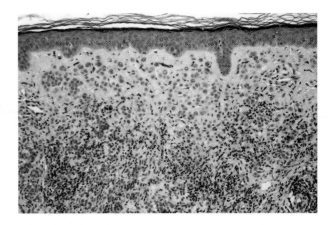

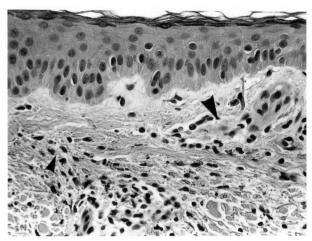

18.16 Pityriasis lichenoides et varioliformis acuta

♦ lymphocytic vasculitis which involves the superficial and deep dermal vessels, resulting in an inverted wedge of lymphocytes extending from the dermo-epidermal junction to the reticular dermis

♦ marked exocytosis of lymphocytes

♦ extravasated red cells in dermis and epidermis

♦ vacuolar degeneration of basal cells and occasional necrotic keratinocytes and colloid bodies

♦ focal hyperkeratosis and parakeratosis with entrapped erythrocytes

♦ generalized eruption primarily on the trunk and extremities, especially in children and young adults, consisting of crops of reddish-brown scaly papules that may develop central vesiculation and hemorrhagic necrosis leading to ulceration; heal with small depressed scars or varioliform scars

♦ many cases clear within 6 months, but may become chronic and recurrent

♦ clinical differential diagnosis: varicella; leukocytoclastic vasculitis; and insect bites

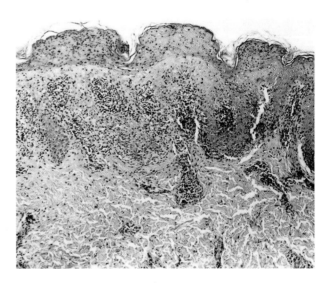

18.17 Pityriasis lichenoides chronica

♦ less intense lymphocytic infiltration and less extra-vasation of red cells in chronic lesions
♦ basal cell necrosis and colloid bodies are subtle
♦ pigmentary incontinence and dermal melanophages are present
♦ clinical correlation is often required if the histologic changes are subtle
♦ chronic eruption consisting of reddish-brown papules with an adherent scale that, when gently scraped off, reveals a shiny brown surface
♦ usually heals with postinflammatory hyperpigmentation
♦ clinical differential diagnosis: psoriasis; pityriasis rosea; and secondary syphilis

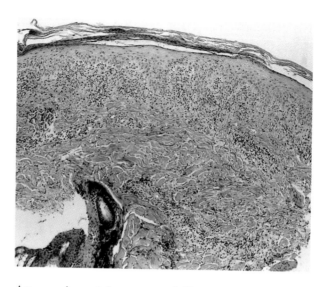

NEUTROPHILIC INFILTRATION

Neutrophilic granulocytes, polymorphonuclear (PMN) leukocytes, or neutrophils are known as acute inflammatory cells because they are seen in the early phase of inflammation. They respond to activated complement and various chemotactic factors, and contain myeloperoxidase, acid hydrolase, neutral protease, and lysozyme, which are bactericidal. Neutrophils are also capable of phagocytosis.

Neutrophilic infiltration of the dermis occurs in three main types of disease: suppurative infections of the skin; tissue necrosis due to ischemia and destructive or ischemic tumor growth; and immunologic disorders, such as dermatitis herpetiformis, pyoderma gangrenosum, and vasculitis.

An angiocentric neutrophilic infiltrate favors vasculitis whereas extensive epidermal necrosis with thrombi in dermal vessels suggests necrosis. Fungal and bacterial infections often lead to dermal abscesses and pseudoepitheliomatous epidermal hyperplasia.

As several of the neutrophilic dermatoses may have similar histologic findings, clinical pathologic correlation is usually necessary to arrive at the correct diagnosis. On occasions, however, even the clinical presentation is similar. Sweet's syndrome, for example, may be difficult to differentiate both clinically and histologically from acute pyoderma gangrenosum, cellulitis, or erythema elevatum diutinum.

Differential diagnoses

Superficial angiocentric neutrophilic infiltration

Leukocytoclastic vasculitis	19.1
Disseminated intravascular coagulation	19.2
Septicemia	19.3

Deep dermal and subcutaneous angiocentric neutrophilic infiltration

Polyarteritis nodosa	19.4
Thrombophlebitis / Trousseau's syndrome	19.5

PMNs diffusely in the dermis

Ischemia	19.6
Cellulitis / erysipelas	19.7

SUPERFICIAL ANGIOCENTRIC NEUTROPHILIC INFILTRATION

19.1 Leukocytoclastic vasculitis

♦ all of the vessels in the papillary dermis are involved and infiltrated by neutrophils

♦ nuclear fragments (arrows) from degenerated neutrophils are seen even in early lesions of only a few hours' duration; this is the most reliable finding

♦ extravasation of red cells is usually extensive

♦ endothelial cell nuclear swelling, and fibrinoid necrosis of blood vessel walls and thrombi (upper picture) may or may not be obvious; this full-blown lesion (lower picture) shows relatively normal-looking capillaries

♦ vessels in the mid- and lower dermis are involved in lesions of some duration; arteries in the lower dermis and subcutis are not involved

♦ a result of immune complex-mediated neutrophil-induced dermal vessel damage

♦ palpable purpura is the clinical hallmark; lesions, usually < 1 cm in diameter, often occur in crops particularly on the limbs; may have nodules, hemorrhagic bullae, and/or ulcerations

♦ may be associated with fever, myalgias, and arthritis

♦ may be secondary to infections, drugs, collagen–vascular disease, cryoglobulinemia, inflammatory bowel disease, and malignancy

♦ may be mistaken for dermatitis herpetiformis, ischemia, cellulitis, EED, and DIC on microscopy but, clinically, these conditions are different

♦ clinical diagnosis is usually confirmed by histopathology

♦ skin involvement may or may not be associated with systemic vasculitis

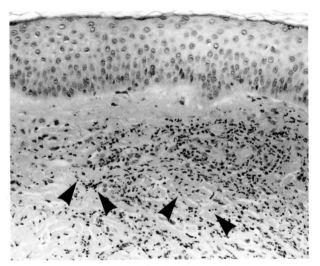

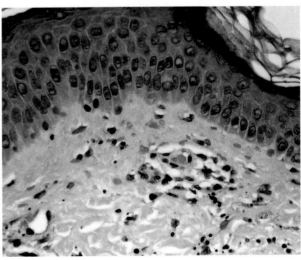

19.2 Disseminated intravascular coagulation

♦ fibrin thrombi are seen in many of the dermal vessels (large arrow)

♦ diffuse extravasation of red cells (small arrow)

♦ neutrophilic infiltration is usually less dense compared with lesions of allergic vasculitis

♦ histologic appearance is identical to those of **thrombotic thrombocytopenic purpura** and **cryoglobulinemia**

♦ clinical history needed: sudden onset of large areas of bruising and hemorrhagic bullae, bleeding from multiple sites, hypotension, high fever, and widespread intravascular coagulation and clotting abnormalities

♦ may be secondary to infections such as Gram-negative sepsis, varicella, or hypovolemic or cardiogenic shock

♦ often fatal

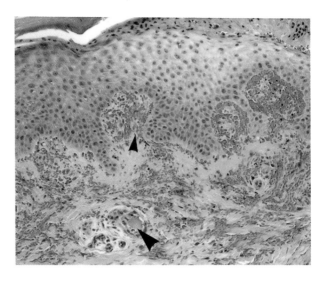

19.3 Septicemia

♦ histologic changes are similar to those of DIC, and septic thrombi are common in the vascular lumina

♦ Gram staining as well as bacterial culture should be carried out to identify organisms

♦ *Neisseria meningitidis, Pseudomonas,* and *Vibrio vulnificus* are pathogens of cutaneous septicemic vasculitis

♦ patient is usually gravely ill with a clinical diagnosis of meningitis, ecthyma gangrenosum, or a history of having eaten raw seafood

DEEP DERMAL AND SUBCUTANEOUS ANGIOCENTRIC NEUTROPHILIC INFILTRATION

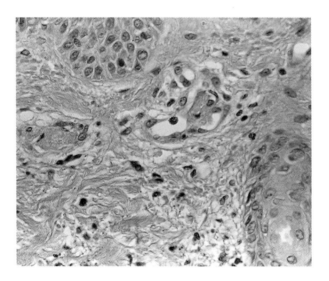

19.4 Polyarteritis nodosa (PAN)

♦ this shows inflammation of a muscle-type artery with recognizable tunica media in the deep dermis

♦ neutrophilic infiltration of the vessel wall is associated with fibrinoid necrosis of the artery (arrow)

♦ thrombus in the vascular lumen, and extravasated red cells and neutrophilic exudates in the tunica adventitia are seen

♦ multiple-section biopsy may be needed to demonstrate these features because of the focal nature of the inflammation

♦ large punctate cutaneous ulcers, gangrene, or livedo reticularis with ulcerating nodules primarily on legs

♦ 1/5–1/2 of cases have cutaneous lesions, and 3/4 cases have renal involvement

♦ may affect heart, eyes, joints, and peripheral and CNS

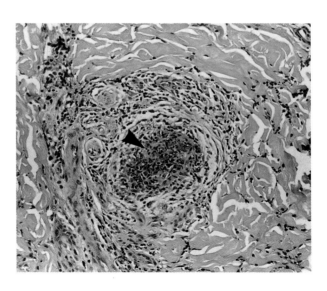

19.5 Thrombophlebitis

♦ neutrophils are abundant especially in newer lesions

♦ thrombosed veins are located in subcutaneous tissue

♦ veins of the lower extremities often have a thick medial muscular layer with lumina larger than the arteries

♦ longer-standing lesions show recanalization of the vessel lumina, and endothelial cell and fibroblast proliferation

♦ superficial migratory thrombophlebitis may be associated with Behçet's disease or visceral carcinoma, particularly pancreatic cancer (**Trousseau's syndrome**)

♦ superficial migratory thrombophlebitis should stimulate a search for underlying malignancy

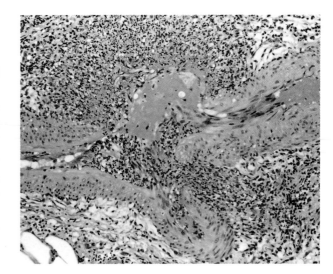

PMNs DIFFUSELY IN DERMIS

19.6 Ischemia

♦ margination and transmigration of neutrophils around dermal vessels in areas of ischemic necrosis and diffusely in the dermis

♦ thrombi in dermal vessels (arrow)

♦ full-thickness necrotic epidermis separating from dermis

♦ may resemble leukocytoclastic vasculitis histologically, but tissue necrosis is often extensive and vascular insufficiency is usually clinically distinct from vasculitis

♦ clinically manifested as severe pain, edema, and limb cyanosis

♦ prolonged ischemia, as in atherosclerosis, may lead to necrosis and gangrene

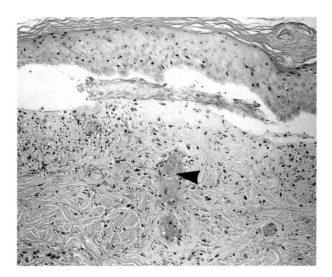

19.7 Cellulitis

♦ acute inflammation of the dermis and subcutis with edema and diffuse neutrophilic infiltration

♦ no vasculitic changes; leukocytoclasis is uncommon

♦ erythema, warmth, induration, and tenderness ± vesicles, bullae, pustules, and epidermal necrosis; often associated with fever, lymphadenopathy, leukocytosis and elevated erythrocyte sedimentation rate

♦ caused by numerous bacteria, particularly group A streptococci, although it is usually difficult to isolate the organisms unless there is a site of trauma, ulceration, or pyoderma

♦ **erysipelas** is a type of cellulitis that has well-demarcated borders (in cellulitis, the borders are usually irregular and ill-defined as the inflammation is usually deeper) and lymphatic involvement, and is typically located on the face or lower leg

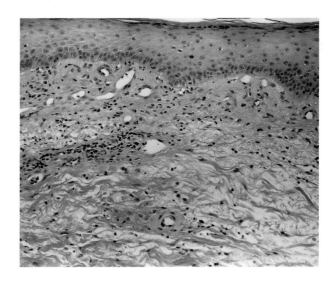

19.8 Non-clostridial necrotizing fasciitis

♦ diffuse neutrophilic infiltration of the dermis with extensive tissue necrosis and ulceration; microscopic appearance is not diagnostic

♦ rapidly spreading, life-threatening, soft-tissue inflammation and subsequent fascia necrosis due to group A β-hemolytic streptococci, staphylococci, or Gram-negative or mixed anaerobic bacteria

♦ often a history of minor trauma; initially, disproportionately intense pain with few cutaneous findings, then acute illness due to rapidly progressing cellulitis with anesthetic bullae and extensive gangrene

♦ early diagnosis is essential to reduce mortality

♦ **Fournier's gangrene** is a form of necrotizing fasciitis that starts in the perineum and genitalia

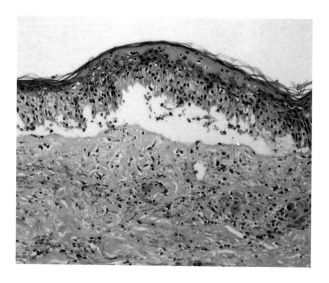

19.9 Acute febrile neutrophilic dermatosis (Sweet's syndrome)

♦ moderate to dense neutrophil infiltrate in the dermis

♦ nuclear fragments may be seen, but no fibrinoid necrosis of the vessels

♦ a few intact capillaries are seen here

♦ extravasation of red cells is less common than in leukocytoclastic vasculitis

♦ clinically, crops of painful erythematous plaques ± surface vesiculopustules primarily on the upper body, especially the face

♦ marked peripheral neutrophilia is common

♦ more common in women

♦ as with pyoderma gangrenosum and Behçet's disease, there may be pathergy

♦ bullous lesions are more often associated with myeloproliferative disorders, occurring in 10–15% of cases of Sweet's syndrome

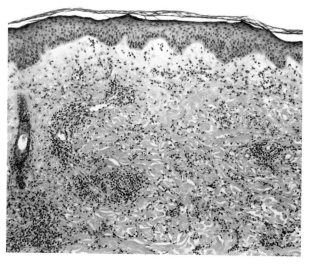

♦ clinically, lesions differ from the palpable purpuric lesions of leukocytoclastic vasculitis, which show angiocentric inflammation; however, both conditions may have fever, myalgias, and arthralgias

♦ clinical differential diagnosis: erythema multiforme (lymphocytic rather than neutrophilic infiltrate); erythema elevatum diutinum (not painful, no fever); gyrate erythema; cellulitis (border usually not elevated or sharply demarcated, as in Sweet's syndrome); granuloma faciale (not painful, with eosinophils); infections (such as orf, tinea faciale); erythema nodosum (lower legs, panniculitis); and pyoderma gangrenosum

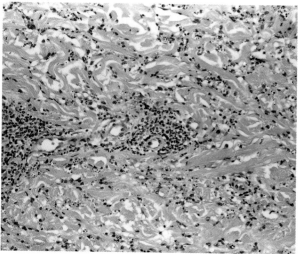

19.10 Erythema elevatum diutinum (EED)

♦ chronic form of neutrophilic vasculitis

♦ likened to an exploding grenade, dermis is filled with neutrophils and nuclear fragments due to leukocytoclasis

♦ histiocytes and eosinophils are common, as seen in acute allergic vasculitis

♦ marked spongiosis of the overlying epidermis and exocytosis of neutrophils (upper picture)

♦ capillary proliferation is marked; capillary lined by endothelial cells with abnormal nuclei (middle picture)

♦ later stage of disease (lower picture) shows homogenization of dermal collagen and fibrosis `

♦ foamy histiocytic cells (arrow) and extracellular lipid deposition are present

♦ symmetric, persistent, violaceous to brown papules, nodules, and plaques on the extensor surfaces of the extremities, typically over joints and, occasionally, on the buttocks, face, and torso

♦ may be associated with monoclonal gammopathy (usually IgA), multiple myeloma, myelodysplasia, and chronic or recurrent infections

♦ differs clinically from leukocytoclastic vasculitis in that the acute inflammatory lesions of EED are followed by formation of fibrous nodules whereas leukocytoclastic vasculitis resolves without sequelae

♦ clinical differential diagnosis: sarcoid; hypertrophic lichen planus; Sweet's syndrome (leukocytosis, fever); and granuloma annulare (necrobiotic granuloma with mucin)

19.11 Granuloma faciale

♦ microscopically similar to EED

♦ another form of chronic leukocytoclastic vasculitis

♦ mixed heavy infiltrate of neutrophils, eosinophils, and histiocytes in the dermis with vasculitic changes (such as fibrinoid deposits, endothelial cell swelling, thrombi, and extravasation of red cells)

♦ with time, may see fibrosis and fewer inflammatory cells

♦ chronic, single or multiple, reddish-brown plaques almost always located on the face in adults; follicular orifices are often dilated

♦ clinical differential diagnosis: sarcoid; Jessner's lymphocytic infiltrate; lymphocytoma cutis; mycosis fungoides; alopecia mucinosa; B-cell lymphoma; LE; and PMLE

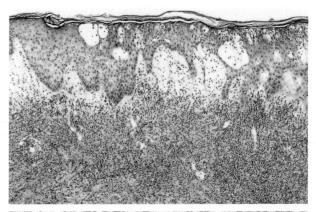

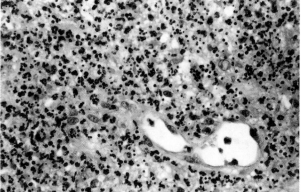

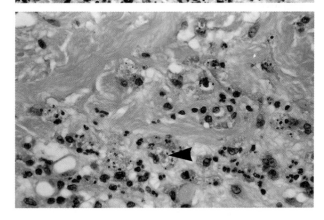

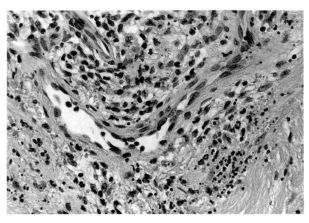

19.12 Pyoderma gangrenosum

♦ dermal necrosis with an abundance of neutrophils on the ulcer floor

♦ lymphocytic vasculitis may be seen in the periphery of the lesion

♦ foreign-body giant cells may be present

♦ fungal and acid-fast bacillary staining, and tissue culture should be considered to rule out deep fungal and mycobacterial infections

♦ clinical correlation essential as there are no diagnostic findings on microscopy

♦ starts as a tender purple papulopustule which quickly ulcerates

♦ ulcer has an undermining dusky-purple border

♦ may have pathergy as seen in Sweet's and Behçet's, and may be associated with inflammatory bowel disease, collagen–vascular disease (particularly rheumatoid arthritis), paraproteinemia, and malignancy

♦ clinical differential diagnosis: carbuncle; Meleney's ulcer; syphilitic gummas; orf; deep fungal and mycobacterial infections; cutaneous amebiasis; spider bite; squamous cell cancer; and factitial ulcers

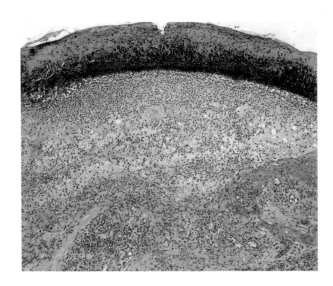

LOCALIZED DERMAL ABSCESSES

19.13 Dermatitis herpetiformis (DH)

♦ this high-power view shows characteristic changes in the skin adjacent to a vesicle

♦ neutrophils are seen at the epidermodermal junction and, although nuclear 'dusts' are noted, they do not surround vessels as in leukocytoclastic vasculitis

♦ microabscesses with neutrophils and neutrophil fragments in papillary dermal tips are highly suggestive of DH

♦ **linear bullous IgA dermatosis**, and some cases of **bullous pemphigoid**, **bullous lupus erythematosus** and **leukocytoclastic vasculitis** may show similar histologic findings

♦ direct immunofluorescence showing IgA deposition in involved and uninvolved skin, including the oral mucosa, helps to differentiate DH

♦ intensely pruritic, erythematous papules and / or vesicles on extensor surfaces, especially over the knees, elbows, buttocks, and nape of neck; intense burning or stinging shortly before the lesions appear; associated with gastric atrophy and hypochlorhydria, thyroid abnormalities, gluten-sensitive enteropathy, *(continued next page)*

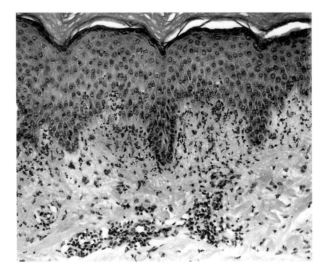

which is usually asymptomatic, and gastrointestinal lymphomas
♦ a confluence of microabscesses in a subepidermal vesicle is seen here
♦ clinical differential diagnosis: dermatitis (spongiosis); neurotic excoriations; scabies (burrows and presence of mites); pemphigoid (linear IgG with direct immunofluorescence); pemphigus (acantholysis, intraepidermal blister); and erythema multiforme (degeneration of basal cell layer, lymphocytic infiltrate)

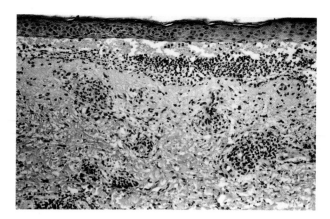

19.14 Dermal abscess
♦ an abscess is a collection of pus cells
♦ this shows an abscess caused by foreign material implanted in the dermis
♦ tender erythematous nodule which becomes fluctuant and may drain pus

19.15 Folliculitis
♦ neutrophilic exudate confined by follicular epithelium in early lesions
♦ rupture of the inflamed follicle releases pus into the dermis
♦ remnants of follicular epithelium and hair in a dermal abscess are indicative of folliculitis
♦ PAS staining after diastase digestion helps to exclude dermatophytic folliculitis
♦ clinically seen as erythematous follicular papules and pustules
♦ may be secondary to bacterial (usually staphylococci) or fungal (such as dermatophytes or *Pityrosporum*) infections, or be sterile (oil and tar folliculitis)
♦ clinical diagnosis is usually not difficult

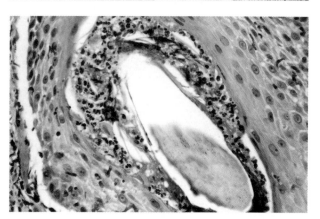

19.16 Majocchi's granuloma
♦ a dermatophytic folliculitis
♦ ulcerated or hyperplastic epidermis showing inflammatory atypia that may be mistaken for invasive squamous cell carcinoma (pseudoepitheliomatous hyperplasia)
♦ granulomatous inflammation with suppuration and heavy neutrophilic infiltration suggests deep fungal infection
♦ species of dermatophytes cannot be distinguished by histologic appearances
♦ clinically, an erythematous nodule with follicular pustules usually on the extremities

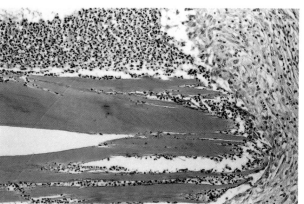

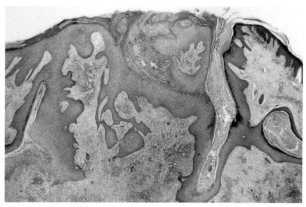

EOSINOPHILIC INFILTRATION

Eosinophils originate from the same stem cell that gives rise to other granulocytes within the bone marrow. Interleukins-1, -3, and -5, produced in the bone marrow, regulate their production.

Interleukin (IL)-5 plays a major role in enhancement of the mature functional activity of eosinophils and acts as a chemoattractant for eosinophils. Mature cells have bilobed nuclei and large refractile eosinophilic granules. These granules contain major basic protein, eosinophilic cationic protein, eosinophil-derived neurotoxin, eosinophil peroxidase, acid phosphatase, and arylsulfatase. Charcot–Leyden crystals (lysophospholipase) are found in non-crystalloid-containing granules, and are also found in basophils.

Eosinophils are present in low numbers in the peripheral blood. They are important in type I hypersensitivity reactions and in the defense against parasitic infections. Their effectiveness depends on their migration into tissues where the contents of their secretory granules are released. Eosinophils respond to platelet-activating factor generated by many cells, IL-5, C3a, C5a, mast cell-derived histamine, leukotriene B_4, and eosinophil chemotactic factor (ECF).

Eosinophils are usually found where there is mastocytosis. Immune-complex deposition is associated with eosinophilia. Eosinophils are capable of down-regulating inflammation by phagocytosing mast cell granules and antigen–antibody complexes.

The density of the eosinophilic infiltrate and whether other cell types are associated help to differentiate among the diseases with eosinophils in the dermis. Eosinophils are recognizable as the cells with bilobed nuclei in black-and-white photographs. In tissue sections stained with H & E, they stand out as cells with brilliant eosinophilic cytoplasmic granules and are therefore easy to detect.

Differential diagnoses

Sparse infiltrate

Urticaria	20.1
Dermatitis	20.2
Drug eruption	20.3
Cutaneous mastocytosis	20.4
Incontinentia pigmenti	20.5
Bullous pemphigoid / herpes gestationis	20.6
Pemphigus vulgaris	20.7

Dense infiltrate

Arthropod bite reaction	20.8
Angiolymphoid hyperplasia with eosinophilia (Kimura's disease)	20.9
Eosinophilic cellulitis (Wells syndrome)	20.10

SPARSE INFILTRATE

20.1 Urticaria

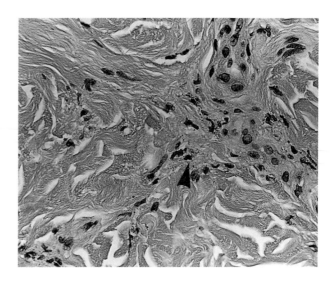

♦ characterized by a sparse dermal infiltrate of eosinophils and lymphocytes; lymphocytes tend to be perivascular whereas eosinophils are often found between dermal collagen fibers

♦ helpful to find degranulated eosinophils (arrow)

♦ well-demarcated, itchy, edematous, circular or serpiginous, blanching, erythematous papules and plaques (wheals) which may have surrounding erythema (flare); clinical diagnosis is usually easy

♦ etiology: allergic; physical (for example, cold, exercise, heat, light, pressure, shear, vibration, water); infectious; systemic disease (such as collagen–vascular, endocrine, neoplasms); mastocytosis; or idiopathic

♦ etiology cannot be discerned on biopsy except when secondary to mastocytosis (increased number of mast cells)

♦ if lesions last > 24 h, a biopsy is necessary to exclude leukocytoclastic vasculitis

20.2 Dermatitis

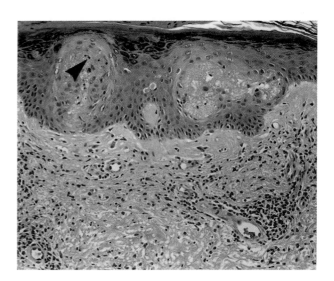

♦ the occasional eosinophil (arrow), recognizable by the bilobed nucleus, is probably related to an increased number of mast cells

♦ eosinophils are usually rare in atopic, allergic, and irritant contact dermatitis; more eosinophils may be seen in lichen simplex chronicus, neurodermatitis, nummular dermatitis, and pityriasis rosea

♦ heavy eosinophilic infiltration is typical of a drug eruption and insect-bite reaction

♦ eosinophils are not usually seen in seborrheic dermatitis or in papulosquamous eruptions such as psoriasis and LE unless there is a superimposed dermatitis

20.3 Drug eruption

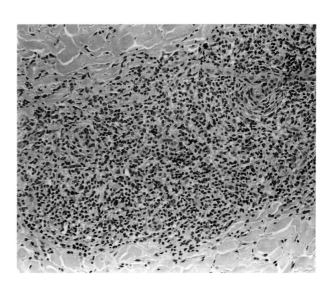

♦ in contrast to dermatitis, a greater number of eosinophils are commonly seen in drug eruptions

♦ diagnosis may be suggested by microscopy, but must be confirmed by patient history and clearing on stopping the causative medication

♦ clinical appearance of drug eruptions may be extremely variable, thus requiring a high index of suspicion

♦ exanthematous and urticarial eruptions are the most common types

20.4 Cutaneous mastocytosis

♦ a few eosinophils (arrow) are often found with mast cells, and there are usually more eosinophilis in urticated lesions (Darier's sign)

♦ papular and nodular lesions usually show an abundance of mast cells, which are rounded and epithelioid with granular cytoplasm so that their identification, even without special stains (such as Bismarck brown or Giemsa), is not difficult

♦ increase in mast cell number is subtle in macular lesions and in telangiectasia macularis eruptiva perstans (see Chapter 21)

♦ clinical presentations include urticaria pigmentosa, solitary cutaneous mastocytoma, telangiectasia macularis eruptiva perstans, diffuse cutaneous mastocytosis, erythroderma, bullous mastocytosis, and xanthelasmoid mastocytosis (see Chapter 21)

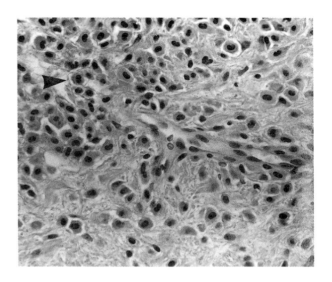

20.5 Incontinentia pigmenti (IP)

♦ linear vesicular dermatitis involving the trunk and extremities, with eosinophilic spongiosis and eosinophils in the dermis in a female infant, should raise the suspicion of this X-linked dominant disease, which is lethal in males

♦ eosinophils may also be seen in some cases of epidermolysis bullosa, which may be mistaken for the vesicular stage of IP; however, the clinical course and distribution of the lesions are different

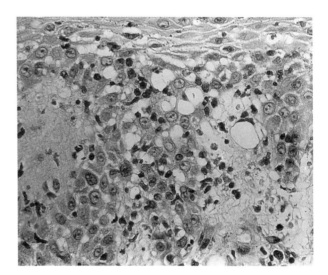

20.6 Bullous pemphigoid

♦ eosinophilic infiltrates are commonly seen in biopsies taken from erythematous urticarial skin

♦ identification of eosinophils in the dermis and in spongiotic epidermis is helpful in differentiating pemphigoid from other blistering diseases

♦ eosinophils may also be present in blister cavities

♦ large, tense, subepidermal blisters on non-inflamed or erythematous urticarial skin; usually affects the elderly

♦ **herpes gestationis** has identical histologic and clinical findings, but affects pregnant women and, occasionally, their offspring

♦ direct immunofluorescence shows linear IgG and / or C3 at the basement membrane zone

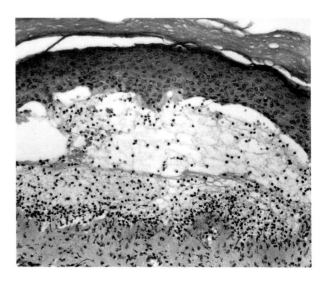

20.7 Pemphigus vulgaris

♦ eosinophilic infiltration of the epidermis and dermis is a characteristic feature of all types of pemphigus

♦ acantholysis confined to the superficial epidermal cell layers (**pemphigus foliaceus**) or the suprabasal layer (**pemphigus vulgaris, pemphigus vegetans**) may result in blister formation

♦ absence of dyskeratosis in most cases

♦ no subepidermal edema or blister

♦ intercellular IgG and / or C3 seen with direct immunofluorescence

♦ flaccid vesicles and mucosal involvement in pemphigus vulgaris; crusted erosions in pemphigus foliaceus and intertriginous papillomatous lesions in pemphigus vegetans

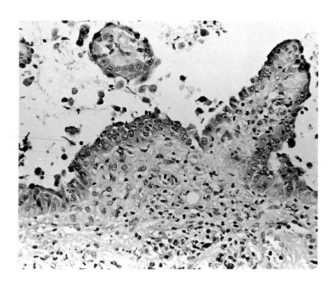

DENSE INFILTRATE

20.8 Arthropod bite reaction

♦ eosinophils are usually seen with heavy lymphocytic infiltration involving the entire dermis and sometimes extending into the subcutis

♦ inflammation involves the entire dermis and may extend into subcutaneous tissue

♦ marked eosinophilia in a typical lesion should be easy to separate from Jessner's

♦ histologic differential diagnosis: lymphomatoid papulosis (pleomorphic lymphoid cells); Hodgkin's lymphoma (Reed–Sternberg cells); and mycosis fungoides (atypical T lymphocytes with epidermotropism); all may show eosinophilic infiltration

♦ clinically, bites are itchy, clustered, erythematous papules with a central punctum and possibly vesicles

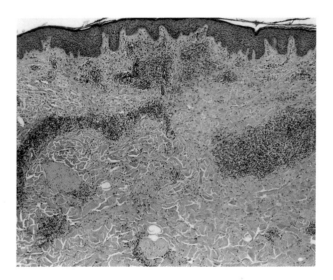

20.9 Angiolymphoid hyperplasia with eosinophilia (Kimura's disease)

♦ disease primarily affecting Orientals; first described by Kimura *et al.* in 1948

♦ nodular proliferations of small to large vessels with large, protuberant endothelial cells which may occasionally be vacuolated

♦ perivascular infiltrate of eosinophils and lymphocytes

♦ occasional luminal obliteration with or without recanalization by endothelial cells surrounding lymphoid follicles

♦ solitary or multiple, subcutaneous or erythematous to violaceous dermal nodules usually on the scalp or face which often bleed with minimal trauma; may persist or spontaneously resolve

♦ clinical differential diagnosis: pyogenic granuloma (ulceration and neutrophils predominate); Kaposi's sarcoma; angiosarcoma (bizarrely shaped vascular channels, spindle cell proliferation, and cytoplasmic vacuoles with eosinophilic inclusions); granuloma faciale (neutrophilic vasculitis and minimal vascular proliferation); lymphoma cutis (few eosinophils)

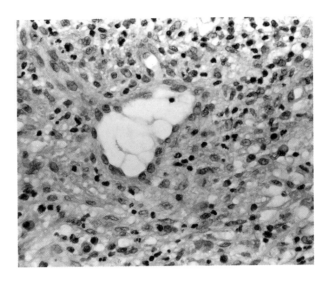

20.10 Eosinophilic cellulitis (Wells syndrome)

♦ described by Wells in 1971 in four patients with recurrent localized swelling of the extremities over a period of years

Phase I

♦ dermal edema and degranulated perivascular eosinophils in the dermis

♦ painful or pruritic erythematous edematous plaques which occasionally may have subepidermal vesicles

♦ half of all patients may have peripheral eosinophilia

Phase II

♦ granulomatous inflammation (upper picture; large arrow) with eosinophils, histiocytes, and giant cells

♦ degranulated eosinophils around collagen fibers give rise to the characteristic 'flame figures' (lower picture, center)

♦ eosinophils are identifiable as cells with bilobed nuclei in black-and-white photographs

♦ 1–3 weeks after phase I

♦ indurated slate-colored skin

♦ lasts 6 weeks

Phase III

♦ as the condition resolves, small granulomas with flame figures and fewer eosinophils are seen

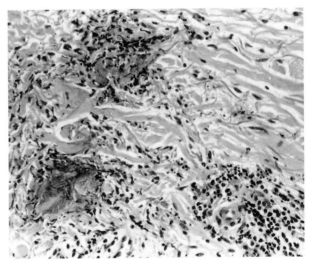

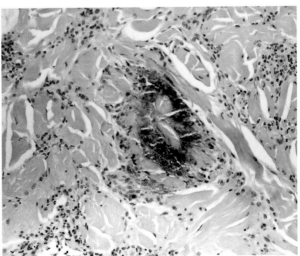

MAST CELL INFILTRATION

Mast cells originate from CD34-positive pluripotential bone marrow progenitor cells. They are normally found scattered in the superficial dermis, and around sensory nerves, blood vessels, and lymphatics, but are not conspicuous in routine H & E sections. Special stains (Leder's, Bismarck brown, Giemsa, toluidine blue) are required to highlight their granules. There are two types of mast cells: those containing only tryptase; and those containing tryptase and chymase. The former predominate in the lung and gastrointestinal mucosa, and the latter in the skin and bowel submucosa.

Cutaneous mast cells produce and release a number of mediators, including histamine, eicosanoids (predominantly prostaglandin D_2 and leukotriene C_4), proteases (tryptase, chymase, and carboxypeptidase), proteoglycans (heparin and chondroitin sulfate), and cytokines, including IL-4, IL-8, and TNF. These mediators locally and systemically affect epithelial and endothelial cells, smooth muscle cells, nerves, and other connective tissue stromal cells. The proximity of mast cells to sensory nerves facilitates neuropeptide (for example, substance P, vasoactive intestinal polypeptide, somatostatin)-induced mast-cell degranulation.

Mastocytosis is characterized by an increased number of mast cells in various organs, particularly the skin. Cutaneous mastocytosis is more common in children whereas systemic mastocytosis is more frequently seen in adults. Systemic mastocytosis refers to involvement of organs other that the skin, regardless of whether there is associated skin involvement. Cutaneous mastocytosis may have the following clinical expressions: urticaria pigmentosa; mastocytoma; telangiectasia macularis eruptiva perstans; diffuse cutaneous mastocytosis; erythroderma; bullous mastocytosis; and xanthelasmoid mastocytosis.

Urticaria pigmentosa accounts for approximately 80–90% of childhood diseases. Onset is typically during the first year of life as symmetric, generalized, non-scaly, brown, monomorphous macules, papules, plaques, or nodules. Darier's sign is diagnostic for mastocytosis, and refers to urtication and sometimes blistering when the lesions are rubbed. Childhood disease usually resolves by adolescence whereas adult disease tends to be chronic in 90% of cases. Approximately one-third of patients with urticaria pigmentosa are adults.

Mastocytoma constitutes around 10% of cutaneous mastocytoses and onsets at birth or in early infancy. Nodules may be solitary or few in number, and are typically reddish-brown, pink, or yellow, and occur on the extremities and / or trunk. Darier's sign is usually positive. Where Darier's sign is positive and the clinical appearance is typical, a biopsy is usually unnecessary to make the diagnosis.

Telangiectasia macularis eruptiva perstans (TMEP) is an uncommon variant primarily in adults, presenting with patchy erythema, macular hyperpigmentation, and telangiectasia usually on the trunk. Darier's sign may be positive. Bone involvement is common in TMEP.

Diffuse cutaneous mastocytosis is characterized by generalized skin infiltration by mast cells. The skin may be leathery and doughy with a yellow-brown *peau d'orange* or cobblestone appearance, or erythrodermic. Pruritus is often intense and blisters frequently develop as a result of pressure or stroking. When blisters predominate, the disease is called **bullous mastocytosis**. Extensive bullae may mimic staphylococcal scalded skin syndrome or erythema multiforme. The bullae are subepidermal and contain mast cells, eosinophils, and neutrophils. Diffuse cutaneous mastocytosis usually onsets during the first month of life with blisters developing in normal-looking skin. The leathery appearance of the skin develops between 1–6 months of age.

Xanthelasmoid mastocytosis onsets before 2 years of age and is characterized by generalized, yellowish, doughy papules and nodules that are 1 mm to 2 cm in diameter. Darier's sign is often negative; this variant usually persists into adulthood.

The histologic diagnosis of mastocytosis is difficult because of the lack of an easy or reproducible technique to quantitate mast cells in tissue sections.

Furthermore, there are no reliable studies of mast cell numbers in normal skin. Clinicopathologic correlation is essential as the histologic findings may be subtle. A few dilated dermal vessels, eosinophils, and mast cells in a perivascular location, for example, are the features of TMEP.

Mast cell infiltration does not invariably indicate mastocytosis. A slight degree of mastocytosis is common in dermatitis. In addition, some tumors (such as neurofibroma, cutaneous myxoma, spindle cell lipoma, and synovial cell sarcoma) are accompanied by a mast cell infiltrate.

Mast cells	21.1

Differential diagnoses

Infiltrative (mastocytosis)

Urticaria pigmentosa /mastocytomas /diffuse cutaneous mastocytosis / erythrodermic mastocytosis / xanthelasmoid mastocytosis /bullous mastocytosis	21.2
Telangiectasia macularis eruptiva perstans	21.3

Mast cell-rich tumors

Neurofibroma	21.4
Cutaneous myxoma	21.5

21.1 Mast cells

♦ normal mast cells may have spindle-shaped or ovoid cell bodies
♦ spindle-shaped mast cells are not unlike fibroblasts seen with H & E staining, although a scant amount of amphophilic granular cytoplasm may be visualized with $\times 400$ magnification (upper picture; mast cells stained with Bismarck brown, arrow)
♦ mast cells in papular and nodular lesions of mastocytosis (lower picture) are always round and epithelioid, with hyperchromatic uniform nuclei and a slight amount of amphophilic granular cytoplasm
♦ their appearance may be mistaken for lymphocytes, nevic cells, or even epithelioid small cell tumors (see Chapters 18, 24, and 27)
♦ cytoplasmic granules may be stained with Bismarck brown, toluidine blue, and Leder's, and have a metachromatic reaction with Giemsa staining
♦ mast cells are negative for leukocyte common antigen and S100 protein

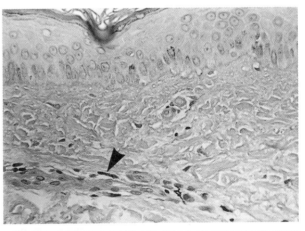
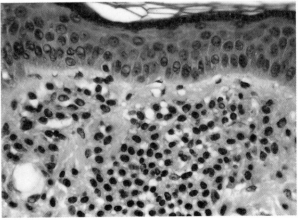

INFILTRATIVE (MASTOCYTOSIS)

21.2 Urticaria pigmentosa

♦ dermal collections of mast cells and a few eosinophils

♦ infiltrates may be sparse to heavy, diffuse or nodular

♦ low magnification shows a histologic appearance reminiscent of dermatitis or intradermal nevus

♦ most common form of mastocytosis

♦ onset is typically during the first year of life as symmetric, generalized, non-scaly, monomorphous brown macules and papules, plaques, or nodules, which may urticate or blister when scratched (positive Darier's sign)

♦ **mastocytomas**, **diffuse cutaneous mastocytosis**, **erythrodermic mastocytosis** and **xanthelasmoid mastocytosis** may be histologically indistinguishable

♦ a subepidermal bulla associated with mast cell and eosinophilic infiltrates is seen in **bullous mastocytosis**

♦ if Darier's sign is positive and the clinical appearance is typical, then there is usually no need to take a biopsy to make the diagnosis

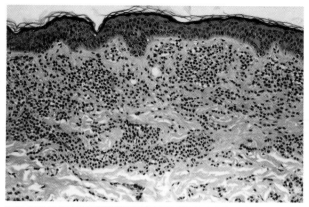

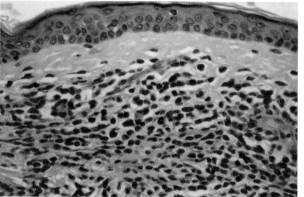

21.3 Telangiectasia macularis eruptiva perstans (TMEP)

♦ mast cells are spindle-shaped, and may be subtle and difficult to identify on routine H & E staining

♦ mast cells are perivascular in location

♦ when a number of mast cells are seen completely surrounding telangiectatic papillary dermal vessels, then TMEP is the probable diagnosis if there is clinical correlation

♦ patchy erythema, macular hyperpigmentation, and telangiectasia usually on the trunk; Darier's sign may be positive

♦ with H & E staining (upper picture), the mast cells (arrows) are difficult to see

♦ with Bismarck brown staining (lower picture), the cytoplasm of mast cells appears light-brown in color (arrows)

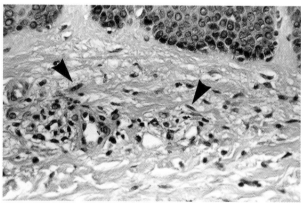

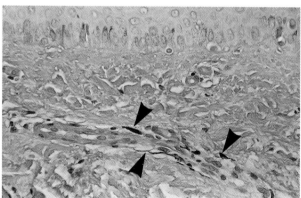

MAST CELL-RICH TUMORS

21.4 Neurofibroma
♦ well circumscribed, but non-encapsulated
♦ thin eosinophilic wavy collagen fibers running in various directions
♦ spindle-shaped cells with elongated nuclei are perineural fibroblasts
♦ randomly scattered mast cells within tumor (arrows)
♦ solitary or multiple skin- or tan-colored papules which may be pedunculated and readily invaginated by the tip of the finger (button-hole sign)
♦ multiple lesions arising in late adolescence in a person with six or more café au lait patches are typical of neurofibromatosis

21.5 Cutaneous myxoma
♦ a mast cell is present (arrow)
♦ myxoid stroma with other spindle-shaped mesenchymal cells (see 17.4 for other features of this tumor)
♦ knowing that mast cells are frequently present in neurilemmoma, cutaneous myxoma, spindle cell lipoma, and synovial cell sarcoma may be helpful in identifying these lesions and differentiating them from other histologically similar tumors

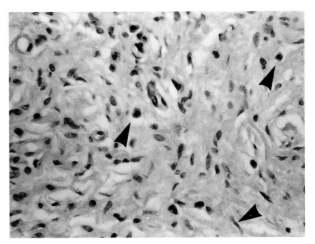
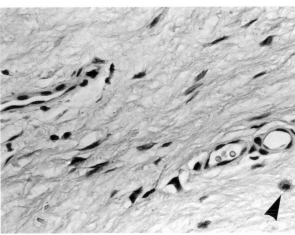

PLASMA CELL INFILTRATION

Plasma cell infiltration is usually not seen in inflammatory dermatoses unless a mucocutaneous area is involved (for example, mucosal lichen planus), or the lesion is excoriated, ulcerated, or impetiginized. A few benign inflammatory conditions of the genitalia, perioral skin, and mucosa refer to plasma cells in their names, such as plasma cell orificial mucositis (other names for this condition include the anatomic structure: balanitis circumscripta plasmacellularis; vulvitis circumscripta plasmacellularis; plasma cell gingivitis; circumorificial plasmacytosis; and plasmacytosis mucosae). Inflammation that is plasma cell-rich is characteristic of spirochete infections.

In contrast to inflammatory dermatoses, inflammatory infiltrates associated with regressing nevi, precancerous lesions, and skin cancers (such as actinic keratosis, Bowen's disease, basal cell carcinoma, squamous cell carcinoma, and melanoma) often contain numerous plasma cells, suggesting a possible role of humoral antibody production in these lesions.

Primary plasmacytoma of the skin is extremely rare. The diagnosis of cutaneous plasmacytoma, whether primary or metastatic, should be supported by immunohistochemical demonstration of light chain restriction and electrophoresis. A plasma cell variant of cutaneous lymphoid hyperplasia has also been described.

Plasma cells

22.1

Differential diagnoses

Non-infectious inflammatory dermatoses

Spirochete infection

Non-plasma cell skin tumors

Plasma cell proliferation

22.1 Plasma cells

♦ clock-face eccentric nucleus
♦ amphophilic cytoplasm with perinuclear halos representing the Golgi apparatus (small arrow)
♦ Russell bodies are eosinophilic, homogeneous, round, PAS-positive, diastase-resistant bodies seen in cytoplasm or outside of plasma cells that are actively synthesizing antibodies (large arrow)
♦ Dutcher bodies are similar eosinophilic inclusions seen in the nucleus
♦ both Russell and Dutcher bodies are accumulations of antibodies
♦ methyl green–pyronine stains the cytoplasm
♦ antibodies to κ and λ light chains help to determine clonality in neoplastic proliferation
♦ plasma cells are leukocyte common antigen-negative

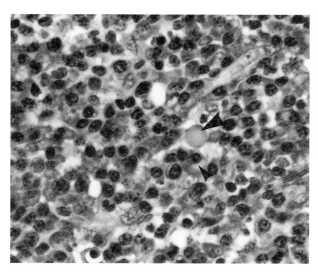

NON-INFECTIOUS INFLAMMATORY DERMATOSES

22.2 Mucosal lichen planus

♦ a few plasma cells may be seen with the band-like lymphocytic infiltration in mucosal lesions
♦ erosion and ulceration may mask the basal cell degeneration and band-like infiltration
♦ focal parakeratosis is not uncommon
♦ consider syphilis in high-risk patients
♦ oral lichen planus may present as reticulated white keratotic papules, or vesiculobullous, erosive, or atrophic lesions

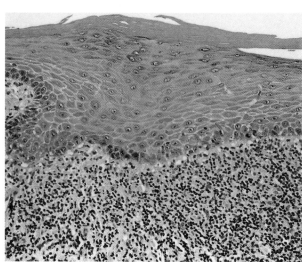

22.3 Balanitis circumscripta plasmacellularis (Zoon's balanitis)

♦ dense infiltrate of plasma cells in lamina propria

♦ secondary bacterial infection probably explains the neutrophilic infiltration; yeasts cells are not present

♦ usually abundant hemosiderin demonstrable with iron staining

♦ chronic, well-demarcated, asymptomatic, erythematous, shiny, moist macule, which may show purpuric cayenne-pepper spots on the glans penis and adjacent prepuce

♦ similar histology in **vulvitis circumscripta plasmacellularis** (brick-red, glistening, fine papules and erosions on the vulva)

♦ clinical differential diagnosis: Bowen's disease; Paget's disease; and pemphigus

♦ biopsy is essential to confirm the diagnosis and to rule out the other clinical diagnoses, which all have distinctive histopathologic features

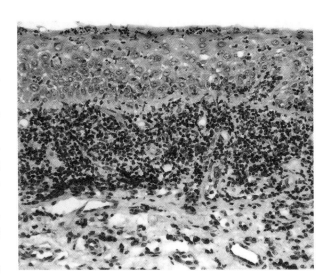

SPIROCHETE INFECTION

22.4 Chancre of primary syphilis

♦ primary mucosal lesions tend to show heavy plasma cell infiltration

♦ acanthosis at the margin with a central ulcer

♦ may show endothelial cell proliferation and swelling

♦ silver stains (Steiner, Warthin–Starry) or dark-field examination demonstrate spirochetes in most primary lesions

♦ develops at the site of inoculation; classically, a single painless ulcer with raised indurated edges and a smooth clean base; when pressure is applied, a scant serous exudate filled with spirochetes is seen

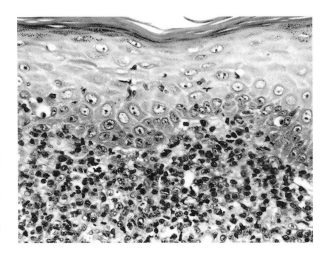

22.5 Secondary syphilis

♦ secondary syphilis involving the lip is shown here

♦ secondary lesions may be non-specific, lichenoid, pustular, or granulomatous

♦ presence of plasma cells in a cutaneous inflammatory infiltrate should raise the suspicion of syphilis

♦ spirochetes may be seen in around 30% of secondary lesions with silver staining

♦ histologically may mimic lichenoid dermatitis and pityriasis lichenoides et varioliformis acuta

♦ variable clinical presentation, but usually generalized and often papulosquamous, with a predilection for the palms and soles

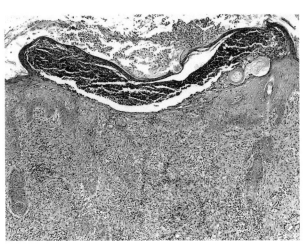

22.6 Erythema chronicum migrans (ECM)

♦ lichenoid inflammatory infiltrate consisting of plasma cells, lymphocytes, and eosinophils around superficial and deep dermal vessels is seen; appearance may be non-specific

♦ silver stains (Steiner, Levaditi's, Warthin–Starry) may be used to demonstrate spirochetes; biopsy should be taken from the periphery of the lesion to increase the chances of finding the organism

♦ infectious organism is *Borrelia burgdorferi*, transmitted by the painless bite of an infected *Ixodes* tick; ECM arises around the tick bite as a large, firm, bluish-red, non-scaly ring around a central punctum; secondary lesions without a central punctum may develop

♦ ECM is the first stage of Lyme disease; stage II: fever, lymphadenopathy, headache, myalgia, arthralgias, and atrioventricular blocks; stage III: arthritis, paresthesias, memory loss, acrodermatitis chronica atrophicans, morphea, and lichen sclerosus

NON-PLASMA CELL SKIN TUMORS

22.7 Syringocystadenoma papilliferum

♦ dense plasma cell infiltration of the fibrous stroma surrounding epithelial tubules and lumina is highly characteristic of this benign tumor of adnexal glandular origin

♦ solitary papule or plaque, or linear papules, usually on the scalp at birth or in early childhood; may develop in nevus sebaceous

♦ plasma cells are seen in many other common cutaneous neoplasms (such as ulcerated basal cell and squamous cell carcinomas)

PLASMA CELL PROLIFERATION

22.8 Plasma cell variant of benign cutaneous lymphoid hyperplasia

♦ rarely, benign cutaneous lymphoid hyperplasia may show a predominantly plasma cell proliferation that may be mistaken for low-grade mantle-zone cutaneous MALT-type lymphoma

♦ the nodule seen here has a well-demarcated smooth margin

(continued next page)

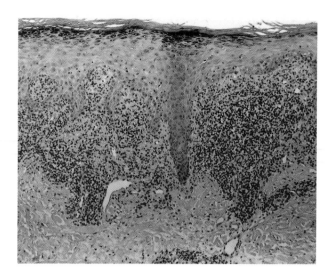

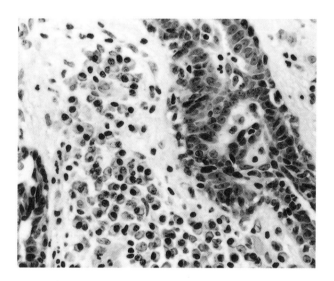

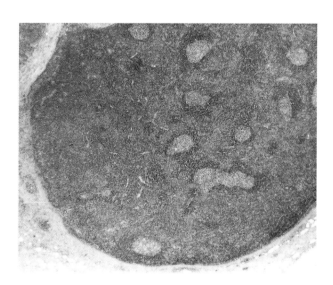

♦ a uniform plasma cell infiltrate with a few eosinophils and lymphocytes in the dermis is seen here

♦ binucleated cells (arrow), and Russell and Dutcher bodies may be present, but with minimal nuclear enlargement and / or pleomorphism

♦ cytologic features are often unreliable in plasma cell-rich lesions; immunohistochemistry is required to exclude monoclonality

♦ formalin-fixed tissue may be used to demonstrate cytoplasmic immunoglobulins

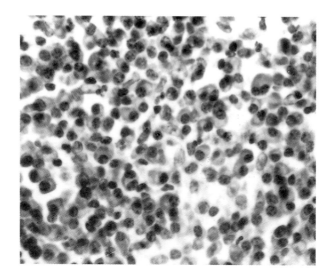

22.9 Cutaneous plasmacytoma

♦ sheets and clusters of plasma cells are seen in the dermis and subcutis with very few other cell types

♦ a slight degree of nuclear enlargement and hyperchromasia is usually observed

♦ cytologic atypia and nuclear pleomorphism are often slight

♦ unlike reactive plasma cell proliferation or marginal-zone (MALT-type) lymphoma, the infiltrate is almost entirely of plasma cells with few other types of inflammatory cells

♦ light chain exclusion and monoclonality may be demonstrated by immunohistochemistry in most lesions

♦ specific cutaneous involvement in multiple myeloma is uncommon but, when present, it is usually an extension of an underlying osseous lesion; extramedullary cutaneous plasmacytoma is less common

♦ clinically presents as multiple or, occasionally, solitary dusky-red, violaceous, or sometimes flesh-colored nodules on the trunk, extremities, and face

♦ plasmacytomas may be the initial manifestation of multiple myeloma

♦ plasmacytomas without evidence of systemic myeloma may be associated with increased serum IgA

♦ non-specific cutaneous lesions associated with multiple myeloma include amyloidosis, xanthomas, opportunistic infections, pyoderma gangrenosum, leukocytoclastic vasculitis, Sweet's syndrome, Raynaud's phenomenon, and cryoglobulinemic purpura

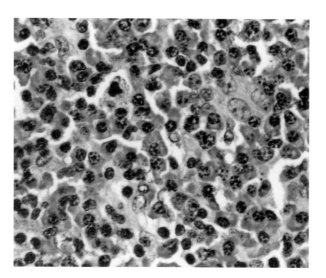

GIANT CELL INFILTRATION

Giant cells are large cells with abundant cytoplasm and multiple nuclei. They are easily discernible at scanning magnification. Giant cells may be lymphocytic, histiocytic, epithelial, mesenchymal, or melanocytic in origin. Their nuclear and cytoplasmic features are often distinctive. The differential diagnosis can be considerably reduced by recognizing the specific types of giant cells.

Giant cells are seen in various inflammatory and neoplastic lesions. Those with uniform nuclei tend to be seen in inflammatory or benign lesions. Touton giant cells, with their peripheral wreath-like arrangement of uniform nuclei, are easy to identify and are seen in xanthomas, juvenile xanthogranuloma, dermatofibroma, and nevocellular nevus. Giant cells with a horseshoe-shaped nuclear configuration are common in mycobacterial and deep fungal infections. Foreign-body giant cells have numerous uniform nuclei scattered throughout the cytoplasm. They are not only seen in foreign-body reactions, but also in benign fibrous papule. Giant cells with cytoplasmic inclusions are typically seen in sarcoidosis, annular elastolytic granuloma, and reticulohistiocytic granuloma.

Giant cells in inflammatory conditions are usually associated with granulomatous inflammation. In addition to identification of the different types of giant cells, the histologic diagnosis is greatly assisted by categorizing the type of granulomatous inflammation: epithelioid; caseating; suppurative; or vasculitic. Necrobiotic granulomas have focal alteration or degeneration of collagen, and a few giant cells may be present. Examples of necrobiotic granulomas include granuloma annulare, necrobiosis lipoidica, and rheumatoid nodule (discussed in Chapter 17).

Epithelioid granulomas have also been referred to as sarcoidal or 'naked' granulomas. A circumscribed nodule with necrosis is seen. There is usually an abundance of epithelioid histiocytes and few lymphocytes. Sarcoidosis is the prototype, although tuberculosis, tuberculids (such as lichen scrofulosorum, erythema induratum), aquarium

granuloma due to *Mycobacterium marinum*, leprosy, deep fungal infections (for example, sporotrichosis, cryptococcosis, coccidioidomycosis, North American blastomycosis), leishmaniasis, tertiary syphilis, foreign-body granulomas (secondary to silica, beryllium, zirconium, or tattoo pigment), acne rosacea, metastatic Crohn's disease, and cheilitis granulomatosa (Melkersson–Rosenthal syndrome) may show similar inflammation.

Caseating granulomas involve coagulative necrosis without suppuration. Some may show caseation macroscopically. Cellular details and intact nuclei are lost, and eosinophilic granular material with nuclear fragments may be seen. The presence of necrosis within an epithelioid granuloma should suggest tuberculosis or atypical mycobacterial infections. Sarcoid and lupus miliaris disseminatus faciei (a type of granulomatous acne rosacea) may occasionally show necrotizing granulomatous inflammation.

Suppurative granulomas show acute inflammation with neutrophils and sometimes abscess formation. There is no vasculitis. Suppurative granulomatous inflammation may be seen in mycetoma, botryomycosis (usually due to staphylococci or possibly *Pseudomonas aeruginosa*), cat-scratch, tularemia, lymphogranuloma venereum, granuloma inguinale, North American blastomycosis, chromomycosis, paracoccidioidomycosis, coccidioidomycosis, pseudofolliculitis barbae, hidradenitis suppurativa, acne conglobata, perifolliculitis capitis abscedens et suffodiens, and pilonidal cysts. The deep fungal infections are often histologically distinguishable on the basis of spore diameter (rare 4–6-mm spores in sporotrichosis; 6–12-mm pigmented spores in chromomycosis; 6–20-mm spores in paracoccidioidomycosis which may occasionally show a characteristic 'ship's-wheel' appearance due to multiple budding yeast forms on the parent cell; 8–15-mm thick-walled spores in North American blastomycosis; and 30–60-mm spores with 2–5-mm endospores in coccidioidomycosis).

Granulomatous dermatitis with vasculitis is seen in Wegener's granulomatosis, lymphomatoid granulomatosis, temporal arteritis (giant cell arteritis), and Churg–Strauss syndrome (allergic granulomatosis). The vessel walls show inflammation and the endothelial cells may be swollen, necrotic, or proliferating. Thrombosis and / or fibrin deposition in vessel walls are required before a diagnosis of vasculitis can be made. Foreign-body giant cells are commonly seen in these conditions. In Wegener's granulomatosis, granulomas are seen in the upper and lower respiratory tract, small arteries and veins, and kidneys. Skin lesions are unusual and show necrotizing vasculitis and / or necrotizing granulomas with giant cells. The inflammatory infiltrate contains neutrophils, lymphocytes, and histiocytes, and giant cells surround the areas of necrosis. A deep dermal vasculitis with fibrinoid necrosis of the vessel wall, atypical lymphocytes with large hyperchromatic nuclei, and occasional giant cells or epithelioid nodules are seen in lymphomatoid granulomatosis. Patchy granulomatous inflammation throughout the arterial wall is seen in temporal arteritis. Asthma, eosinophilia, and small artery and vein vasculitis are features of Churg–Strauss syndrome. Unlike the other conditions mentioned above, eosinophils are a prominent histologic feature of Churg–Strauss syndrome.

Giant cells with pleomorphic nuclei are usually neoplastic. Many tumors, including carcinomas, sarcomas, lymphomas, and melanomas, occasionally have tumor giant cells interspersed among other neoplastic cells. As the tumor giant cells are often similar to the latter in appearance, the cellular background in such tumors is also of diagnostic importance.

Foreign-body giant cell	23.1
Giant cells with wreath-like nuclear configuration	
Xanthelasma / xanthomas	23.2
Juvenile xanthogranuloma	23.3
Dermatofibroma	23.4
Nevocellular nevus	23.5
Giant cells with horseshoe-shaped nuclear configuration	
Aquarium granuloma	23.6
Sporotrichosis	23.7
Lupus miliaris disseminatus faciei	23.8
Giant cells with uniform, but scattered, nuclei	
Benign fibrous papule of the face	23.9
Foreign-body reaction	23.10
Giant cells with cytoplasmic inclusions	
Sarcoidosis	23.11
Annular elastolytic granuloma	23.12
Multicentric reticulohistiocytosis / reticulohistiocytoma / reticulohistiocytic granuloma	23.13
Tumor giant cells with pleomorphic nuclei	
Squamous cell carcinoma	23.14
Anaplastic large cell lymphoma of the skin / lymphomatoid papulosis	23.15
Spitz nevus	23.16
Malignant melanoma	23.17
Atypical fibroxanthoma	23.18
Malignant fibrous histiocytoma	23.19
Dermatofibroma with monster cells	23.20

23.1 Foreign-body giant cell

♦ typical giant cells (arrows) in a foreign-body granuloma reacting to the vegetal cells of a wooden splinter

♦ giant cells have multiple, round, uniform nuclei scattered throughout their cytoplasm

♦ on occasions, the type of foreign body is identifiable on histology: tattoo pigment is usually coarse; hair cortex and medulla are seen in a pilonidal sinus; silica appears as refractile crystals; talc appears as glassy, white, refractile birefringent crystals; starch resembles an ovoid, basophilic, polarized Maltese cross; and paraffinomas have a Swiss-cheese appearance

♦ examination of granulomas under polarized light is invaluable

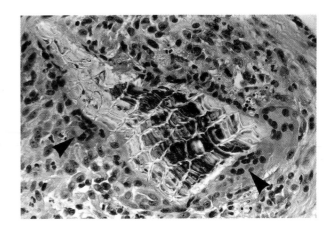

GIANT CELLS WITH WREATH-LIKE NUCLEAR CONFIGURATION

23.2 Xanthelasma

♦ Touton giant cells are typically, though not exclusively, present

♦ typical Touton giant cells have wreath-like nuclei surrounding a central eosinophilic homogeneous cytoplasm

♦ foamy histiocytes lie more superficially, and there is no dermal fibrosis in xanthelasma

♦ a granulomatous dermal reaction with elastosis should raise the possibility of granulomatous mycosis fungoides

♦ **xanthomas** may be eruptive, tuberous, tendinous, planar, mucosal, or intertriginous, and are usually associated with disorders of lipoprotein metabolism, content, or structure

♦ **xanthelasma** are yellow papules around the eyes

♦ the yellow color is due to the lipid in the foam cells

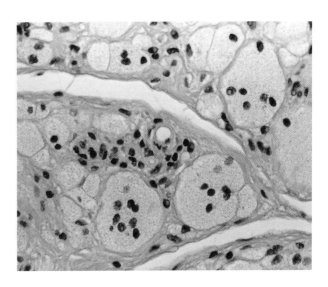

23.3 Juvenile xanthogranuloma

♦ the number of giant cells is dependent on the duration of the lesion

♦ more mature lesions tend to show numerous Touton-type giant cells, as seen here; at such low magnification, the giant cells appear as rings because of their wreath-shaped nuclei

(continued next page)

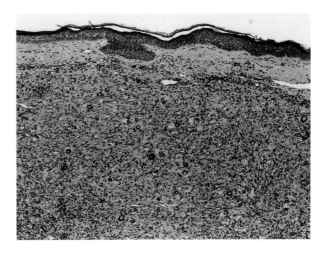

♦ a Touton giant cell at high magnification; the eosino-philic homogeneous cytoplasm in the cell center is surrounded by a ring of nuclei; the peripheral cyto-plasm is foamy

♦ solitary or multiple, yellow to orange, asymptomatic papules and nodules seen typically on the head and neck of infants and children

♦ spontaneously disappear within 3–6 years

♦ may have extracutaneous lesions especially in the eye

♦ adults may also be affected

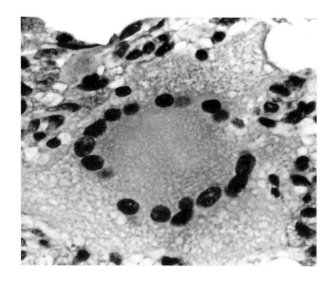

23.4 Dermatofibroma

♦ occasionally, dermatofibromas may show foamy histio-cytes and Touton giant cells

♦ Touton giant cells with cytoplasmic iron pigment are most commonly present in dermatofibromas; hemo-siderin granules (arrows) may be highlighted by iron staining

♦ spindle-shaped fibroblastic cells may not be prominent in this type of cellular dermatofibroma (see 32.3)

♦ cellular dermatofibroma is often vascular and hemor-rhagic, the so-called siderotic dermatofibroma

♦ epidermal hyperplasia with pigmentation is often seen (so-called dirty fingers)

♦ single or multiple, firm, reddish-brown papules or nodules with ill-defined borders and a dimple or button sign, seen most usually on the extremities

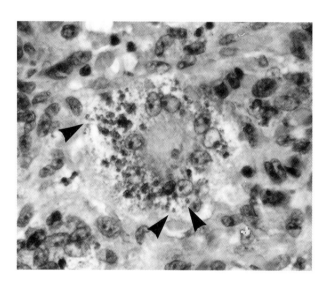

23.5 Nevocellular nevus

♦ giant cells of melanocytic origin have rounded uniform nuclei and pale cytoplasm that often contains intra-cytoplasmic melanin pigment (arrows)

♦ in contrast to giant cells seen in melanoma, giant cells in nevocellular nevus do not show atypia

♦ nevic giant cells may or may not show special nuclear patterning

♦ when there is nuclear organization, the nuclei may have a wreath-like arrangement

♦ melanocytic giant cells are seen primarily in longstand-ing benign compound or intradermal nevi

♦ presence of melanocytic giant cells has been consid-ered a reassuring sign of a benign nevus

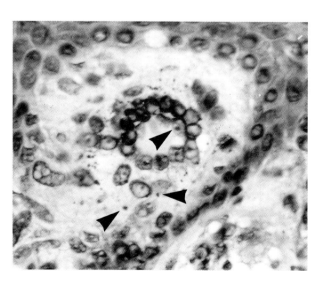

GIANT CELLS WITH HORSESHOE-SHAPED NUCLEAR CONFIGURATION

23.6 Aquarium granuloma
♦ in this example secondary to *Mycobacterium marinum*, Langhans' giant cells have multiple U-shaped nuclei and faintly eosinophilic cytoplasm (small arrow)
♦ nuclear fragments of neutrophils (large arrow); presence of neutrophils and necrotic foci strongly suggest an infectious cause; staining for acid-fast bacilli and fungi should be routine
♦ identification of acid-fast bacilli requires special stains; organisms are difficult to find especially where there is a marked granulomatous host response (see abundance of bacilli in lepromatous **leprosy**, another mycobacterial infection with a minimal host response compared to tuberculoid leprosy, which has few organisms); an oil-immersion lens is recommended when searching for acid-fast bacilli

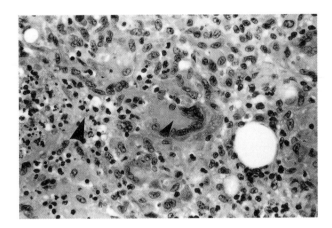

23.7 Sporotrichosis
♦ fungal spores (arrows) within the cytoplasm of a Langhans' giant cell, although spores are often not visible
♦ special stains, such as Ziehl–Neelsen, Fite (stains atypical mycobacteria, but not *Sporothrix*), and PAS with diastase (stains *Sporothrix* spores), are indicated when Langhans' giant cells are seen with neutrophils and tissue necrosis
♦ cutaneous lymphatic variety, the most common presentation, starts as a crusted, ulcerated, nodule typically on the hand; within a few days, multiple subcutaneous nodules appear in a linear arrangement up the arm along the lymphatics; cannot be distinguished clinically from aquarium granuloma
♦ culture for fungi and atypical mycobacteria (a differential diagnosis) is required

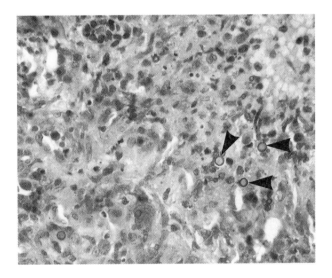

23.8 Lupus miliaris disseminatus faciei
♦ form of granulomatous acne rosacea that is a caseating granuloma on histology
♦ characteristic central eosinophilic necrosis is surrounded by epithelioid histiocytes where Langhans' giant cells may be seen
♦ the clinical appearance is distinctive; lesions are papular and grouped on the face
♦ eyelids and upper lip are typical sites; spontaneous regression is sometimes observed
♦ given the characteristic clinical appearance, special stains for organisms are usually not indicated

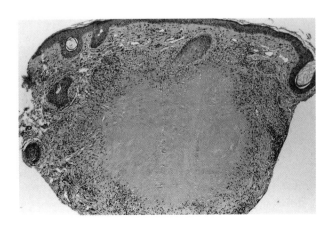

GIANT CELLS WITH UNIFORM, BUT SCATTERED, NUCLEI

23.9 Benign fibrous papule of the face

♦ reactive mesenchymal cells and fibroblasts may be multinucleated

♦ such fibroblastic giant cells are common in this disease

♦ dilated dermal vessels and other spindle-shaped fibroblasts are present

♦ usually seen as a firm, pink, tan- or flesh-colored papule 2–3 mm in diameter on the nose

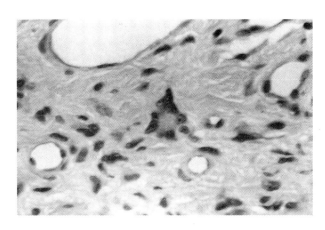

23.10 Foreign-body reaction

♦ many round nuclei are scattered throughout the cytoplasm of the foreign-body giant cell

♦ foreign material is often found in the cells, although the nature of the material is not always identifiable by morphology

♦ cytoplasmic vacuoles contain eosinophilic linear and curve-shaped material (arrow), which is probably keratin from a ruptured epidermal cyst

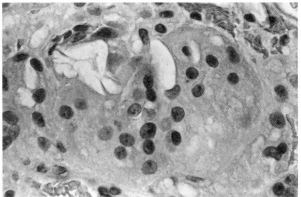

GIANT CELLS WITH CYTOPLASMIC INCLUSIONS

23.11 Sarcoidosis

♦ non-caseating granulomas, and nodular collections of epithelioid histiocytes and lymphocytes are seen throughout the dermis (upper picture)

♦ granulomas do not have central necrosis

♦ overlying epidermis is of the usual thickness (epidermal hyperplasia seen in deep fungal infections)

♦ neutrophilis are few in number in non-infectious granulomas

♦ giant cells in sarcoid often have characteristic cytoplasmic inclusions

♦ an asteroid body is a star-shaped, refractile, eosinophilic inclusion (lower picture)

(continued next page)

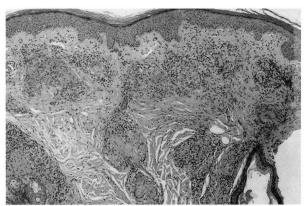

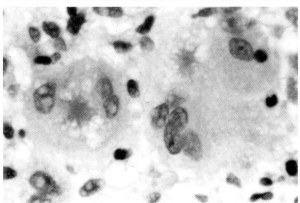

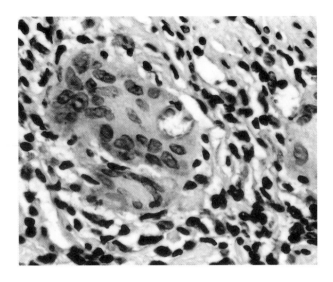

♦ a calcific inclusion, the so-called Schaumann's body, is seen here in a sarcoidal giant cell

♦ as with asteroid bodies, these are commonly, but not exclusively, found in sarcoidosis

♦ as necrotic granulomata may be seen in sarcoid, an infectious process should be excluded clinically and on histopathology by using special stains

♦ idiopathic systemic granulomatous inflammation seen more commonly in blacks

♦ firm papules, plaques, and nodules most commonly seen on the face, rimming an opening such as the nose or eyes, and on the extremities, buttocks, and shoulders

♦ may be annular, erythrodermic, hypopigmented, ulcerated, psoriasiform, or present as scarring alopecia

♦ cutaneous sarcoidosis is commonly found in old scars

♦ may involve any organ

♦ bilateral hilar adenopathy, pulmonary interstitial fibrosis, and uveitis are commonly associated

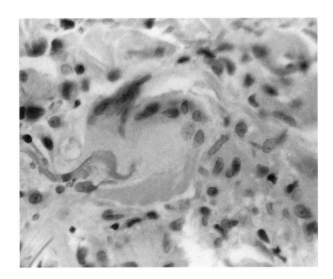

23.12 Annular elastolytic granuloma

♦ 'Miescher's granuloma' and 'actinic granuloma' are other names for this annular lesion of the head and neck

♦ many consider this to be a distinct entity whereas others believe it is a form of granuloma annulare occurring in elastotic skin

♦ no necrobiosis or mucin; collagen fibers are normal outside of the lesion, but thinned and running parallel to the skin surface in the center

♦ intracellular elastin in giant cells is frequently observed and asteroid bodies may be seen

♦ clinical differential diagnosis: sarcoidosis; granuloma annulare; and necrobiosis lipoidica

23.13 Multicentric reticulohistiocytosis

♦ well-circumscribed, non-encapsulated, dermal nodule

♦ unlike other lesions of cutaneous histiocytes, cells have a homogeneous eosinophilic ground-glass cytoplasm

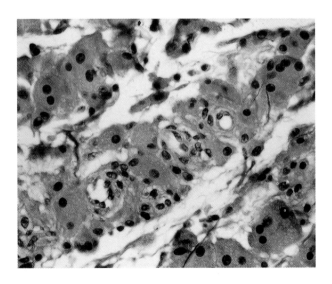

♦ cytoplasmic granules are seen with PAS staining after diastase digestion

♦ **reticulohistiocytoma** refers to a solitary lesion, **reticulohistiocytic granuloma** to multiple lesions, and **multicentric reticulohistiocytosis** to a multisystem disorder characterized primarily by a papulonodular skin eruption and polyarthritis

♦ histologic appearances are identical in these three entities

TUMOR GIANT CELLS WITH PLEOMORPHIC NUCLEI

23.14 Squamous cell carcinoma

♦ neoplastic keratinocytes with enlarged hyperchromatic nuclei and syncytial cell bodies are seen here

♦ carcinomatous giant cells are usually not difficult to distinguish

♦ such giant cells are commonly seen in less differentiated squamous cell carcinoma

♦ clinically seen as an indurated, flesh-colored to reddish-brown, hyperkeratotic, scaly papule or nodule with or without ulceration on sun-exposed skin

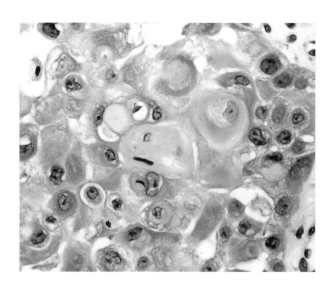

23.15 Anaplastic large cell lymphoma of the skin

♦ binucleate tumor giant cells are reminiscent of Reed–Sternberg cells, but primary cutaneous Hodgkin's disease is extremely rare

♦ sheets of atypical CD30 (Ki-1+) lymphocytes with numerous mitoses

♦ anaplastic large-cell lymphoma may be histologically identical to histiocytic type A **lymphomatoid papulosis** (LyP)

♦ LyP is seen most commonly in the fourth decade and characterized by crops of erythematous to violaceous papules and nodules that may ulcerate and form crusts; lesions regress spontaneously, although the disease is often chronic; 10–20% may develop malignant lymphoma

♦ anaplastic large cell lymphoma resembles LyP clinically, although the lesions are generally larger, fewer, and persistent

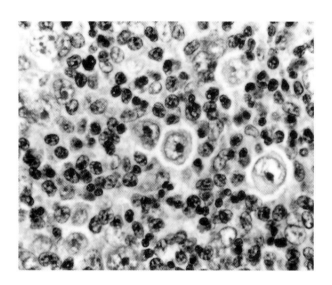

23.16 Spitz nevus

♦ cellular pleomorphism in Spitz nevus is well recognized

♦ occasional multinucleated melanocytic giant cells in a Spitz nevus may have a large vesicular nucleus and prominent nucleoli (arrow)

♦ giant cells are usually not a diagnostic problem as they are seen accompanied by similarly pleomorphic spindle and epithelioid melanocytes

♦ pink/red to tan papules or nodules which may occur anywhere on the skin, but are seen especially on the face, trunk, or legs in children

♦ clinical differential diagnosis: pyogenic granuloma (endothelial proliferation in some capillary lumina)

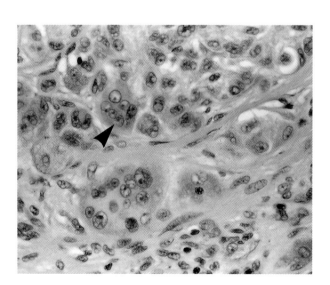

23.17 Malignant melanoma

♦ tumor giant cells are common and show a striking degree of cytologic atypia

♦ melanoma cells tend to have dense, darkly eosinophilic, homogeneous cytoplasm

♦ presence of melanin pigment always helps to differentiate from non-melanocytic tumors

♦ cytoplasmic pseudoinclusions are common in epithelioid melanocytes

♦ asymmetric tumor with an irregular border and variegated color

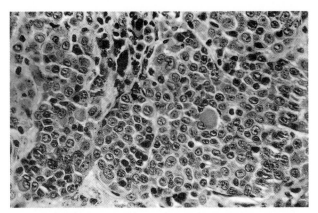

23.18 Atypical fibroxanthoma

♦ numerous sarcomatous spindle and multinucleated tumor cells and giant cells showing an extreme degree of pleomorphism

♦ frequently abnormal mitotic figures

♦ atrophic epidermis often with no Grenz-zone

♦ bizarre tumor cells positive for CD68, but negative for S100 protein and cytokeratin

♦ polypoidal solitary nodule 1–2 cm in diameter, usually found in actinically damaged skin (particularly the nose, cheek, and ear) of elderly persons

♦ indolent, locally aggressive, tumor with minimal risk of distant metastases

♦ clinical and histologic differential diagnoses: spindle cell squamous cell carcinoma (cytokeratin-positive); spindle cell melanoma (S100 protein-positive)

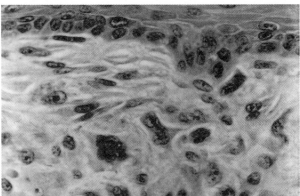

23.19 Malignant fibrous histiocytoma (MFH)

♦ sarcomatous spindle cells in a storiform arrangement

♦ tumor giant cells commonly have hyperchromatic pleomorphic nuclei and abundant eosinophilic cytoplasm

♦ two types of tumor giant cells are found

♦ osteoclastic giant cells (upper picture) are typically found in great numbers in giant cell variant

♦ a prototypical tumor giant cell (lower picture) of high-grade sarcoma, often seen in the pleomorphic type

♦ differentiation from other benign reactive giant cells is seldom a challenge; this type of bizarre tumor giant cells may also be seen in liposarcoma and atypical fibroxanthoma of the skin

♦ most common soft tissue sarcoma in adults

♦ skin involvement is usually secondary to a large, deeply located, fascial or subcutaneous tumor

♦ often a large and poorly demarcated tumor with rapid growth on the thigh and buttock in 50–70-year-olds

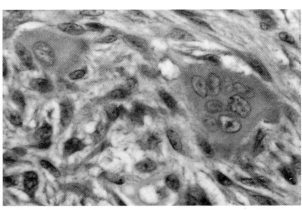

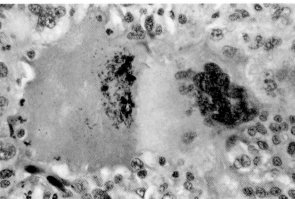

23.20 Dermatofibroma with monster cells

♦ rarely, giant cells with atypical nuclei may be seen even in benign fibrous histiocytomas of the skin (dermatofibromas)

♦ these atypical giant cells are not associated with either other atypical tumor cells or intense mitotic activity

♦ atypical giant cells have been described with cellular or **deep penetrating dermatofibroma** and **giant cell fibroblastoma**

♦ fibrohistiocytic tumors of the skin that are confined to the dermis are usually benign despite the occasional atypical cells or mitotic figures (see 23.18)

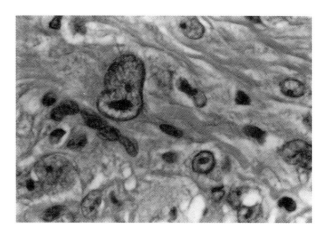

EPITHELIOID CELL TUMORS

The term 'epithelioid' describes a round to ovoid cell that has ample cytoplasm and is thus easily seen at low power. The cell is similar to an epithelial cell (for example, squamous, transitional) in appearance only. Distinctive keratinization and glandular differentiation are rarely observed. The term is used descriptively to facilitate microscopic diagnosis and not necessarily to imply epithelial origin. Melanocytes located in the dermis, for example, frequently have an epithelioid appearance with a central nucleus and peripheral pale-staining cytoplasm. Dermal lesions consisting of epithelioid cells need to be differentiated from true epithelial neoplasms.

Nevocellular lesions are common tumors containing epithelioid cells and should always be considered when epithelioid cells are present within the dermis. The concurrent presence of epithelioid cell nests along the epidermodermal junction and in the dermis is strongly suggestive of a nevocellular lesion. Careful attention paid to the architectural and cytologic features, presence or absence of ulceration, number of cells in mitosis, and desmoplastic reaction should help to distinguish benign from malignant lesions.

Other infiltrative cells in the dermis that may have an epithelioid histologic appearance include true epithelial tumors, large cell lymphomas, and some uncommon infiltrative histiocytic and connective tissue tumors. Immunohistochemical stains are invaluable in difficult cases. The typical panel includes leukocyte common antigen (lymphomas), S100 protein (melanocytic lesions and tumors of Langerhans cells), CD68 (fibrohistiocytic tumors), cytokeratin (most epithelial tumors), and vimentin (melanocytic tumors, epithelioid sarcomas, and cutaneous meningiomas).

Epithelioid cells in a Spitz nevus	24.1

Differential diagnoses

Metastatic / recurrent melanoma	24.2
Spitz nevus	24.3
Nevocellular nevus	24.4
Cutaneous meningioma	24.5
Metastatic breast carcinoma	24.6
Anaplastic large cell lymphoma	24.7
Langerhans cell histiocytosis	24.8
Reticulohistiocytoma / reticulohistiocytic granuloma / multicentric reticulohistiocytosis	24.9
Epithelioid cell dermatofibroma	24.10

24.1 Epithelioid cells in a Spitz nevus

- these dermal nevic cells are epithelioid with abundant, thick, homogeneous, and often faintly eosinophilic cytoplasm, an appearance similar to that of an epithelial cell
- cells of diverse origin may be epithelioid; without further histochemical and immunohistochemical staining, it may be impossible to make a definitive diagnosis
- histochemical stains to consider when epithelioid cells are present in the dermis should include PAS with and without diastase, or a mucin stain; melanin and iron will stain if brown pigment is present
- immunohistochemical stains to consider include cytokeratin, (epithelial) vimentin, S100 protein (strong reaction with melanocytes and weak staining with Langerhans cells), and leukocyte common antigen

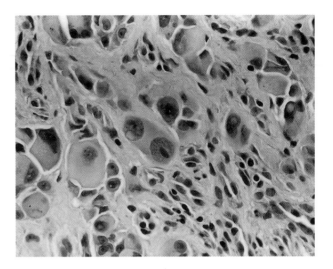

24.2 Metastatic / recurrent melanoma

- epidermal origin or involvement may not be present in metastatic or recurrent melanoma, as seen here
- infiltrating melanomatous cells in the dermis are sometimes epithelioid (as here), although elongated spindle cells may also be present
- unlike benign intradermal nevi, melanoma cells tend to occur in sheets and clusters that displace, rather than lie between, collagen fibers
- larger vesicular nuclei with prominent nucleoli
- occasional melanomas may show only a slight degree of cytologic atypia, and mitoses may not be numerous
- look for fibrous and inflammatory reactions
- S100 protein and melanoma-associated antigen may help to confirm the diagnosis

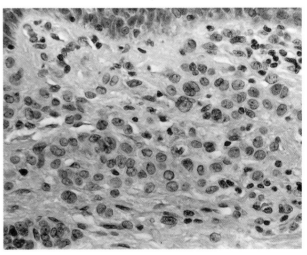

24.3 Spitz nevus

- these intradermal epithelioid cells have large pleomorphic nuclei and nucleoli, and are difficult to distinguish from melanoma when viewed in isolation
- excessive emphasis on abnormal cytologic features, seen under high-power, of the nevic cells in a Spitz nevus is probably the only reason for its being mistaken for a melanoma, yet this diagnostic error is frequently committed by the pathologist

(continued next page)

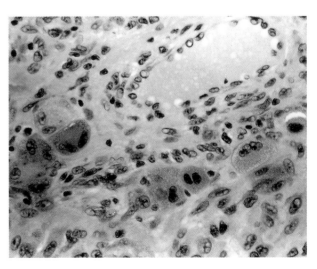

♦ low magnification of a nevus from a 6-year-old shows that it is papular, exophytic, and symmetric

♦ helpful clues that suggest a Spitz nevus include smaller size (usually <6 mm) and presence in children (these are uncommon on sun-exposed skin in the elderly)

♦ melanomas may be small and seen in children

♦ most Spitz nevi are papular compound nevi, minimally pigmented or pink/red due to telangiectatic vessels in the papillary dermis

♦ Kamino bodies (degenerated squamous cells, eosinophilic globules) are more common in Spitz nevi

♦ consider melanoma when the mitotic rate is >1/mm² and abnormal mitotic figures are present

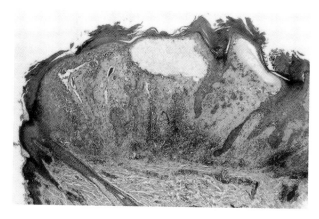

24.4 Nevocellular nevus

♦ type B nevic cells in the superficial dermis are epithelioid and have uniform round nuclei with occasional nuclear cytoplasmic pseudoinclusions (see Chapter 27 for the different types of nevic cells)

♦ moderate to abundant eosinophilic cytoplasm

♦ variable amounts of melanin granules

♦ no nuclear atypia

♦ uniformly brown or flesh-colored papule

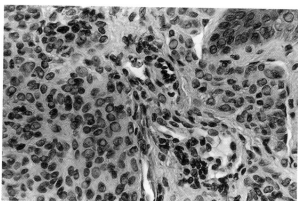

24.5 Cutaneous meningioma

♦ scalp tumor usually arising from ectopic meningothelial cells

♦ a small percentage is due to direct invasion of the scalp by an aggressive intracranial meningioma

♦ lesional cells shown here are epithelioid with rounded uniform central nuclei and scanty cytoplasm

♦ histologic appearance is remarkably like that of nevic cells if the whorl-like cell arrangement is ignored

♦ occasional cells may have pseudonuclear inclusions, as seen in nevic cells

♦ meningothelial cells (lower picture) exhibit an infiltrative growth pattern

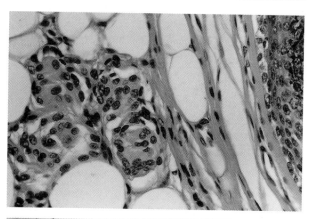

♦ meningothelial cells are S100 protein-negative and cytokeratin-negative, but positive for vimentin

♦ differential diagnosis: melanocytic lesions; and metastatic carcinoma

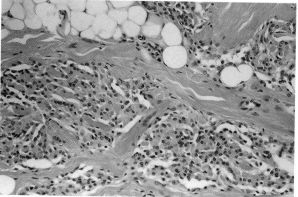

24.6 Metastatic breast carcinoma

- ♦ carcinoma refers to malignancy of epithelial cells; metastatic carcinoma must be in the differential diagnosis of atypical epithelioid cell infiltrates
- ♦ pleomorphic tumor cells are seen in most cases, although metastatic lobular carcinoma of the breast often shows small uniform tumor cells not unlike a congenital intradermal nevus
- ♦ look for cytoplasmic vacuoles and 'Indian-file' appearance (arrow) typical of metastatic breast carcinoma
- ♦ skin biopsy may detect occult malignancy
- ♦ primary tumors that may present with skin metastases include renal cell carcinoma, breast carcinoma, thyroid carcinoma, and small-cell carcinoma of lung
- ♦ flesh-colored erythematous to violaceous tumor / nodule ± ulceration in proximity of the underlying primary tumor or elsewhere (commonly the scalp)

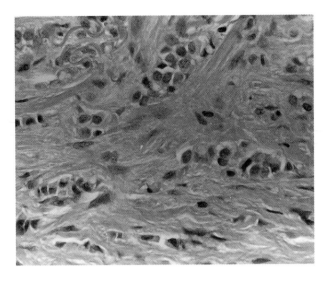

24.7 Anaplastic large cell lymphoma

- ♦ large arrow shows overlying epidermal cells; small arrow shows a tumor cell undergoing mitosis
- ♦ narrow rim of cytoplasm has a readily recognizable epithelioid appearance
- ♦ tumor cells are typically Ki-1 (CD30) antigen-positive
- ♦ spectrum of lymphoproliferative T-cell disorders includes anaplastic large cell lymphoma, regressing atypical histiocytosis, and lymphomatoid papulosis
- ♦ usually, large tumors and nodules on the extremities; nodal involvement and prognosis are variable
- ♦ most common cutaneous lymphoma in HIV-positive patients

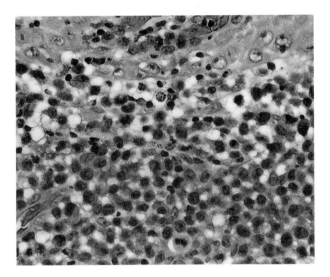

24.8 Langerhans cell histiocytosis

- ♦ epithelioid histiocytes are seen intraepidermally and within the superficial dermis
- ♦ histiocytic cells have pale-staining cytoplasm and kidney- or bean-shaped nuclei
- ♦ three forms: Letterer–Siwe (proliferative); Hand–Schüller–Christian (xanthomatous); and eosinophilic granuloma (granulomatous)
- ♦ all show proliferation of histiocytes with slightly twisted-looking nuclei
- ♦ PAS-positive cytoplasm
- ♦ characteristic Birbeck granules on electron microscopy
- ♦ S-100 protein- and CD1a (OKT6)-positive cells
- ♦ suspect in children with a persistent, reddish-brown, scaly eruption, particularly with associated purpura, ulceration, hepatomegaly, or systemic infection

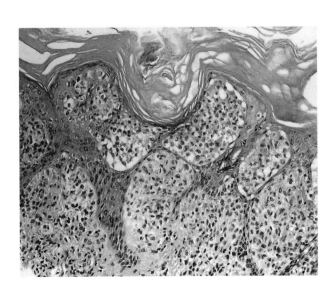

24.9 Reticulohistiocytoma

♦ dermal collections of multinucleated giant cells with an abundance of finely granular eosinophilic cytoplasm (mitochondria)

♦ granules are PAS-positive and diastase-resistant

♦ giant cells have scalloped cytoplasmic outlines

♦ transitional tri- and binucleate as well as single-nucleate histiocytes

♦ S-100 protein- and CD1a (OKT6)-negative; no Birbeck granules

♦ **reticulohistiocytoma** is a solitary lesion

♦ **reticulohistiocytic granuloma** has an identical histopathologic appearance, but lesions are multiple

♦ **multicentric reticulohistiocytosis** also has the same microscopic appearance, but is a multisystem disease with papulonodules and polyarthritis

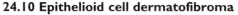

24.10 Epithelioid cell dermatofibroma

♦ rarely, dermatofibromas consist only of epithelioid histiocytic cells; as the typical spindle-shaped fibroblasts and / or foamy histiocytic cells are absent, recognizing a dermatofibroma may be difficult

♦ knowledge of such a histologic variant and exclusion of other epithelioid lesions are key points for a correct diagnosis

♦ histologic variant only; there are no special clinical features

♦ single or multiple, firm, reddish-brown papule(s) or nodule(s) with ill-defined borders that fade into the surrounding skin

♦ usually present on the extremities, especially the legs of women

24.11 Epithelioid hemangioma

♦ reactive inflammatory lesion with heavy infiltration of lymphocytes, plasma cells, and eosinophils

♦ proliferation of dermal vessels lined by epithelioid endothelial cells (arrow) that are prominent because of the increased amount of cytoplasm

♦ lesion is identical to so-called **histiocytoid hemangioma** and **angiolymphoid hyperplasia with eosinophilia**

♦ single or multiple erythematous to violaceous nodules typically on the scalp or face, which often bleed with minimal trauma

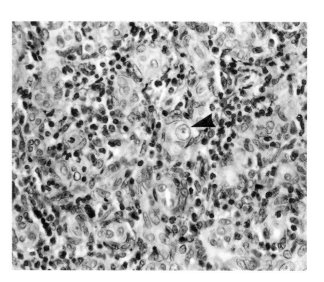

24.12 Epithelioid angiosarcoma

♦ tumor cells may be epithelioid, as shown here

♦ formation of neoplastic vascular channels may not be readily recognizable in epithelioid angiosarcoma

♦ CD34 is a more reliable marker for angiosarcoma than factor VIII

♦ dark red plaque with satellite nodules on the face and scalp; a tumor of the elderly

♦ epithelioid sarcoma may have epithelioid cells; it is a firm slow-growing nodule(s) on the extremities, often annular, and may be ulcerated

♦ histologic differential diagnosis: malignant melanoma; atypical fibroxanthoma of the skin; and spindle cell squamous carcinoma

♦ clinical differential diagnosis: sporotrichosis; mycobacterial infections

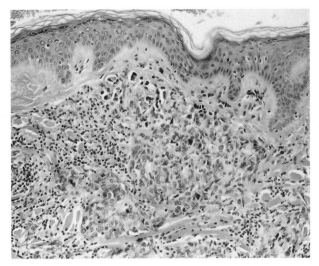

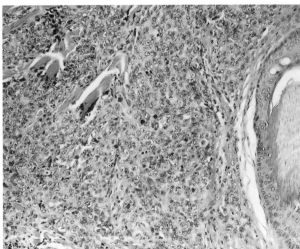

BASALOID AND SMALL CELL TUMORS

Basaloid cells, as the name implies, resemble cells of the basal layer of the epidermis. Basal cells are the stem cells of the epidermis. They are columnar to cuboidal in shape with oval to elongated nuclei and a slight amount of basophilic cytoplasm. Basal cells are interconnected by desmosomes (as intercellular bridges) which are not usually as apparent under routine microscopy as those seen between the more superficial squamous cells. Indeed, the absence of obvious intercellular bridges together with the tendency of basal cells to palisade are useful features to look for when deciding whether a given tumor is basal or squamous in origin.

Multiple basal cell carcinomas (BCCs) of varying histologic subtypes may be seen in the basal cell nevus syndrome and Bazex's syndrome. Both have an autosomal-dominant inheritance. In the former, multiple BCCs, palmar and plantar pits, skeletal and central nervous system abnormalities may be seen. In the latter, multiple BCCs occur in association with follicular atrophoderma, which appears as 'ice-pick' marks and hypo- or anhidrosis.

As the cells of the basal layer are also the embryologic precursor of the skin, it is not surprising that BCCs have a cytology similar to that of the basaloid component of skin appendage tumors and may exhibit hair (trichoepithelioma) or glandular differentiation (eccrine spiradenoma).

With their high nuclear:cytoplasmic ratio and smaller cell size, basal cell tumors also histopathologically resemble the so-called small blue cell tumors, which traditionally include lymphomas and neuroectodermal neoplasms, such as neuroblastomas and Merkel cell tumors. Small cell sarcomas are extremely rare in the skin.

Merkel cells are non-dendritic, non-keratinocytic, epithelial cells which function as slow-adapting type I mechanoreceptors located in the basal or suprabasal layers of the epidermis, or in association with hair follicles. They may also be found singly in the dermis, particularly during fetal life. On light microscopy, they are difficult to identify and often mistaken for melanocytes and Langerhans cells. Electron microscopy shows membrane-bound dense-core neurosecretory granules 80–120 nm in diameter peripherally located in the cytoplasm, occasional intranuclear rodlet structures, paranuclear clusters of intermediate filaments, and desmosomes without attached tonofilaments connecting the cells to neighboring keratinocytes. Merkel cells contain intermediate keratin filaments of simple epithelial type, but not prekeratins as found in stratified squamous epithelium.

Positive staining for neuron-specific enolase (NSE), low-molecular-weight cytokeratins, and negative staining for leukocyte common antigen and S100 protein help confirm the diagnosis of Merkel cell carcinoma. NSE is a marker for neuroendocrine tumors including Merkel cell carcinoma, oat cell carcinoma, carcinoid, and neuroblastoma. Merkel cell carcinomas may also show positive staining for chromogranin, a secretory protein in dense-core granules, and a variety of neuropeptides, including vasoactive intestinal polypeptide (VIP), calcitonin, corticotropin (ACTH), met-enkephalin, gastrin, and somatostatin. Oat cell carcinoma, carcinoid and neuroblastoma may also be revealed by chromogranin staining, but not VIP. Monoclonal antibody staining to cytokeratins 8, 18, and 19 differentiates Merkel cell carcinoma from neuroblastoma, eccrine carcinoma, melanoma, and lymphoma, and neurofilament protein markers may also stain Merkel cell carcinomas. Vimentin, desmin, glial fibrillary acidic protein, leukocyte common antigen and S100 markers are absent although, rarely, S100 may be weakly positive. Leukocyte common antigen is present in lymphoma, but not in any of the other tumors with similar histologic appearances. Similarly, S100 protein is often present in melanomas, but is almost always absent in Merkel cell carcinomas.

Metastatic breast and gastric carcinoma in the skin may present with small neoplastic cells containing only slight amounts of cytoplasm, although cytoplasmic mucin vacuoles and signet-ring cells are often seen under high magnification. These tumors are cytokeratin- and carcinoembryonic antigen (CEA)-positive. Metastatic carcinomas often spread *via* the lymphatics, leading to either an Indian-file appearance due to strands of small cells between collagen bundles, or cell masses within lymphatics. Mast cells seen under low power may mimic small cell tumors, but their granules are easily identifiable with Leder's or Bismarck brown staining.

Differential diagnoses

Nodular histologic pattern

Pilomatricoma (calcifying epithelioma of Malherbe)	25.1
Nodular (solid) basal cell carcinoma	25.2
Adenoid basal cell carcinoma	25.3
Trichoepithelioma	25.4
Trichoblastoma	25.5

Infiltrative histologic pattern

Other small-cell tumors of the skin

NODULAR HISTOLOGIC PATTERN

25.1 Pilomatricoma
(calcifying epithelioma of Malherbe)

♦ well-circumscribed, often encapsulated, tumor showing hair matrix cell differentiation

♦ hair matrix cells are basophilic and basaloid (arrow)

♦ abrupt tricholemmal keratinization without a granular layer

♦ keratinized eosinophilic ghost cells have distinct cell borders and central non-staining areas ('ghost' nuclei; lower picture)

♦ central areas are often calcified

♦ foreign-body giant cells are present in the surrounding dermis

♦ usually seen in the head and neck of children as a firm to stone-hard, lobular, deep dermal or subcutaneous nodule with a positive tent sign

♦ children usually have no other types of acquired epidermal cysts

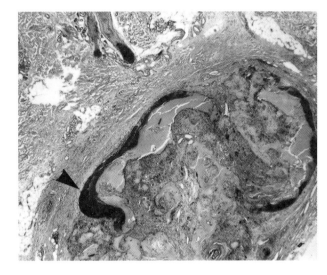

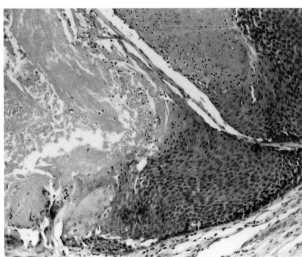

25.2 Nodular (solid) basal cell carcinoma (BCC)

♦ nodular variant is most common (± 60%) type of BCC
♦ distinct peripheral palisading layer suggestive of slow non-aggressive growth
♦ nests usually show retraction (fixation artifact) away from the surrounding stroma, which may contain acid mucin
♦ pink or red translucent papule or nodule with telangiectasia, rolled raised border, and often ulcerated center (rodent ulcer)
♦ pigmented BCCs may be mistaken for melanoma clinically

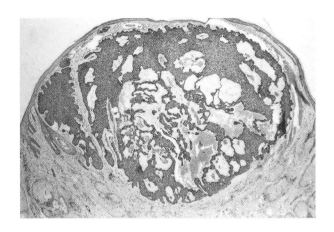

25.3 Adenoid basal cell carcinoma (BCC)

♦ adenoid BCC shows complex tubular / ribbon-like formations of basalis cells reminiscent of adenoid cystic carcinoma
♦ 'tubules' are one to a few cells in thickness
♦ peripheral palisading is inconspicuous
♦ may be mistaken for eccrine tumors, especially eccrine spiradenoma although, unlike the latter, all BCCs show high apoptotic and mitotic activity
♦ no true glands; less retraction artifact than nodular type
♦ same clinical presentation as nodular BCC

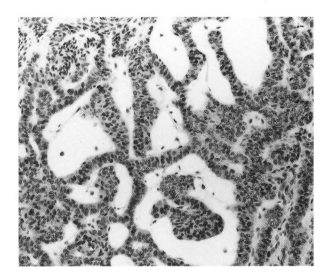

25.4 Trichoepithelioma

♦ basaloid cells are organized into lobules surrounded by uniform, laminated, fibrous tissue layers, unlike the disorganized desmoplastic stroma in BCCs
♦ small keratin cysts and foreign body-type granulomatous inflammation are common findings
♦ may be difficult to distinguish from keratotic BCC, but single-cell necrosis, numerous mitoses, and clefts between tumor cells and stroma are suggestive of BCC

(continued next page)

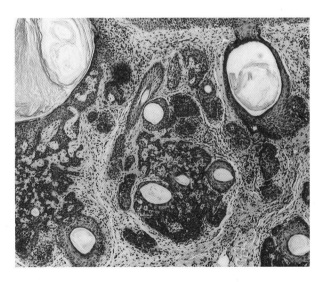

- lace-like cell cords are often seen between keratin cysts, as shown here; the tumor cell clusters are interconnected
- flesh-colored firm papules on the face, particularly in the nasolabial folds
- multiple tumors are often due to autosomal-dominant inheritance
- may be associated with cylindroma and apocrine adenoma

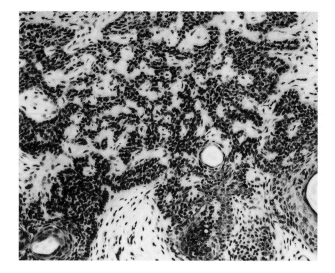

25.5 Trichoblastoma

- large deep-seated tumors composed of basaloid cells
- keratinization of tumor cells is infrequent; when present, keratinization is abrupt and tricholemmal
- characteristic tadpole-like structures reminiscent of hair germ cells are readily identifiable
- surrounded by mesenchyme analogous to developing hair follicles
- no retraction artifact, unlike BCC
- clinically nondescript nodules
- diagnosis is usually made by microscopy

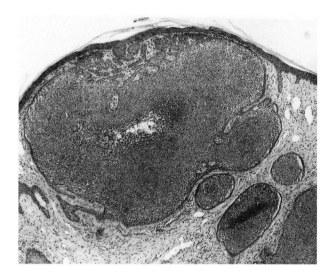

INFILTRATIVE HISTOLOGIC PATTERN

25.6 Desmoplastic trichoepithelioma

- narrow strands of double rows of basaloid cells infiltrating a fibrotic dermis (arrow)
- resembles a morpheic BCC microscopically and clinically, but with minimal apoptotic and mitotic activity, as expected with hamartomatous growth
- may have calcification and foreign-body granulomatous formation
- associated with intradermal nevus in some cases

(continued next page)

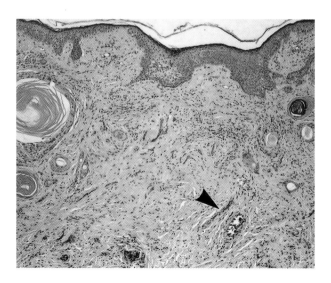

- hard annular papule with depressed non-ulcerated center seen on the face, particularly in women
- may have pinpoint milia at the periphery
- may be solitary or multiple
- multiple lesions may be sporadic or inherited
- clinical differential diagnosis: BCC; granuloma annulare (necrobiosis); and sebaceous hyperplasia (hyperplastic sebaceous gland)

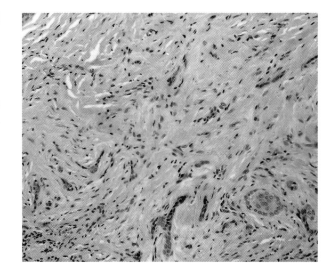

25.7 Morpheic (sclerosing) basal cell carcinoma (BCC)

- morpheic BCC has an abundant, dense, fibrous stroma which compresses the basal cells into thin elongated strands which are often only one cell thick; groups of cells often show branching
- minimal or no retraction artifact is seen
- as the name suggests, resembles a plaque in morphea
- indurated (due to the fibrous stroma) white to ivory tumor with ill-defined borders
- biologically aggressive variant that is frequently deceptively small and superficial clinically, but is often deep with finger-like projections extending well beyond the apparent border of the lesion

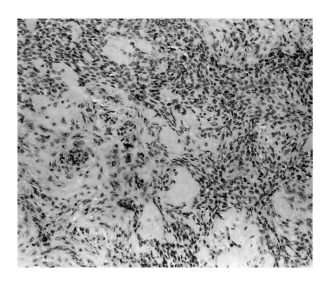

25.8 Superficial multifocal basal cell carcinoma (BCC)

- characterized by multiple, minimally invasive, nests of basal cells
- diagnosis is suggested at low power by multiple hyperchromatic foci in the lower epidermis, which also shows underlying cleft artifacts
- as with other types, often prominent solar elastosis
- usually seen on the trunk and extremities as a flat, erythematous, sometimes translucent, macule or patch up to several centimeters in diameter, with telangiectasia and scaling
- extends peripherally and remains superficial
- recurrences are common, particularly at the periphery
- clinical differential diagnosis: psoriasis; dermatitis; and Bowen's disease; should be considered in a refractory dermatitic or psoriasiform lesion

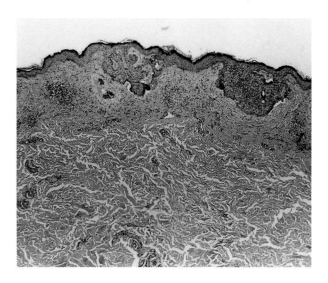

25.9 Neuroendocrine carcinoma of the skin (Merkel cell carcinoma; trabecular cell carcinoma; cutaneous APUDoma; or primary small-cell carcinoma of the skin)

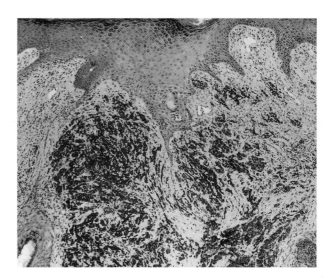

- fairly uniform cells with hyperchromatic nuclei, inconspicuous nucleoli, and scant cytoplasm (as with other neuroendocrine small-cell carcinomas, such as metastatic small-cell bronchogenic carcinoma, metastatic carcinoid, and metastatic neuroblastoma)
- pleomorphic tumor cells arranged in sheets with irregular and anastomosing trabeculae, rosettes, and pseudoglandular formations; abundant cell necrosis and mitosis
- 'ball-in-mitt' arrangement of cells is characteristic (one or two crescent-shaped cells wrapped around a central, round, tumor cell)

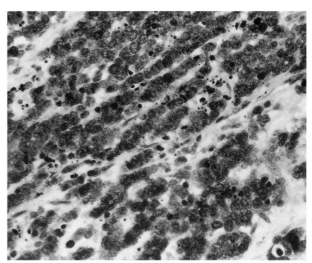

- features on electron microscopy: dense-core cytoplasmic granules, occasional intranuclear rodlets, perinuclear aggregates of intermediate filaments, and intercellular desmosomes, but not in all tumors
- special stains may help to differentiate from other basophilic tumors (NSE-positive, chromogranin-positive, VIP-positive, anticytokeratin-positive, and antineurofilament-positive)
- solitary reddish-blue nodule with telangiectasia ± ulceration on the head and neck in elderly persons; no distinctive clinical features
- local recurrences and metastases are common
- clinical differential diagnosis: BCC; SCC; pyogenic granuloma; melanoma; lymphoma; and metastatic carcinoma
- diagnosis usually made histologically after exclusion of other small-cell tumors in other sites
- histopathologic features are identical to metastatic small-cell carcinoma of the lung so that chest radiography is always indicated

OTHER SMALL-CELL TUMORS OF THE SKIN

25.10 Metastatic neuroblastoma

♦ appearance on light microscopy is identical to that of Merkel cell carcinoma

♦ contains dense-core neurosecretory granules, but perinuclear intermediate filaments are absent; neuroblastoma is NSE-positive and cytokeratin-negative

♦ cellular rosettes (arrow) are typical of neuroblastoma

♦ metastatic cutaneous nodules occur in approximately one-third of neonatal cases, primarily on the trunk and extremities

♦ firm blue-gray papules or nodules with central blanching which develop an erythematous halo 2–3 min after stroking, then return to their original blue-gray color 1–2 h later

♦ clinical differential diagnosis: congenital TORCH infections; cavernous hemangiomas; histiocytosis; leukemia; and lymphoma

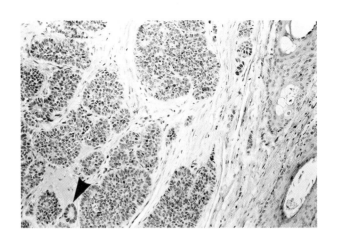

25.11 Metastatic breast carcinoma

♦ a common tumor; cutaneous metastases on chest wall are not uncommon

♦ low-grade breast carcinoma of no special type, and invasive lobular carcinoma often showing small bland tumor cells with minimal cytologic atypia

♦ may be mistaken for congenital dermal nevus except for the high cell density, as seen here

♦ more careful examination should reveal other malignant features, including dark-staining nuclei with molding, cells in narrow files, intracytoplasmic vacuoles, and the occasional mitosis

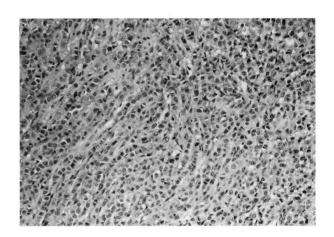

25.12 Small cell melanoma

♦ may present with small tumor cells and minimal cytologic atypia

♦ look for atypical melanocytic hyperplasia in the overlying epidermis; however, this is not seen in metastatic lesions and is often absent in recurrent lesions

♦ S100 protein-, melanoma-associated antigen-, and vimentin-positive

♦ asymmetric, irregularly contoured, pigmented lesion

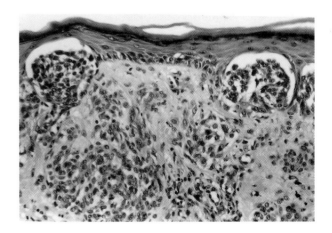

25.13 Eccrine spiradenoma

♦ **eccrine spiradenoma**, **dermal cylindroma** and **dermal duct tumor** are some of the more common sweat gland tumors composed of small basaloid cells that may resemble BCC

♦ in general, these eccrine tumors are benign, nodular, and circumscribed

♦ uniform cells are present with few mitoses and apoptotic bodies (unlike BCC, which has an abundance of mitoses and apoptotic cells)

♦ desmoplasia is absent and the surrounding dermis is often hyalinized (cylindroma)

♦ luminal differentiation, as seen here, is usually present if looked for specifically

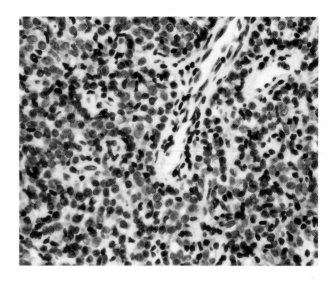

25.14 Small cell lymphoma and leukemia

♦ unlike tumor cells of the large cell lymphomas, which may be epithelioid (see 24.7), tumor cells in low-grade lymphomas or leukemic infiltrates are often small with hyperchromatic nuclei that may be mistaken for other small basaloid tumors

♦ a diffuse, well-differentiated, lymphocytic lymphoma (upper picture) and a myelogenous leukemic infiltrate in the dermis (lower picture)

♦ accurate classification of the lymphomas and leukemias is often impossible from a skin biopsy, and requires examination of peripheral blood films and bone marrow

♦ Leder's stain and stains for myeloperoxidase are useful for demonstrating granulocytic cells

♦ firm, reddish-brown to violaceous macules, papules, nodules, and plaques, which may be purpuric

♦ large cutaneous tumors, frequently on the trunk, are seen with **granulocytic leukemia**

♦ **granulocytic sarcoma**, an erythematous to yellow-green, firm, painless, immobile nodule 1–3 cm in diameter, composed of immature myeloid cells with large oval nuclei is highly specific for acute myelocytic leukemia, and occurs primarily in children and adolescents; granulocytic sarcoma is called **chloroma** when green, the color being secondary to the elevated myeloperoxidase levels in leukemic cells

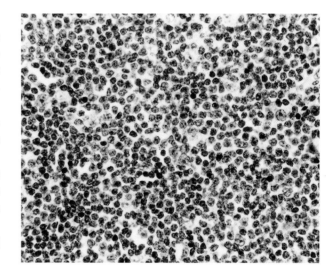

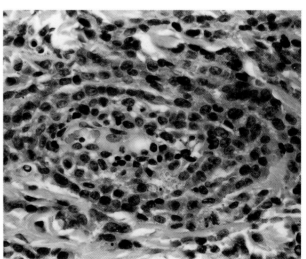

SQUAMOUS CELL TUMORS

Squamous cells are characterized by abundant opaque eosinophilic cytoplasm. The cell border is distinctive and neighboring cells are joined by visible intercellular bridges. There are many tumors of squamous cell origin, both benign and malignant. Histologic features characteristic of a squamous tumor include neoplastic cells with an abundance of eosinophilic cytoplasm, intercellular bridges, keratin cysts and squamous 'pearls' or eddies. Squamous tumors express cytokeratin intermediate filaments, although poorly differentiated squamous carcinoma and spindle cell squamous carcinoma may only express vimentin and not cytokeratin.

Keratin cysts or 'pseudocysts' are the hallmark of seborrheic keratosis, a benign tumor of keratinocytes. Other benign squamous tumors of follicular origin are also cystic with a dilated central opening (such as trichofolliculoma, fibrofolliculoma, dilated pore of Winer, and pilar sheath acanthoma). The finding of fine white hair in the central opening is diagnostic of trichofolliculoma.

Multiple benign tumors of the skin often have an autosomal-dominant inheritance, and may be associated with other cutaneous and internal abnormalities whereas solitary tumors are usually non-hereditary and without other abnormalities. Squamous cell tumors with this genetic pattern include trichilemmoma, fibrofolliculoma, and keratoacanthoma. Other adnexal tumors with this inheritance include trichoepithelioma, trichodiscoma, cylindroma, sebaceous adenoma, and steatocystoma. Non-adnexal examples include neurofibroma, leiomyoma, glomus tumors and clear cell acanthoma. Trichoepitheliomas, trichilemmomas, fibrofolliculomas, trichodiscomas, perifollicular fibromas, and angiofibromas (adenoma sebaceum) present as multiple firm tumors of the face which often cannot be distinguished clinically. Biopsy for histopathologic examination is usually required.

Depending on the location, inverted follicular keratosis, chondrodermatitis nodularis helicis, and proliferating trichilemmal tumor are clinical differential diagnoses for well-differentiated squamous cell carcinoma. Poorly differentiated squamous cell carcinoma needs to be distinguished from atypical fibroxanthoma of the skin, malignant melanoma, and metastatic carcinoma both macro- and microscopically.

Squamous eddies in inverted follicular keratosis	26 .1

Differential diagnoses

26.1 Squamous eddies in inverted follicular keratosis

♦ concentric arrangement of squamous cells forming the so-called pearls or eddies

♦ note the abundant eosinophilic homogeneous cytoplasm

♦ distinctive cell border and intercellular bridges

♦ uniform cells, low nuclear:cytoplasmic ratio, and regular nuclei distinguish this from squamous cell carcinoma

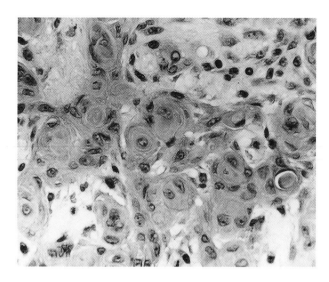

26.2 Inverted follicular keratosis (irritated seborrheic keratosis or follicular poroma)

♦ well-circumscribed benign proliferation of follicular squamous cells extending into the dermis

♦ delayed maturation of peripheral basaloid cells and keratinizing squamous eddies centrally

♦ absence of dysplastic cellular features (such as nuclear enlargement, increased nuclear:cytoplasmic ratio, hyperchromasia)

♦ infrequent mitotic figures

♦ flesh-colored papule with slightly elevated central warty plug seen on the face in middle-aged persons

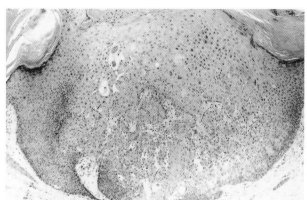

26.3 Seborrheic keratosis

♦ sheets of small uniform round squamous cells with variable amounts of melanin pigment

♦ onion-like lamellation of keratin in recesses and pseudocysts (arrows)

♦ solid or acanthotic type is shown here, but benign squamous proliferation in anastomosing cords (reticulated type) or papillated squamous hyperplasia (papillomatous and hyperkeratotic type) may also be seen

♦ common, exophytic, 'stuck-on', brown, warty papule on the trunk and face in persons >50 years of age; not found on the palms and soles

♦ eruptive and multiple seborrheic keratoses may be associated with internal malignancies (**Leser–Trélat sign**)

♦ histologically similar to **dermatosis papulosa nigra** (1–5-mm dark-brown papules on the face in blacks), **epidermal nevus** (linear warty lesion present at birth or in childhood), and **acanthosis nigricans** (velvety plaque on the neck, axillae, or groin)

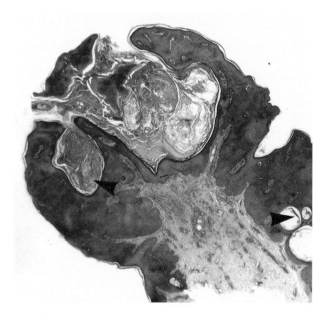

26.4 Trichilemmoma

♦ well-defined endophytic tumor lobules which descend from the epidermal surface and follicular ducts
♦ larger squamous cells with abundant clear cytoplasm
♦ solitary tumor in the middle-aged or elderly, or multiple, 3–8-mm, flesh-colored papules around the mouth, nose, and ears; may have a central hyperkeratotic plug; not usually diagnosed clinically
♦ clinically, solitary lesions may resemble a BCC or wart whereas multiple lesions may mimic trichoepithelioma, adenoma sebaceum fibrofolliculoma, trichodiscoma, or perifollicular fibroma
♦ patients with multiple trichilemmomas have **Cowden's disease**, which may be associated with cutaneous papillomas, fibromas, lipomas, hemangiomas, oral fibromas and papillomas, fibrous hamartomas of the breast, goiter, breast cancer, colonic polyposis and carcinoma, thyroid cancer, and skeletal abnormalities

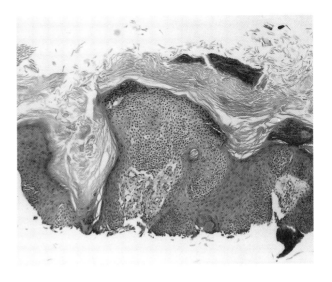

26.5 Trichofolliculoma

♦ dilated follicular infundibulum opening to surface
♦ laminated keratin in dilated follicular opening
♦ radiating rudimentary hair follicles at base of lesion
♦ more follicular differentiation than in fibrofolliculoma with secondary and tertiary hair-containing follicles branching from a central dilated sinus
♦ well-formed, loose, fibrotic surrounding stroma
♦ solitary or multiple, flesh-colored, pearly papules with a central depression containing keratin and/or fine white hairs occurring on the head and neck
♦ presence of white hairs centrally is clinically diagnostic
♦ if white hairs are absent, may be mistaken clinically for BCC

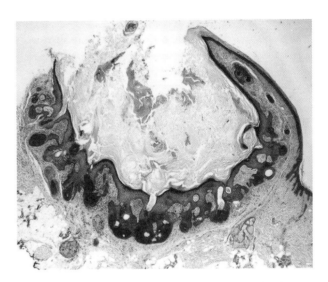

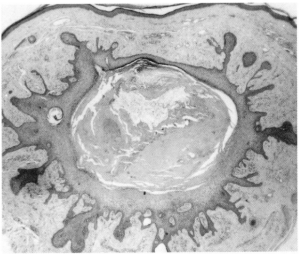

26.6 Fibrofolliculoma

♦ similar to a trichofolliculoma, but with fibrous stromal tissue proliferating within the follicular epithelium

♦ central acanthotic follicular infundibulum containing keratin

♦ multiple, thin, anastomosing bands of basaloid cells extending from the central follicle into the stroma

♦ 2–4 mm in diameter, usually multiple, flesh-colored to white, firm papules, particularly on the face

♦ multiple lesions may be part of the **Birt–Hogg–Dubé syndrome** (multiple fibrofolliculomas, trichodiscomas, perifollicular fibromas, and acrochordons)

♦ indistinguishable clinically from trichodiscoma (proliferation of neural, fibrous, and vascular elements give rise to a tumor with a neuroid appearance) and perifollicular fibroma (fibrous root sheath proliferation without epithelial proliferation)

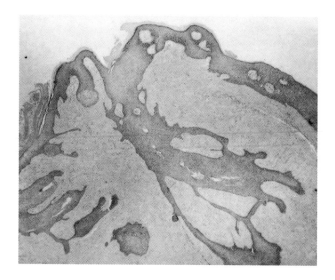

26.7 Dilated pore of Winer

♦ large horn-filled cystic space opening to the surface

♦ lack of prominent fibrous stroma and anastomosing epithelial strands

♦ sebaceous gland lobules and vellus follicles may be attached to the lining epidermis

♦ solitary lesion usually seen in the head and neck areas of male adults

♦ resembles a giant comedo with a brown / black opening on the face

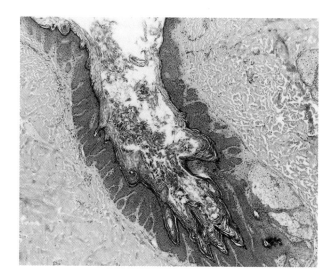

26.8 Pilar sheath acanthoma

♦ dilated infundibulum forming a large cystic cavity plugged with cornified cells

♦ lobulated masses of tumor cells with numerous tiny keratinous cysts radiating from the cavity wall

♦ tumor cells contain glycogen and may show peripheral palisading

♦ usually seen on the upper lip as a small, solitary, flesh-colored papule with a central opening

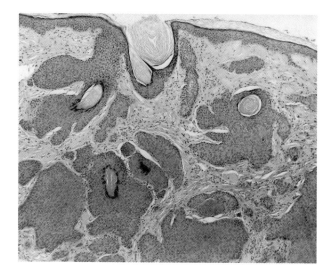

26.9 Nevus sebaceus of Jadassohn

♦ seborrheic keratosis-like squamous lesion (large arrow) consisting of uniform squamous cells with no cytologic atypia
♦ look for rudimentary hair follicles and malformed hair germ cells which may easily be mistaken for BCC (small arrow)
♦ ectopic apocrine glands in deep dermis
♦ may have associated benign (especially syringocystadenoma papilliferum) and malignant skin tumors (especially basal cell carcinoma)
♦ congenital, yellow to orange, hairless, slightly elevated plaque on the scalp or face which becomes larger and warty during adolescence

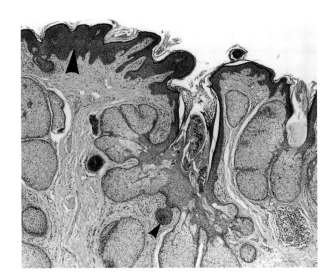

26.10 Proliferating trichilemmal tumor

♦ also called **pilar tumor of the scalp** as approximately 90% of these tumors arise on the scalp and posterior neck
♦ well-demarcated tumor with variable-sized squamous lobules
♦ abrupt transition to amorphous keratin centrally (trichilemmal keratinization, as seen in pilar cysts)
♦ slight nuclear anaplasia and individual cell keratinization
♦ may histologically mimic squamous cell carcinoma, although differs by being sharply demarcated with an abrupt mode of keratinization
♦ may be associated with trichilemmal cysts and are usually seen in older women

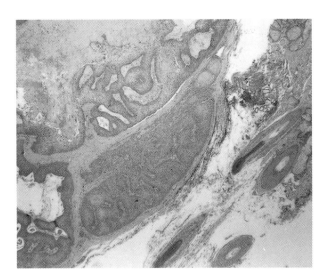

26.11 Keratoacanthoma (KA)

♦ sharply demarcated, symmetric, exo- and endophytic
♦ cup-shaped, keratin-filled, central crater is pathognomonic
♦ crater enclosed by a lip of normal epidermis
♦ squamous cells have abundant glassy cytoplasm
♦ foci of neutrophilic infiltrate within the epidermis and heavy inflammation in the dermis are typical in a regressing lesion
♦ cytologic atypia is usually slight, but marked atypia is sometimes observed and does not imply squamous cell carcinoma
♦ irregular infiltrating dermal interface and cytologic atypia do not necessarily indicate squamous cell carcinoma if the architecture of the lesion is typical

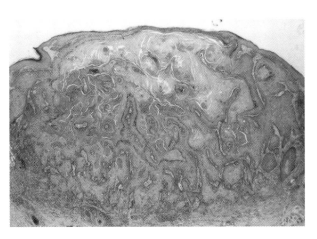

(continued next page)

♦ keratinocytes with abundant 'ground-glass' cytoplasm are seen here

♦ spotty cell necrosis and a neutrophilic infiltrate are characteristic

♦ clinically and histologically may mimic squamous cell carcinoma

♦ rapidly growing tumor nodule with a central depression on sun-exposed skin particularly on the face, forearms, and hands in elderly persons; usually involutes spontaneously within 6 months

♦ usually solitary, although multiple lesions may be seen in the **Ferguson–Smith** (autosomal-dominant inheritance), **Grzybowski** (eruptive lesion 2–3 mm in diameter without a familial pattern), and **Muir–Torre syndromes** (multiple lesions in association with sebaceous neoplasms and visceral cancer, usually of gastrointestinal or urogenital origin)

♦ clinical history of rapid growth and crater-like architecture are the prevailing diagnostic features

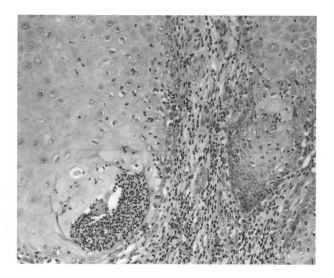

26.12 Squamous cell carcinoma (SCC)

♦ thickened squamous layer with hyperkeratotic surface

♦ irregular, ragged, and infiltrative deep edge

♦ large irregular nuclei with coarse chromatin and prominent nucleoli

♦ variable amounts of keratinization within the tumor

♦ necrosis is often present

♦ poorly differentiated spindle cell squamous carcinoma of the head and neck may be cytokeratin-negative and vimentin-positive, and should be differentiated from atypical fibroxanthoma of the skin (numerous sarcomatous tumor cells and abnormal mitotic figures; cytokeratin-negative and CD68-positive) and desmoplastic melanoma (S100 protein-, melanoma-associated antigen-, and vimentin-positive, and cytokeratin-negative)

♦ indurated, flesh-colored to reddish-brown, hyperkeratotic, scaly papule or nodule with or without ulceration on sun-exposed skin

♦ may also occur in areas of scarring, radiation, and in erythema ab igne

♦ may occur on mucous membranes where it may be associated with tobacco-chewing and erosive lichen planus

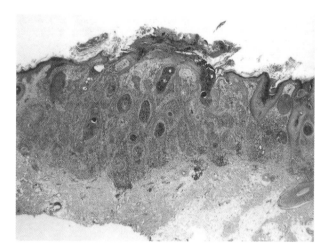

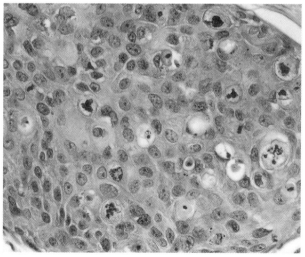

26.13 Verrucous carcinoma

♦ slow-growing, locally aggressive, well-differentiated SCC resembling a giant condyloma both clinically and microscopically, and found on perineal and genital skin; may also be seen on oral mucosa and the sole (**epithelioma cuniculatum**)

♦ well-defined tumor mass showing minimal cellular pleomorphism

♦ downward growth along frontal edge, which advances in a pushing manner

♦ subtle destruction of underlying tissue without ragged tongues of infiltrating malignant cells

♦ difficult histologic diagnosis because of the resemblance to condyloma acuminatum, the apparently relatively benign cytologic features, and minimal dysplasia

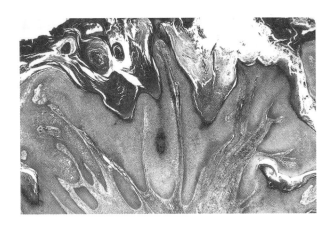

26.14 Metastatic breast carcinoma

♦ metastatic breast carcinoma is seen here in the dermal lymphatic channels

♦ higher-grade breast carcinoma cells are squamous cell-like and may not show their glandular origin

♦ carcinomas in the dermis, especially those within lymphatic channels and without an epidermal origin or associated actinic changes, should raise a suspicion of cutaneous metastasis

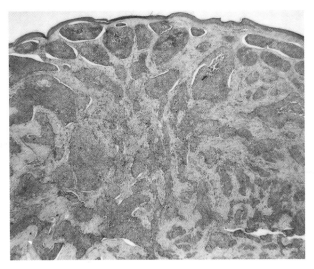

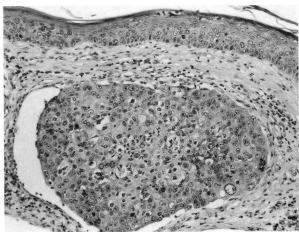

MELANOCYTIC TUMORS

Melanocytes are dendritic cells of neuroectodermal origin. During embryonic life, they migrate to the basal epidermis and hair bulbs in the skin. Dermal melanocytes are believed to be the result of aberrant migration and dislocation of embryologic melanocytes or downward extension of proliferating epidermal melanocytes.

As with intraepidermal melanocytes, dermal melanocytes may be epithelioid or dendritic in histologic appearance (see Chapter 11). The compound, intradermal, and cellular blue nevi are caused by hamartomatous proliferation of epithelioid nevic cells. Dendritic dermal melanocytes form the common blue nevus and the dermal melanocytic hamartomas, such as the nevi of Ito and Ota, and the Mongolian spot. The term 'combined nevus' refers to the coexistence of an epithelioid nevocellular nevus and a blue nevus.

Melanocytic nevi or moles are ubiquitous. The average person bears 25 nevi somewhere on the body. Nevi may be present at birth (congenital) or may appear later in life (acquired). The number of nevi is affected by genetic factors, and the amount of sun-exposure and sunburn. Most nevi develop during the first 30–35 years of life. Pigmented lesions developing after age 40 years should raise suspicion of melanoma.

As a benign nevocellular lesion ages, it undergoes maturation. Nevic cells grow down into the dermis and are morphologically altered. Nevic cells located in the middermis (type B cells) are smaller, round, and resemble lymphocytes whereas those in the lower dermis (type C cells) are spindle-shaped with elongated nuclei and indiscernible cytoplasm. Both types contain little pigment.

Dermal melanocytes are dendritic, fusiform cells with scant cytoplasm and elongated nuclei. Melanomas are malignant tumors of melanocytes. Most melanomas arise *de novo*; only one-third arise in a preexisting nevus. Tumor thickness is the single most important prognostic factor. **Clark** originally described five levels of tumor infiltration:

Level I	Intraepidermal;
Level II	Extension into papillary dermis;
Level III	Involvement of the entire papillary dermis;
Level IV	Involvement of reticular dermis;
Level V	Involvement of subcutis.

The **Breslow** measurement, however, is more accurate as dermal thickness may vary depending on the anatomic location. The Breslow measurement is taken from the top of the granular layer to the deepest tumor cell. Such a measurement is required for every melanoma because both the treatment and prognosis are based on it.

Staging according to the American Joint Committee on Cancer (AJC)

Primary tumor (pT)	TX	Tumor not assessed		
	T0	No evidence of primary tumor		
	Tis	Melanoma in situ (Clark's level I)		
	T	<0.75 mm	5-year survival rate	96%
	T2	0.76–1.49 mm	5-year survival rate	87%
	T3	1.50–3.99 mm	5-year survival rate	66–75%
	T4	>4.0 mm	5-year survival rate	36%

27.1 Dermal epithelioid nevic cells

♦ **type B nevic cells** (large arrow) are located in the middermis
♦ smaller than type A junctional nevic cells
♦ round cells with a small amount of pale cytoplasm and usually very little pigment
♦ **type C nevic cells** (small arrow) are found in the lower reticular dermis
♦ spindle-shaped cells with elongated nucleus and a neuroid appearance
♦ indiscernible cytoplasm with no melanin pigment
♦ nevus with predominantly type C cells is called a neural nevus and resembles a neurofibroma

27.2 Dermal dendritic melanocytes

♦ as seen in this **common blue nevus**, dermal melanocytes are dendritic fusiform cells
♦ scant cytoplasm and elongated nuclei
♦ intracytoplasmic melanin pigment is present in most of the cells

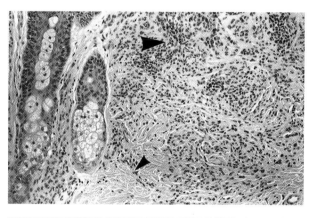
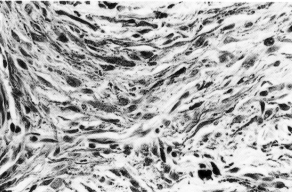

BENIGN HAMARTOMA / PROLIFERATION

27.3 Intradermal nevus

♦ nests, fascicles, and single nevic cells are seen among collagen fibers of the dermis

♦ junctional theques or nests, defined as clusters of more than three nevic cells (epithelioid melanocytes) located at the epidermodermal junction, are absent, but a slight focal increase in the number of normal-looking basal melanocytes is not uncommon

♦ papillated hyperplasia of the overlying epidermis is common

♦ intradermal nevus is unlikely to be malignant; differential diagnoses of recurrent metastases of so-called minimal-deviation melanoma should be considered if atypical dermal nevic cells are observed

♦ uniform, brown or skin-colored papule

♦ skin-colored intradermal nevus may be clinically mistaken for basal cell carcinoma

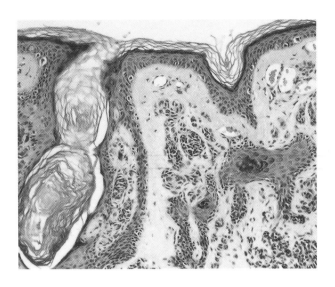

27.4 Acquired compound nevus

♦ nests of nevic cells (epithelioid melanocytes) at the dermoepidermal junction accompanied by a dermal component

♦ dermal nevic cells appear as single cells and in loose clusters

♦ dermal nevic cells are distributed in a plate-like pattern with a flat deep margin, as seen here; nevic cells expand the papillary dermis and do not extend into the reticular or adventitial dermis around adnexal structures

♦ overlying epidermis is often hyperplastic

♦ brown papule occurring anywhere on the body

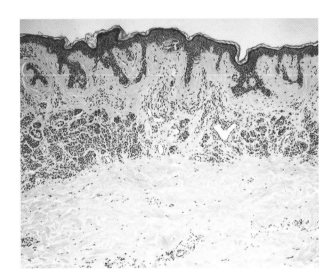

27.5 Congenital nevus

♦ in contrast to the acquired nevus, type C nevic cells are prominent

♦ diffusely infiltrative pattern of nevic cells in the reticular dermis is characteristic

♦ nevic cells are also present in the adventitial dermis and among adnexal structures

♦ often contains darkly pigmented terminal hairs

♦ 1–2% prevalence in the general population

♦ varies from small to large and covers most of the body surface, although 'bathing trunk' and 'glove-and-stocking' type nevi are rare

♦ a giant congenital nevus is >20 cm and carries a 6–10% risk of melanomatous change; alterations in a congenital nevus should be biopsied

♦ removal of a large congenital nevus may not eliminate the risk of melanoma, which is able to develop within the fascia or leptomeninges

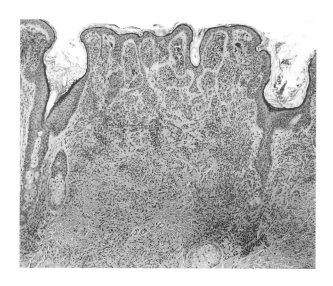

27.6 Deep penetrating nevus

♦ architecture is similar to that of a congenital nevus

♦ a superficial, broad, wedge-shaped edge; nevic cells extend deep to the reticular dermis, and may surround skin appendages, as seen in congenital nevi

♦ nests of nevic cells begin at the dermoepidermal junction; the infiltrative dermal component consists of looser nests and fascicles

♦ individual cells are large, pleomorphic, spindle-shaped, and epithelioid

♦ some cells are heavily pigmented (arrow)

♦ smaller, round, nevic cells are also present

♦ only a slight tendency for cells to become smaller at the base (failure of maturation)

♦ mitoses are rare

♦ unlike melanoma, a desmoplastic and inflammatory reaction should not be present

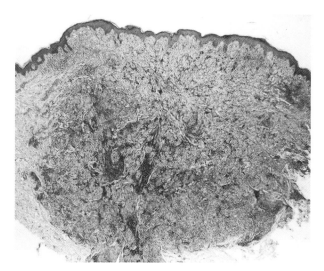

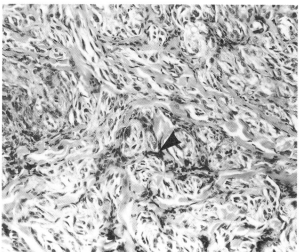

27.7 Pigmented spindle cell nevus

♦ a superficial acquired compound nevus that is heavily pigmented

♦ symmetric pigmented spindle cell nevus (upper picture)

♦ presence of heavily pigmented nevic cells is evident even at low magnification

♦ higher magnification of same lesion (lower picture) reveals spindle-shaped nevic cells

♦ round epithelioid cells (arrow) are, in fact, spindle cells oriented perpendicular to the plane of section (seen end-on and in cross-section, they appear epithelioid)

♦ fascicles of the spindle cells are frequently perpendicular to the skin surface, filling and 'raining down' the papillary dermis

♦ larger pleomorphic cell nuclei and a few normal mitotic figures are to be expected

♦ usually seen in younger persons and presents as a rapidly enlarging dark mole commonly on the lower legs

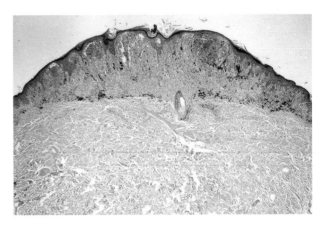

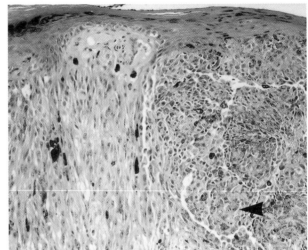

27.8 Halo nevus

♦ nests of nevic cells in the upper dermis ± epidermodermal junction

♦ nevic cells show evidence of nuclear pyknosis and cytolysis

♦ variable amounts of extracellular melanin pigment and presence of melanophages

♦ dense inflammatory lymphoid infiltrate is present among regressing nevic cell nests

♦ may be difficult to identify nevic cells in some lesions; S100 protein staining may be used to highlight nevic cells

♦ pigmented melanocytic nevus with a surrounding depigmented halo; particularly seen on the back usually in young adults

♦ over several months, the central nevus depigments and usually involutes; the surrounding white halo may persist for months to years

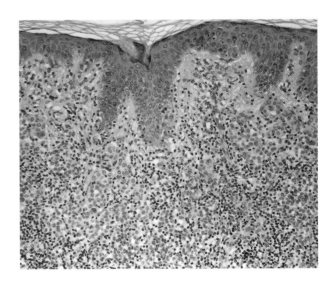

27.9 Spitz nevus (spindle and epithelioid cell nevus)

♦ well-circumscribed and symmetric; most are compound nevi

♦ clefts between junctional nests of melanocytes and keratinocytes are usually present

♦ Kamino bodies (degenerated squamous cells, eosinophilic globules; arrow) in clumps and singly in the epidermis (much more common in Spitz nevi than in melanoma)

♦ melanocytes are spindle-shaped and epithelioid in appearance

♦ cytologic features, including shape, size of cells, and nuclei, may be markedly pleomorphic

♦ multinucleated nevic cells may be present, but the overall microscopic picture is that of regularly irregular cells

♦ upward transmigration of melanocytes within the acanthotic epidermis is subdued; full-blown Pagetoid spread of melanocytes is not observed

♦ a few mitoses may be present, but be wary of abnormal mitotic figures

♦ slight to marked lymphocytic infiltration

♦ typical lesions show telangiectasia and dermal edema with little pigment

♦ intradermal Spitz nevus with a fibrous stroma has been called a **desmoplastic nevus**

♦ histologically may be mistaken for melanoma and the rare melanoma may resemble a Spitz nevus

♦ typically a pink papule on the face, trunk, or extremities, particularly in children

♦ clinically, often mistaken for pyogenic granuloma

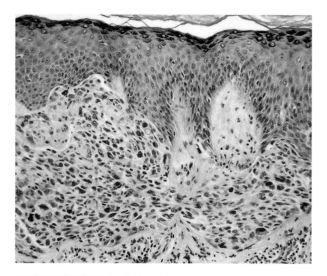

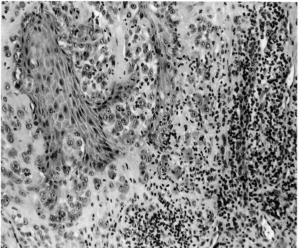

27.10 Atypical (dysplastic) nevus

♦ multiple atypical nevi may be familial or sporadic; atypical nevi appear in adolescence and, unlike common nevi, continue to appear throughout life

♦ 5–10% risk of developing melanoma with multiple dysplastic nevi, and 100% risk if two first- or second-degree relatives have melanoma; changing atypical nevi should be biopsied

♦ histologic diagnosis based on cytologic and architectural atypia, and host response

♦ acanthosis and elongation of rete ridges are common

♦ junctional cell nests fuse laterally, as seen here; the long axis of the junctional cell lies parallel to the skin surface

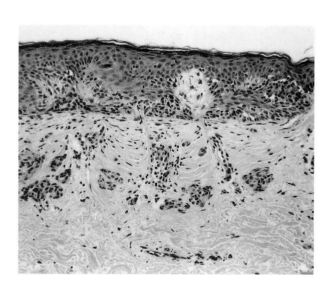

(continued next page)

- cytologic atypia is demonstrated primarily by junctional cells
- atypical nevic cells with a slight degree of histologic (cytologic and architectural) atypia, as seen here
- fibers wrap around the rete ridges in eosinophilic fibrosis whereas, in lamellar fibroplasia, the fibrous tissue runs parallel to the skin surface
- junctional melanocytic hyperplasia at the periphery of the lesion
- lymphocytic dermal infiltrate and prominent vessels
- persons with dysplastic nevi often have >100 nevi compared with the average 25 for common nevi
- dermal nevic cells are small and uniform with a plate-like distribution; the majority (>90%) of atypical nevi are acquired
- clinically, atypical nevi are often large (>8mm) and variably colored, with a slightly elevated center and a border that fades into the surrounding skin
- may be clinically and histologically difficult to distinguish from melanoma

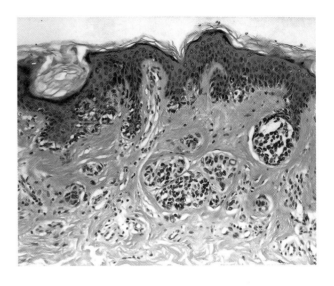

27.11 Common blue nevus

- usually located in the mid- or lower dermis and may extend into the subcutaneum; the blue color is due to the filtering effect of the superficial vascular plexus on the deep-lying melanin pigment
- the superficial blue nevus shown here is, in fact, brown
- dermal melanocytes are arranged as a loose network of spindle cells with dendritic processes
- melanophages are often present (round cells without dendritic processes and packed with coarse granular melanin)
- acquired dark-blue to gray-black papule or nodule which may develop anywhere, but with a predilection for the dorsum of the hands and feet
- **Mongolian spot**, **nevus of Ota** and **nevus of Ito** are common blue nevi present at birth on the buttock, face, and shoulder, respectively

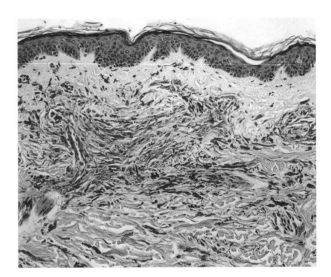

27.12 Cellular blue nevus

♦ similar to common blue nevus, but more cellular, the dermal melanocytes have a greater amount of pale-staining cytoplasm and less melanin

♦ cells resemble type C cells of a nevocellular nevus, as seen here

♦ generally a greater degree of cytologic and nuclear pleomorphism

♦ marked cytologic atypia and increased mitotic activity should raise suspicion of malignant transformation

♦ coexistence of a nevocellular nevus and a blue nevus is termed a **combined nevus**

♦ clinically similar to common blue nevus, but larger (1–3 cm)

♦ usually found on the buttocks, or over the sacrum or coccyx

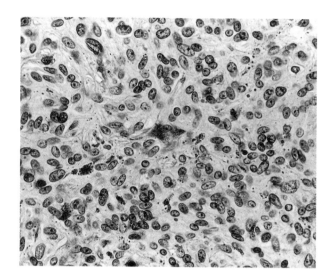

MALIGNANT PROLIFERATION

27.13 Lentigo maligna melanoma

♦ neoplastic melanocytes in the dermis may show only slight cytologic atypia and invasive spindle cells (arrow)

♦ spindle tumor cells are common; dermal invasion is always associated with some degree of desmoplastic reaction and inflammation

♦ epidermal involvement is often lentiginous; neoplastic melanocytes may be confined to the basal and lower squamous cell layers; full-blown Pagetoid spread is frequently absent

♦ finding dermal elastosis is helpful, and junctional or compound nevi should be suspected in elastotic skin in elderly persons

♦ progression from lentigo maligna is gradual, often taking 10–15 years

♦ irregularly pigmented patch with induration and/or papulonodules on sun-exposed skin, particularly the face, in elderly persons

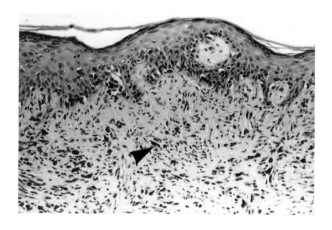

27.14 Superficial spreading melanoma

♦ a melanoma with prominent radial growth and intraepidermal lateral extension of neoplastic melanocytes

♦ radial intraepidermal growth extending for more than three rete ridges from the invading tumor (vertical growth)

♦ Pagetoid invasion (arrow) of overlying epidermis by neoplastic nevic cells is usually present unless the lesion is a recurrence of a metastasis

(continued next page)

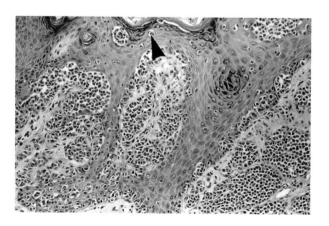

- in addition to Pagetoid spread, cellular pleomorphism, fine 'gold-dust' type of cytoplasmic melanin pigmentation, and abnormal mitotic figures are probably the most helpful microscopic features to confirm the melanomatous nature of a lesion
- invasive nevic cells are often seen in tight nests in the dermis in contrast to benign type C cells that diffusely infiltrate the dermis
- most common type of melanoma
- asymmetric tumor with irregular border and variegated coloration
- radial growth gives rise to macular areas and irregular borders whereas elevation of the lesion indicates vertical growth and dermal invasion
- most commonly seen on the lower legs in women and upper back in men

27.15 Nodular melanoma

- vertical-growth phase of atypical epithelioid melanocytes predominates in the nodular tumor seen here
- radial-growth phase is restricted and generally does not exceed three rete ridges from the invasive dermal component; thus, the lateral margins of the tumor are sharply defined (upper picture)
- medium- and high-power views (middle and lower pictures) demonstrate the cytologic features of melanoma cells
- malignant melanocytes are arranged in alveolar groups and solid sheets
- slight to moderate amount of eosinophilic cytoplasm (epithelioid) with or without cytoplasmic melanin pigmentation, large pleomorphic vesicular nuclei, prominent nucleoli, nuclear pseudoinclusions (arrow), and frequent mitoses
- ulceration of surface epidermis indicates a poor prognosis
- Pagetoid spread may be absent, especially in ulcerated lesions
- **polypoidal** or **pedunculated melanoma** is an aggressive variant of nodular melanoma
- all nodular and polypoidal melanomas are at least Clark level III despite any obvious exophytic nature
- blue / black nodule ± ulceration

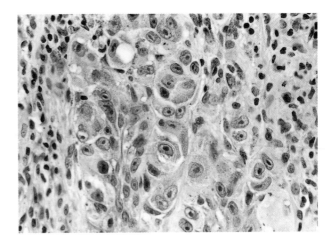

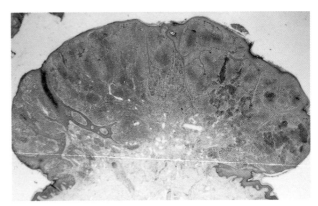

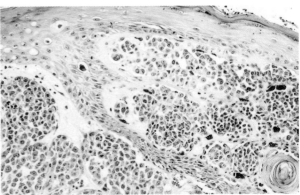

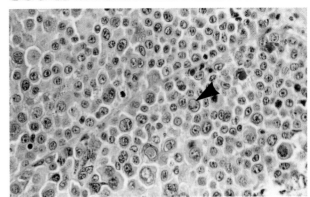

27.16 Acral lentiginous melanoma

♦ infiltrating, dermal, melanomatous cells are frequently spindle-shaped

♦ intraepidermal growth is often lentiginous

♦ common in blacks and Asians

♦ clinically resembles a superficial spreading melanoma on the soles and around the nails

♦ aggressive type of melanoma

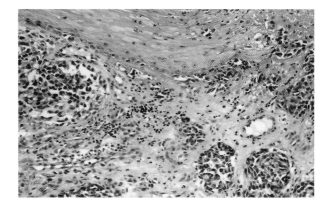

27.17 Metastatic / recurrent melanoma

♦ metastatic and recurrent melanoma cells may show minimal pleomorphism and no evidence of melanocytic hyperplasia or dysplasia in the overlying epidermis

♦ metastatic small-cell carcinomas and lymphomas are the main histologic differential diagnoses (see 24.1, 24.2, and 25.12)

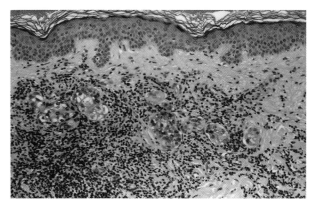

ECCRINE AND PSEUDOECCRINE TUMORS

Glandular tumors of the dermis may be primary or secondary and benign or malignant. The majority of primary glandular tumors of the skin are benign tumors. True eccrine glandular tumors have glands with cuboidal cells forming double-layered lumina and a PAS-positive diastase-resistant cuticle along the luminal margin of the lining cells. Apocrine glandular tumors have characteristic glands with eosinophilic cells showing decapitated secretion whereas sebaceous tumors demonstrate lobular masses of cells with central nuclei and foamy lipidized cytoplasm, but no well-formed glands or ductular structures.

Eccrine glandular cells undergoing adenomatous proliferation often exhibit clearing of the cytoplasm. The name 'clear cell hidradenoma' was coined to describe such a benign adenoma of eccrine glandular origin. Clear cell dermal tumors, however, do not always arise from the eccrine glands. Cytoplasmic clearing may be due to the accumulation of fat (adipocyte), glycogen (squamous cell) or mucin (glandular cell), or combinations of all three. The nature of the clear substance(s) is usually readily apparent with ancillary histochemistry. PAS with and without diastase highlights mucin and glycogen, respectively. Fat is not usually demonstrable as it is leached out by routine processing, but it may be specifically tested for in fresh, frozen, or formalin-fixed tissue that has not been infiltrated with paraffin.

Knowing the nature of cytoplasmic clearing is helpful in arriving at a diagnosis; for example, the clear cells of a renal cell carcinoma stain for glycogen and / or fat, but never mucin whereas the clear cells of a nodular hidradenoma are strongly PAS-positive and diastase-sensitive. Degenerative changes within melanosomes explain the cytoplasmic clearing seen in balloon melanocytes. Melanocytes and nevic cells do not usually stain positively for fat, mucin, or glycogen.

Carcinoembryonic antigen (CEA) is found in adnexal sweat gland neoplasms, and in extramammary and mammary Paget's disease, but not in tumors of basal cells, squamous cells, or melanocytes. S-100 protein is found in eccrine, but not apocrine, secretory epithelium, and is also present in melanocytes, Langerhans cells, Schwann cells, and their associated neoplasms. Eccrine spiradenoma and eccrine acrospiroma may stain for S-100 protein, but eccrine poroma and syringoma do not. Epithelial membrane antigen is present in eccrine and apocrine glands, but not in their ducts.

Malignant eccrine tumors are rare. Nuclear pleomorphism, prominent nucleoli, increased nuclear: cytoplasmic ratio, more frequent mitoses, and vascular and / or perineural invasion suggest a malignant tumor.

A cutaneous metastasis from an adenocarcinoma is usually associated with nuclear and cytologic atypia as well as glandular complexity. Common tumors metastatic to skin include adenocarcinomas of the breast, colon, and lung. Occasionally, nonglandular primary epidermal carcinomas (such as adenoid squamous cell carcinoma and adenoid basal cell carcinoma) may masquerade as adenocarcinomas by forming gland-like spaces (pseudoglands) secondary to cystic degeneration or acantholysis.

Eccrine ducts in syringoma	28.1

Differential diagnoses

Benign eccrine tumors

Eccrine hidrocystoma	28.2
Syringoma	28.3
Chondroid syringoma (mixed tumor of the skin)	28.4
Clear cell (nodular) hidradenoma	28.5
Eccrine spiradenoma	28.6
Eccrine poroma	28.7
Syringofibroadenoma	28.8
Papillary eccrine adenoma	28.9

Malignant eccrine tumors

Eccrine adenocarcinoma	28.10
Sclerosing sweat gland carcinoma (microcystic adnexal carcinoma, syringoid eccrine carcinoma, sclerosing sweat gland carcinoma)	28.11
Aggressive digital papillary adenocarcinoma	28.12
Mucinous (colloid) eccrine adenocarcinoma	28.13
Adenoid cystic eccrine adenocarcinoma	28.14

Pseudoeccrine tumors

Metastatic colonic adenocarcinoma	28.15
Adenoid basal cell carcinoma	28.16
Adenoid squamous cell carcinoma	28.17

Other clear cell tumors of the skin

Balloon cell nevus	28.18
Xanthoma	28.19
Sebaceous carcinoma of Meibomian gland	28.20
Metastatic renal cell carcinoma	28.21
Metastatic gastric carcinoma	28.22

28.1 Eccrine ducts in syringoma

♦ luminal and ductal structures are lined by a double-layered, low, cuboidal epithelium
♦ PAS-positive diastase-resistant cuticle lines the lumen
♦ clear cell change of the ductal epithelium and clear cell syringoma have both been described

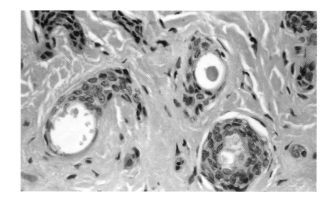

BENIGN ECCRINE TUMORS

28.2 Eccrine hidrocystoma

♦ cystic space lined by a double-layered epithelium which does not show decapitated secretion
♦ one or a few translucent bluish papule(s) 1–3 mm in diameter on the face
♦ number of lesions may increase in the summer

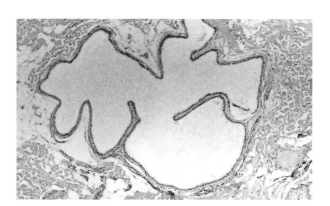

28.3 Syringoma

♦ multiple, small, intradermal ducts composed of a double layer of flattened cells in a fibrous stroma
♦ many ducts have typical comma or tadpole shapes
♦ occasionally, the inner layer is composed of clear glycogenated cells (clear cell variant)
♦ some ducts are filled with keratin or amorphous debris; their rupture may induce a foreign body-type reaction with multinucleated giant cells
♦ usually multiple, yellowish to flesh-colored, small papules primarily on the lower eyelids in women, typically commencing at puberty, although more develop during adulthood

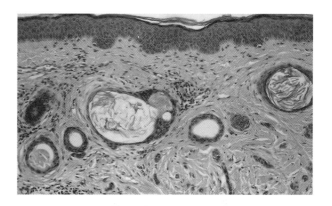

28.4 Chondroid syringoma
   (mixed tumor of the skin)

♦ cartilaginous appearance of the stroma
♦ chondrocyte-like cells in small lacunae surrounded by a homogeneous eosinophilic matrix
♦ ductules and lumina are lined by a double-layered epithelium
♦ ductules may have comma or tadpole shapes
♦ outer myoepithelial cell layer
♦ histologically identical to pleomorphic adenoma of the salivary gland; thus, a deep lesion at the angle of the jaw is more likely to be a mixed tumor of the parotid gland
♦ firm nodule on the head or neck

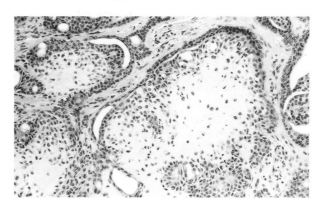

28.5 Clear cell (nodular) hidradenoma

♦ well-circumscribed, often encapsulated, eccrine gland adenoma

♦ cells with clear cytoplasm (glycogen) and a small dark nucleus are frequently seen, hence the tumor's name

♦ cystic spaces are common (solid cystic hidradenoma)

♦ tubular lumina are lined by cuboidal cells

♦ areas of squamous differentiation may be present

♦ focal eosinophilic hyalinized stroma

♦ may or may not be connected to the epidermis; lesions connected to the epidermis have been referred to as **eccrine acrospiromas**

♦ usually a solitary, firm nodule which may be ulcerated

♦ marked cytologic atypia, infiltrative cell growth, numerous mitoses (1–2 figures per high-power field), and focal necrosis suggest malignancy

♦ malignant counterpart is rare and usually arises *de novo*

♦ most commonly located on the scalp, face, or anterior trunk

♦ more common in women in the fourth decade of life

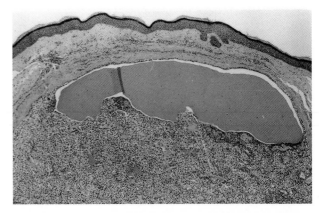

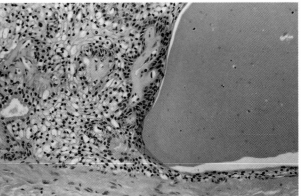

28.6 Eccrine spiradenoma

♦ composed of a few well-demarcated nodules (upper picture)

♦ uniform, small basaloid cells with dark nuclei and scant cytoplasm arranged in thin anastomosing cords

♦ two cell types are apparent under higher power

♦ peripheral cells have small dark nuclei and scant cytoplasm

♦ central cells have paler nuclei and slightly more eosinophilic cytoplasm

♦ occasional tubular and luminal formations with a PAS-positive cuticle lining the lumen and a double-layered epithelium, histologic features characteristic of all eccrine adenomas

♦ often eosinophilic, PAS-positive, diastase-resistant, granular material within the lumina

♦ focal cellular atypia, infiltrative growth, and mitotic activity should raise the possibility of malignant transformation, which is rare

♦ malignant eccrine spiradenoma *de novo* is exceedingly rare

♦ solitary, but occasionally multiple, painful, firm nodule(s) usually arising in early adulthood

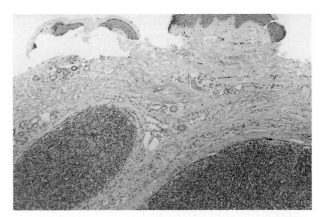

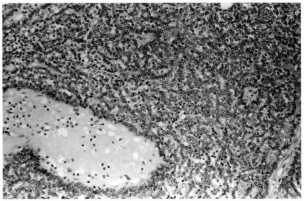

28.7 Eccrine poroma

♦ large anastomosing cords of cuboidal cells that are slightly smaller than the surrounding epidermal cells

♦ occasional luminal differentiation; some tumors exhibit cystic spaces lined by a PAS-positive, diastase-resistant, eosinophilic cuticle

♦ sharp border between the tumor and stroma

♦ intraepidermal poroma is termed **hidroacanthoma simplex** and a completely intradermal tumor is called **dermal duct tumor (Winkelmann)**

♦ cytologic atypia and infiltrative cell growth should suggest malignant transformation and **porocarcinoma**

♦ red, solitary, sessile or pedunculated tumor usually on the sole or palm in middle-aged persons; two-thirds of cases involve the sole

♦ surface may be smooth or keratotic, and there may be a surrounding hyperkeratotic epidermal collar

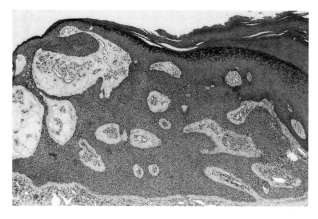

28.8 Syringofibroadenoma

♦ resembles a poroma, with downgrowths of poromatous squamous cells compressed into narrow cords by the surrounding fibrous stroma, as seen here

♦ microscopic appearance is also similar to a fibroepithelial polyp of Pinkus except that the epithelial cells are often glycogenated and have a clear cytoplasm

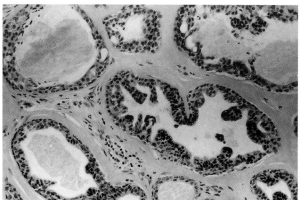

28.9 Papillary eccrine adenoma

♦ as seen here, there is circumscribed proliferation of well-differentiated eccrine ducts

♦ hyperplastic ductal epithelial cells form small intraductal papillary projections

♦ stratification of ductal epithelial cells, nuclear pleomorphism, mitotic figures, and poorly formed ductal structures should raise the possibility of aggressive digital eccrine adenoma / adenocarcinoma

♦ uncommon, solitary, nodular tumor that occurs mainly on the hands or feet (see 28.12)

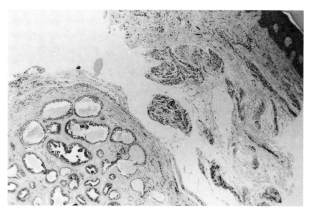

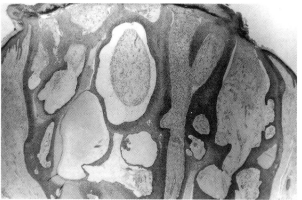

MALIGNANT ECCRINE TUMORS

28.10 Eccrine adenocarcinoma

♦ eccrine adenocarcinoma is composed of neoplastic glandular cells forming elongated tubules and glands, some of which have discernible lumina

♦ low-power view (upper picture) shows a dermal tumor composed of infiltrating glandular structures

♦ neoplastic openings (lumina; lower picture, arrow) of these glandular structures seen under higher power

♦ remnants of benign eccrine glands may or may not be found in the vicinity of the tumor

♦ differentiation from metastatic adenocarcinoma is difficult or impossible without exclusion of primary carcinoma elsewhere in the body

♦ histologic variants include malignant counterparts of benign eccrine adenomas, such as **malignant poroma (eccrine porocarcinoma)** and **malignant spiradenoma**, usually arising from malignant transformation of long-standing poroma and spiradenoma

♦ other malignant eccrine tumors resembling morphologically benign adenomas, but usually arising *de novo*, include **malignant syringoma, malignant nodular hidradenoma (clear cell eccrine carcinoma)**, and **aggressive digital papillary adenocarcinoma**

♦ further histologic variants of eccrine malignancies without benign equivalents are **mucinous eccrine carcinoma** and **adenoid cystic eccrine carcinoma**

♦ solitary nodular, noduloulcerative, or infiltrative plaque usually on the extremities or head in older persons

♦ diagnosis usually made histologically and not clinically

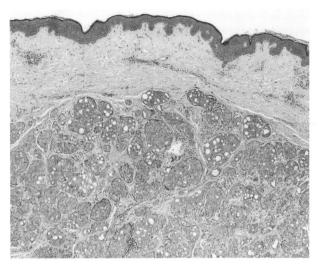

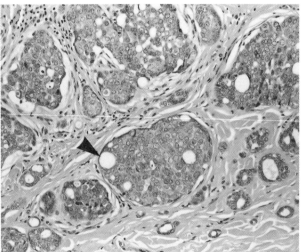

28.11 Sclerosing sweat gland carcinoma (microcystic adnexal carcinoma, syringoid eccrine carcinoma, sclerosing sweat gland carcinoma)

♦ superficial glands similar to syringoma with tadpole-shaped figures

♦ may have nests of squamous to basaloid cells and cysts similar to trichoepithelioma

♦ variable ductal differentiation

♦ no striking pleomorphism or nuclear atypia

♦ infrequent mitotic figures

♦ sclerotic stroma

(continued next page)

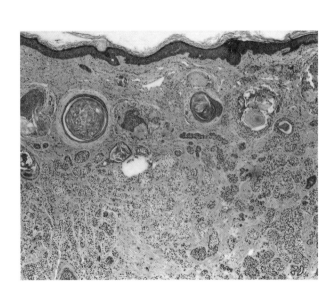

- ♦ perineural invasion common
- ♦ invades deeply, typically into the subcutis
- ♦ histologic differential diagnosis: desmoplastic tricho-epithelioma; syringoma; perineural invasion, and subcutaneous infiltration indicate a diagnosis of sclerosing sweat gland carcinoma; CEA is present in syringoma and sclerosing sweat gland carcinoma, but not in trichoepithelioma; horn cysts are present in desmoplastic trichoepithelioma and sclerosing sweat gland carcinoma, but not in syringoma
- ♦ slow-growing, commonly recurring, flesh-colored indurated plaque, nodule, or cystic tumor with a predilection for nasolabial area and periorbital skin, although it may occur in the axillae and on the buttocks

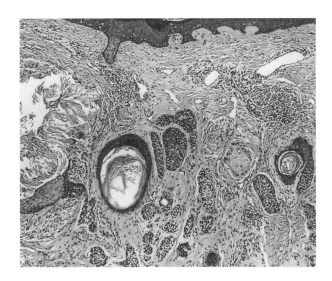

28.12 Aggressive digital papillary adenocarcinoma

- ♦ infiltrative, rather than encapsulated, growth pattern compared with papillary eccrine adenoma (see 28.9)
- ♦ ductal structures are less differentiated and cytologic atypia is easily discernible, as seen here
- ♦ all digital lesions with a significant degree of histologic atypia should be regarded as a potentially malignant tumor capable of destructive local growth
- ♦ enlarging nodule on a digit usually seen in white males
- ♦ tumor of the fingers and toes, but may involve the palms and soles
- ♦ prone to recurrence and pulmonary metastases
- ♦ radical surgery may be necessary for high-grade adeno-carcinomas

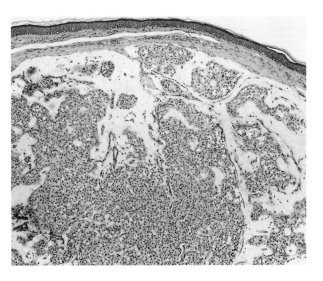

28.13 Mucinous (colloid) eccrine adenocarcinoma

- ♦ characterized by small glandular 'islands' which appear to be floating in large pools of mucin
- ♦ thin fibrous septa separate the mucin pools into com-partments
- ♦ mucin is PAS- and colloidal iron-positive, diastase- and hyaluronidase-resistant, and stains with alcian blue at pH 2.5, but not at 0.4
- ♦ alcian blue staining becomes negative with sialidase (neuraminidase), suggesting that the mucinous mate-rial is a non-sulfated mucoprotein, probably sialo-mucin
- ♦ cells exhibit minimal to moderate atypia

(continued next page)

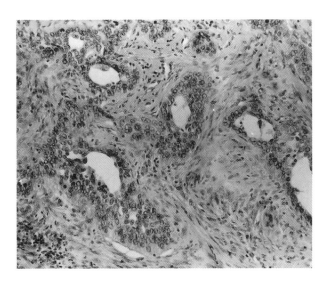

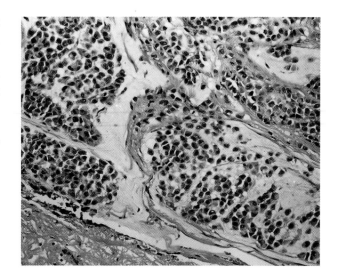

♦ may be histologically indistinguishable from metastatic mucinous carcinoma from the gastrointestinal tract, breast, salivary gland, lacrimal gland, and bronchus
♦ in contrast to mucinous eccrine adenocarcinoma which typically affects the face and scalp, metastatic colonic carcinoma usually involves the anterior abdominal wall
♦ reddish dome-shaped nodule with a predilection for the face or scalp
♦ cut surface has a gelatinous or mucoid appearance

28.14 Adenoid cystic eccrine adenocarcinoma

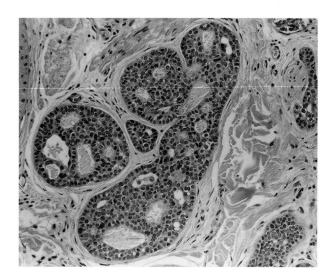

♦ rare form of primary eccrine adenocarcinoma that has low malignant potential
♦ morphologically resembles adenoid cystic carcinomas of salivary glands and mucosae
♦ cylinders of cells present a cribriform cross-sectional appearance, as seen here
♦ acid mucin is present in the glandular openings
♦ prominent hyaline basement membrane around the cell clusters
♦ usually some degree of cytologic atypia, including nuclear hyperchromasia, pleomorphism, and obvious apoptotic bodies, as seen here
♦ perineural invasion is a common finding in adenoid cystic carcinomas at all anatomical sites, as seen here
♦ more common in middle-aged to elderly women
♦ predilection for the trunk, scalp, and extremities
♦ painful plaques or nodules

PSEUDOECCRINE TUMORS

28.15 Metastatic colonic adenocarcinoma

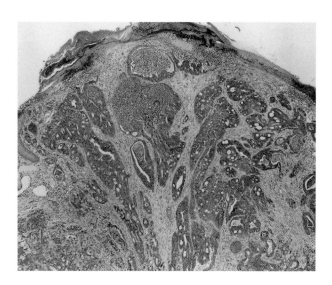

♦ an ulcerated skin nodule with neoplastic atypical glandular structures invading the dermis, as seen here
♦ differentiated neoplastic glands favor colonic, bronchial, or ovarian primary sites, but clinical information is often necessary
♦ adenocarcinomas of the lung, breast, colon, stomach, and oral cavity commonly metastasize to skin

(continued next page)

♦ high-power view of the glands shows that they are composed of columnar cells with pleomorphic hyperchromatic nuclei, as seen here

♦ necrotic cell debris is seen in the lumina of the glands

♦ origin of the primary tumor may not be obvious on histology alone, although particular features – neoplastic glands with tall columnar cells (seen here) typical of colonic carcinomas, signet-ring cells commonly seen in metastatic gastric adenocarcinoma, and narrow cell columns typical of metastatic breast carcinoma – may provide clues

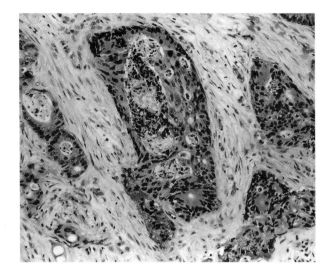

28.16 Adenoid basal cell carcinoma

♦ infiltrative ribbon-like formations of basaloid cells, one to several cells thick, are typical of adenoid BCCs

♦ illusion of a gland-like lumen may be due to a circular arrangement of the ribbon formations, or cell necrosis in the center of the tumor cell mass

♦ lack of CEA staining, unlike eccrine tumors

♦ pink, translucent papule with telangiectasia, rolled borders, and a tendency to ulcerate occurring on sun-exposed skin

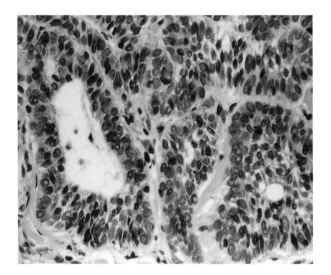

28.17 Adenoid squamous cell carcinoma

♦ infiltrating lobular or alveolar formations of loosely cohesive aggregates of malignant squamous cells

♦ intercellular bridges can be seen

♦ individual cell keratinization may be extensive

♦ spaces between cells are due to loss of intercellular cohesion, resulting in a pseudoglandular appearance

♦ lack of CEA staining, unlike eccrine tumors

♦ flesh-colored to reddish-brown, hyperkeratotic, scaly papulonodule which may be ulcerated

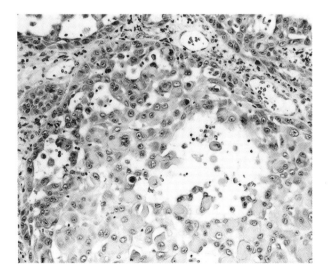

OTHER CLEAR CELL TUMORS OF THE SKIN

28.18 Balloon cell nevus
♦ nevus composed almost entirely of balloon cells, which are large cells with bland nuclei and voluminous pale-staining cytoplasm
♦ melanin pigment may be seen in the occasional balloon cell
♦ heavy pigmentation is present in dermal melanophages
♦ benign nevocellular architecture is retained
♦ characteristic, easily recognizable nevic cells are usually present
♦ lack of CEA staining, unlike eccrine tumors, although S-100 protein may be present in both types of tumors
♦ no distinguishing clinical features to differentiate from other benign melanocytic nevi

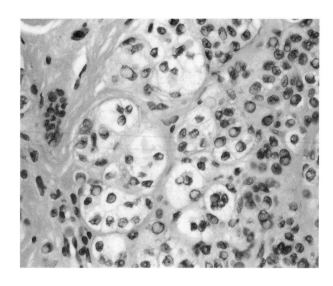

28.19 Xanthoma
♦ small central nuclei
♦ cell margin is well-defined
♦ microvesicular cytoplasm rather than complete clearing
♦ yellow papules and plaques resulting from abnormal lipoprotein metabolism, content, or structure
♦ yellow color of lesions is due to lipid in foam cells
♦ **xanthoma** may be eruptive, tuberous, tendinous, planar, mucosal, or intertriginous
♦ **xanthelasma** are yellow papules found around the eyes

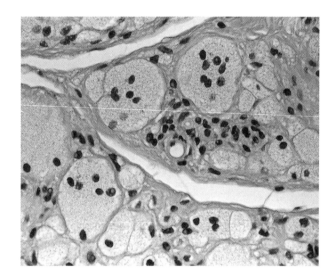

28.20 Sebaceous carcinoma of Meibomian gland
♦ malignant cells are loaded with lipid
♦ cytoplasm is microvesicular as in xanthomatous cells rather than with complete clearing as in glycogenated squamous cells
♦ yellowish-white eyelid nodule that may ulcerate
♦ upper eyelid is involved twice as often as the lower lid, probably due in part to the greater number of Meibomian glands in the former
♦ often associated with recurrence and widespread metastases
♦ clinical differential diagnosis: chalazion; basal cell carcinoma; squamous cell carcinoma; and metastatic tumors

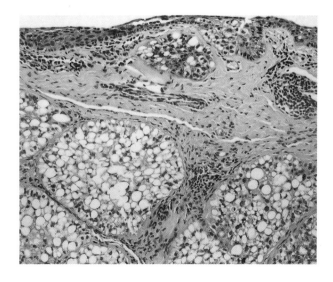

28.21 Metastatic renal cell carcinoma

♦ intradermal aggregates of clear cells (intracellular glycogen) arranged in small sheets or somewhat gland-like structures
♦ nuclei show variable atypia and are centrally placed
♦ may be highly vascularized and show prominent central necrosis
♦ cells with granular cytoplasm often coexist
♦ one or more erythematous, polypoid lesions resembling pyogenic granuloma, often in a person with a history of renal mass

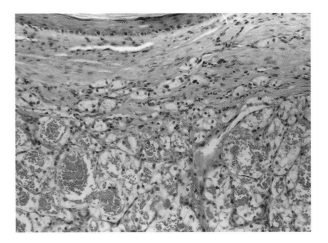

28.22 Metastatic gastric carcinoma

♦ signet-ring cells are malignant adenocarcinomatous cells with mucin-filled, optically clear, cell bodies
♦ as seen here, infiltrating signet-ring cells in the dermis contain hyperchromatin, eccentric nuclei (arrow), and large cytoplasmic vacuoles
♦ mucin is epithelial, and the cytoplasm is mucin carmine- and PAS-positive, and diastase-resistant
♦ signet-ring cells are characteristic of metastatic diffuse-type gastric carcinoma (linitis plastica) and lobular carcinoma of the breast
♦ adenocarcinomas from other body sites rarely give rise to cutaneous metastases with an abundance of signet-ring cells

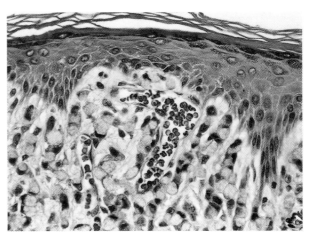

APOCRINE TUMORS

Apocrine differentiation is characterized by 'decapitation' secretion of cells with abundant eosinophilic cytoplasm and a uniform, centrally placed, nucleus. As with other sweat gland tumors, a vast majority of apocrine tumors are benign adenomas with luminal or ductal structures lined by a double-layered epithelium. Apocrine tumors may have cystic, glandular and, less commonly, papillary histologic appearances.

As apocrine glands are normally present in the skin of the axilla, anogenital region, external ear, eyelid, and breast, apocrine tumors are often found at these locations. Fox–Fordyce disease is a follicular eruption in women with itchy papules primarily in the axillae as the result of occlusion and rupture of the apocrine glands. Apocrine adenocarcinoma is also most commonly found in the axillae. Hidradenoma papilliferum arises almost exclusively in the vulval and perineal skin of women.

Ectopic apocrine glands and syringocystadenoma papilliferum are often associated with nevus sebaceus of Jadassohn, a hamartoma usually seen on the scalp or face. Cylindroma, apocrine adenoma, and apocrine hidrocystoma are all located on the scalp or face.

Malignant apocrine tumors are extremely rare. Malignant transformation of cylindromas is suggested by loss of hyaline sheaths, anaplastic cells with nuclear pleomorphism, numerous mitotic figures, loss of peripheral palisading, stromal invasion, and focal necrosis. Nuclear pleomorphism, hyperchromasia, mitoses, stromal invasion, and necrosis are also features of apocrine adenocarcinoma.

29.1 Decapitated secretion and apocrine cells
♦ abundance of granular eosinophilic cytoplasm, which is the secretory product
♦ fragmentary loss of cytoplasm along the luminal cell surface gives rise to the characteristic 'decapitation' secretion (arrow)

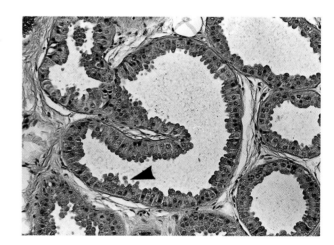

SIMPLE CYSTS

29.2 Apocrine hidrocystoma
♦ one or more cystic spaces lined by typical apocrine cells with eosinophilic cytoplasm
♦ many cells exhibit decapitation secretion
♦ similar to eccrine hidrocystoma, this is a cystic non-neoplastic change of the apocrine gland
♦ usually solitary, bluish papule on the face
♦ similar cystic dilatation of the apocrine glands with superimposed inflammation may be seen in **Fox–Fordyce disease** and **hidradenitis suppurativa**

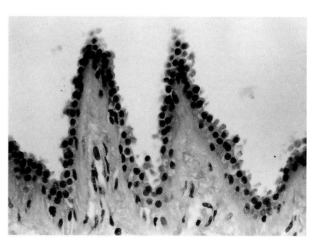

ADENOMATOUS HYPERPLASIA

29.3 Apocrine adenoma
♦ rare tumor consisting of dermal and subcutaneous lobular masses of apocrine cells
♦ histologic appearance may vary from a solid lesion to cystic proliferation of the apocrine epithelium, as seen in **apocrine cystadenoma** (upper picture), and of the apocrine tubules, as seen in **tubular adenoma** (lower picture)
♦ outer myoepithelial cells (arrow) are small, cuboidal, or flattened, and lack an eosinophilic cytoplasm
♦ inner epithelial cells are columnar and eosinophilic, and demonstrate characteristic decapitated secretion
♦ apocrine cystadenoma is common in the head and neck region whereas the rare tubular adenoma is seen mostly in anal and axillary skin
♦ **ceruminous adenoma** of the external ear canal is a benign apocrine adenoma

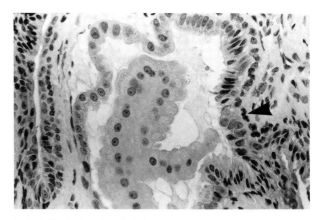

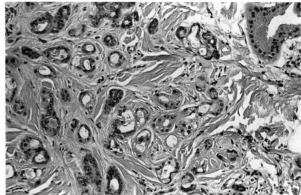

PAPILLARY / CYSTIC TUMORS

29.4 Hidradenoma papilliferum
♦ encapsulated dermal adnexal tumor showing apocrine differentiation
♦ tubules, papillary fronds, and glands are present in varying proportions
♦ lumina are lined by an outer basal cell layer and an inner layer of apocrine cells, many of which show decapitation secretion
♦ most of the lesions are covered on the surface by intact skin, but show no evidence of an epidermal origin
♦ the very occasional lesion appears to extend upwards, and the adenomatous epithelium is continuous with the epidermis
♦ malignant transformation has never been documented
♦ asymptomatic, small, flesh-colored papule seen only in women and almost exclusively on the labia majora or perineal skin

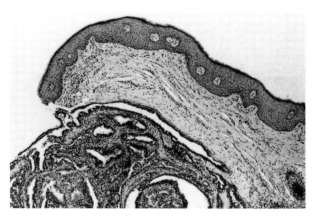

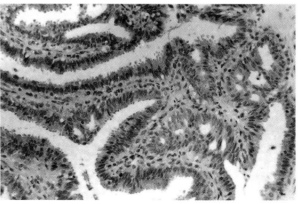

29.5 Syringocystadenoma papilliferum

♦ characterized by cystic invaginations of epidermis into dermis

♦ connected to the skin surface in most cases

♦ in deeper portions of the invaginations, multiple papillary fronds are lined by a double layer of cells

♦ surface cell layer is formed by columnar cells with eosinophilic cytoplasm, often with decapitation secretion

♦ inner cells are cuboidal with bland nuclei and scant cytoplasm

♦ stroma is rich in plasma cells

♦ solitary plaque or papule, or linear papules most frequently on the scalp or face at birth or in early childhood; increased size at puberty

♦ may develop in 10–20% of cases of sebaceous nevi

♦ malignant transformation is very uncommon

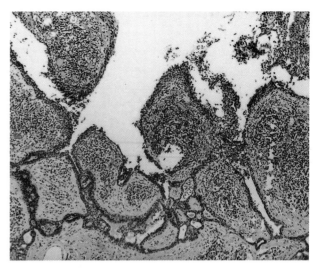

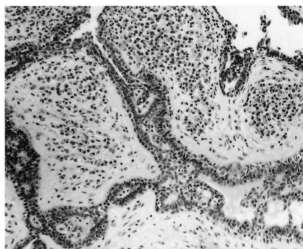

JIGSAW-PUZZLE TUMOR NODULES

29.6 Cylindroma

♦ also known as 'turban tumor' or 'Spiegler's tumor'

♦ the only apocrine tumor showing a solid jigsaw-puzzle pattern of tight-fitting cell cylinders surrounded by a hyaline basement membrane

♦ each aggregate comprises an outer dark-staining cell layer with peripheral palisading, and larger, pale-staining, centrally placed cells

♦ occasional aggregates have a central lumina lined by a double-cell layer; the inner cell layer exhibits decapitation secretion, which may be subtle

♦ unencapsulated, but well-demarcated, dermal tumor with a cylindroma (seen here, on left) coexisting with a rounded nodule of eccrine spiradenoma (on right); such an association has been described

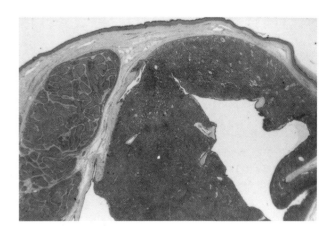

(continued next page)

- PAS-positive, diastase-resistant, hyaline material is commonly seen within the cell masses (arrow)
- overlying epidermis is often stretched and atrophic
- malignant transformation, rare in this tumor, is suggested by infiltrative growth across the hyaline basement membrane and increased mitoses
- pinkish-red, smooth-surfaced, usually multiple papulo-nodule(s) typically on the scalp or face in women, although they may occur on the trunk and extremities
- may be pedunculated and have surface telangiectasia
- multiple lesions may cover the entire scalp, and have an autosomal-dominant inheritance and an association with multiple trichoepitheliomas

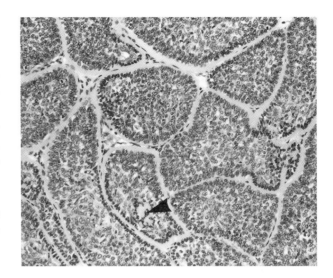

MALIGNANT CYTOLOGY

29.7 Apocrine adenocarcinoma

- a very rare tumor
- diagnosis is not difficult in well-differentiated tumors in which the neoplastic cells form abundant glands and show typical apocrine cytology (eosinophilic granular cytoplasm and decapitation secretion)
- poorly differentiated tumors may be difficult to recognize as having apocrine lineage
- PAS-positive, diastase-resistant, iron-positive granules (not present in eccrine carcinoma)
- glycogen, characteristic of eccrine carcinoma, is usually absent
- may histologically resemble metastatic breast carcinoma, but mature apocrine glands, a transitional zone between normal and neoplastic glands, and intra-cytoplasmic iron granules favor primary apocrine adenocarcinoma
- painless, flesh-colored, red, or violaceous, firm or cystic nodule most commonly located in the axilla
- commonly metastasizes
- clinical differential diagnosis: epidermal or pilar cyst; keloid; sarcoid; hemangioma; and cutaneous metastasis

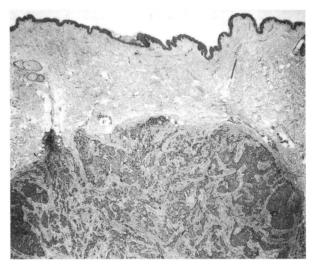

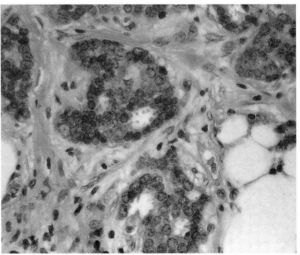

SEBACEOUS TUMORS

Sebaceous cells (from the Latin word *sebum* which means 'suet') are lipid-containing cells found in sebaceous glands. Sebaceous glands are composed of a single peripheral layer of small flattened basal cells surrounding the inner lipid-containing cells. These inner cells disintegrate and their debris is exuded as sebum from the duct. Sebum primarily comprises squalene, wax esters, and triglycerides as well as small amounts of sterols and sterol esters. More than one layer of non-lipidized outer germinative cells should suggest hyper- or neoplastic change.

Sebaceous glands are found everywhere on the skin except the palms and soles. In most areas, they are connected to and drain into the proximal follicular infundibulum. Follicles with large sebaceous glands and fine vellus hairs are called the 'sebaceous follicles'. In the mucous membranes, and nipple and areolar skin, sebaceous glands are independent of follicular structures. The face and scalp have the most numerous and largest sebaceous glands. At the midface, sebaceous follicles predominate, with approximately 900 sebaceous glands / cm^2 whereas the extremities have an average of <100 glands / cm^2. Larger glands tend to have deeper lobules, and the junction of the sebaceous duct with the hair canal is also usually deeper. Sebaceous glands of the lips and buccal mucosa enlarge at puberty and may become visible as Fordyce's spots. Sebaceous glands are also present on the labia minora, internal fold of the prepuce (glands of Tyson), eyelids (Meibomian glands and glands of Zeis), and parotid glands.

Sebaceous hyperplasia is a common condition, particularly on the forehead of men >50 years of age. Sebaceous gland neoplasms are uncommon, but are usually located on the eyelid, face, or scalp.

Sebaceous gland	30.1

Differential diagnoses

Non-neoplastic lesions

Fordyce's spots	30.2
Sebaceous hyperplasia	30.3

Benign neoplasms

Nevus sebaceus of Jadassohn (infantile stage)	30.4
Nevus sebaceus of Jadassohn (adolescent stage) / linear sebaceous nevus syndrome	30.5
Nevus sebaceus of Jadassohn (adult stage)	30.6
Sebaceous adenoma / Torre's syndrome	30.7
Sebaceous epithelioma / Muir–Torre syndrome	30.8

Malignant neoplasms

Sebaceous carcinoma	30.9
Meibomian gland carcinoma	30.10

30.1 Sebaceous gland

- most sebaceous glands empty into hair follicles; they are found everywhere except on the palms and soles
- free sebaceous glands independent of follicular structures are present in nipple and areolar skin
- sebocytes have lipid-laden cytoplasm and central pyknotic nuclei
- germinative cells of the sebaceous gland are seen as a single peripheral layer of cells with basophilic non-lipidized cytoplasm (small arrow)
- holocrine-type of gland in which secretion is effected by disintegration of the cell (large arrow) through lysosomal activation

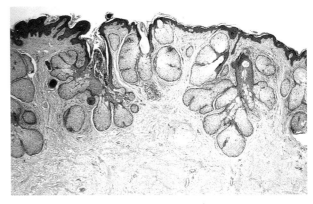

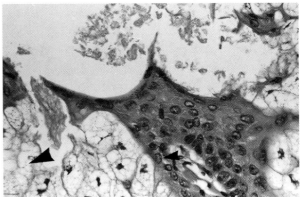

NON-NEOPLASTIC LESIONS

30.2 Fordyce's spots

- squamous buccal mucosa (arrow)
- normal mature sebaceous glands seen on microscopy
- represents a physiological variant of sebaceous gland development
- small white-to-yellowish macules or barely elevated, grouped, papules on the lips and buccal mucosa
- diagnosis is usually made clinically

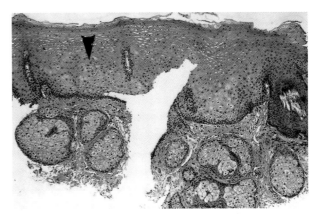

30.3 Sebaceous hyperplasia

- resembles an enlarged gland with numerous lobules grouped around a single dilated duct opening to the skin surface
- no associated hair follicle
- single or multiple yellow papules with central umbilication at the site of ductal opening
- usually seen on the face, particularly on the forehead of persons age > 50 years
- diagnosis is usually made clinically
- clinical differential diagnosis: basal cell carcinoma, especially if prominent blood vessels are present at the margins of the lesions; histologically, it is not difficult to distinguish the two conditions

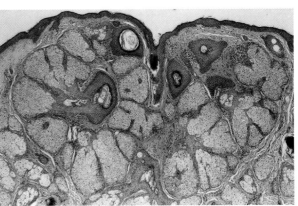

BENIGN NEOPLASMS

30.4 Nevus sebaceus of Jadassohn (infantile stage)

♦ this is a hamartoma of the skin involving not only the sebaceous glands, but also apocrine glands, hair follicles, and epidermis

♦ note the paucity of terminal hair follicles

♦ follicles that are present are malformed with a large hair bulb in the dermis (arrow)

♦ epidermal hyperplasia is minimal during infancy

♦ diagnosis may be missed without attention paid to maldeveloped follicles or ectopic apocrine glands

♦ yellow-to-orange, hairless, slightly elevated plaque present at birth on the scalp or face

♦ most common cause of localized congenital alopecia

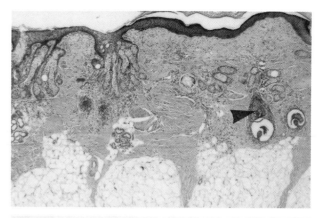

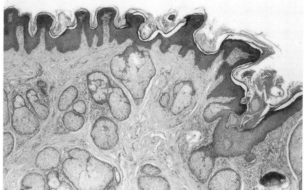

30.5 Nevus sebaceus of Jadassohn (adolescent stage)

♦ during adolescence, the nevus usually enlarges and becomes warty due to epidermal hyperplasia and enlargement of sebaceous glands

♦ look for malformed hair follicles and ectopic apocrine glands to confirm the diagnosis

♦ may be associated with mental retardation, epilepsy, cerebrovascular malformations and cortical abnormalities, ocular abnormalities, and skeletal deformities (**linear sebaceous nevus syndrome**)

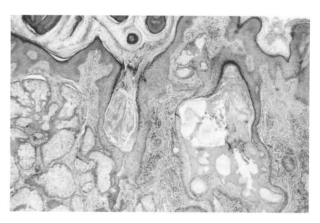

30.6 Nevus sebaceus of Jadassohn (adult stage)

♦ papillomatous epidermis and hyperplastic sebaceous glands are prominent histologic features

♦ further growth of the lesion is often due to the development of benign or malignant tumors

♦ syringocystadenoma papilliferum is the most common benign adnexal tumor (about 20% of lesions), and basal cell carcinoma (arrow) is the most common malignant tumor (approximately 10% of cases) to arise in a nevus sebaceus

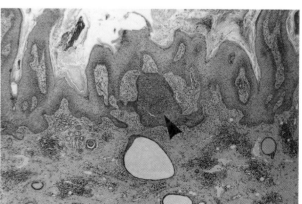

30.7 Sebaceous adenoma

♦ sharply defined, incompletely differentiated, dermal lobules of irregular size and shape encased in fibrotic stroma (upper picture)

♦ two cell types: basaloid germinative cells in several layers at the periphery; and sheets of mature sebaceous cells

♦ differentiated sebocytes outnumber germinative cells in most areas of the lesion

♦ no significant atypia in either cell type (lower picture)

♦ larger nests of sebocytes may demonstrate central cysts secondary to disintegration of sebaceous cells (arrow)

♦ foci of keratinized squamous cells may be present

♦ smooth, firm, usually solitary papule which may be pedunculated, on the face and scalp of adults

♦ if multiple, consider **Torre's syndrome** (multiple sebaceous hyperplasia, adenomas, epitheliomas and carcinomas, keratoacanthomas, and visceral carcinomas)

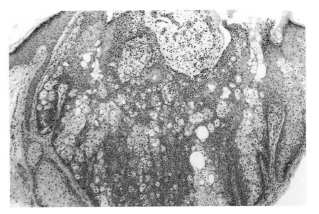

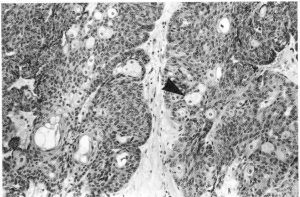

30.8 Sebaceous epithelioma

♦ irregularly shaped cell masses in the dermis with sebaceous cells admixed with > 50% undifferentiated basaloid germinative cells

♦ central hemorrhage and 'pushing' margins are seen (upper picture)

♦ significant aggregates of mature sebaceous cells predominantly in the papillary dermis

♦ ratio of differentiated to basaloid cells may vary from region to region within a particular lesion; diagnosis is based on the overall impression

♦ lesser degree of infiltration and cellular atypia (lower picture) differentiates epithelioma from carcinoma

♦ may have associated epidermal changes, including thinning, ulceration, and an epidermal connection to the underlying sebaceous epithelioma

♦ may have cystic area due to holocrine degeneration of sebaceous cells, or cystic spaces lined by eosinophilic cuticle, suggesting sebaceous duct differentiation

♦ solitary or occasionally multiple yellow nodules and plaques with a rolled pearly border and possibly ulceration usually on the face and scalp; may arise in a nevus sebaceus

♦ diagnosis is rarely made clinically; solitary sebaceous epithelioma is usually recognized as a BCC clinically

♦ behaves like a BCC, and multiple lesions may be associated with **Muir–Torre syndrome**

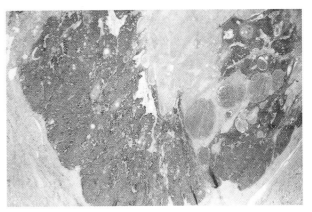

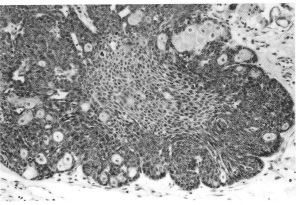

MALIGNANT NEOPLASMS

30.9 Sebaceous carcinoma

- ◆ a large dermal tumor nodule with a necrotic center (upper picture)
- ◆ invasive sheets and lobules of malignant cells are in the dermis
- ◆ most tumor cells are squamoid or basaloid in appearance (lower picture)
- ◆ variable degrees of sebaceous differentiation, indicated by cytoplasmic lipidization (arrow)
- ◆ cellular pleomorphism is usually marked, and mitotic figures are frequent
- ◆ may be associated with **Torre's syndrome** (multiple sebaceous hyperplasia, adenomas, epitheliomas and carcinomas, keratoacanthomas and visceral carcinomas)

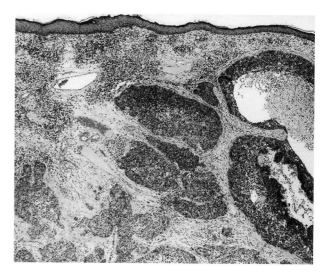

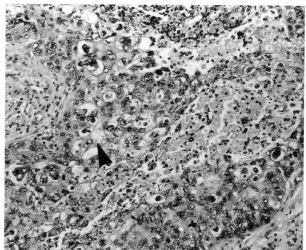

30.10 Meibomian gland carcinoma

- ◆ ulcerated nodule usually on the eyelid, where they originate from Meibomian glands, which are sebaceous glands
- ◆ Pagetoid spread of the tumor cells may be seen in the overlying conjunctival squamous epithelium (arrow)
- ◆ note the marked cytologic atypia of the tumor cells and the lipidized cytoplasm
- ◆ differentiation from basal cell carcinoma is important because of the more aggressive behavior; eyelid sebaceous carcinoma (**Meibomian carcinoma**) is often associated with widespread metastases whereas lesions arising elsewhere usually are not

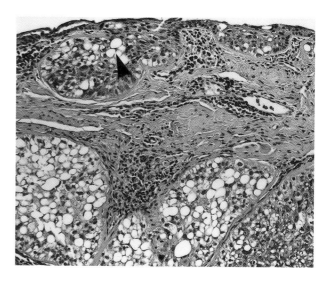

LYMPHOMAS AND LEUKEMIAS

As alluded to in Chapter 18, distinguishing reactive lymphoid proliferations from cutaneous lymphoma or leukemia may be difficult. Immunohistochemical and / or gene-rearrangement studies may be required to assess clonality. Reactive infiltrates tend to be top-heavy (bulk of the cells is superficial) whereas those which are malignant tend to be bottom-heavy. There may be transitional forms between the clearly benign at one end of the spectrum and the clearly malignant at the other. Lymphomatoid papulosis (LyP), a benign condition, and primary cutaneous CD30+ anaplastic large cell lymphoma (ALCL) are at opposite ends of the range of primary cutaneous CD30 (Ki-1+) lymphoproliferative disorders. In between the two, there are borderline cases of uncertain malignant potential, reflected in such terms as 'pleomorphic giant LyP', 'LyP diffuse large-cell type', 'regressing atypical histiocytosis', and 'regressing-phase anaplastic lymphoma'. Both LyP and CD30 (Ki-1+) anaplastic large cell lymphoma share similar cytologic and immunophenotypical characteristics although, compared with LyP, the lesions of ALCL are usually fewer, larger, and more persistent, with sheets of anaplastic large lymphocytes rather than single cells or small cell clusters.

Primary cutaneous lymphomas are usually of T-cell origin. The most common T-cell lymphoma is mycosis fungoides. T-cell lymphomas are never seen with a follicular or nodular pattern, although non-neoplastic follicles may be admixed with the lymphomatous infiltrate. Primary cutaneous B-cell lymphomas are less common, and are usually of the diffuse large B-cell type or low-grade lymphomas of skin-associated lymphoid tissue (SALTomas).

Most secondary lymphoid malignancies are of B-cell lineage and may represent a manifestation of either lymphoma or leukemia. Skin involvement is seen in around 5% of nodal B-cell lymphomas. The malignant lymphomatous infiltrate may occur in sheets and invade the dermis diffusely. Nodular and follicular patterns may also be seen and secondary cutaneous follicular lymphoma representing metastasis from a nodal follicular lymphoma has a poorer prognosis than primary cutaneous follicular lymphoma. Malignant cells in primary cutaneous SALTomas with a follicular pattern express bcl-2 protein, but are not characterized by the t(14;18) translocation typical of nodal follicular lymphomas.

Leukemia cutis is usually secondary to dissemination of systemic leukemia to skin and is associated with a poor prognosis. It generally develops several months after the diagnosis of systemic leukemia but, occasionally, may precede the diagnosis. The morphology of the cells in the skin as well as in the bone marrow and peripheral blood often correlates with the type of leukemia, although typing is more accurate if based on bone marrow and peripheral blood smear cytochemical and cytomorphologic studies. Gene-rearrangement studies of cutaneous leukemic infiltrates may also show the characteristic genetic features of the leukemia [for example, rearrangement of the T-cell receptor gene and monoclonal integration of human T-cell leukemia virus I into the host genome in adult T-cell leukemia / lymphoma, and demonstration of t(15;17) translocation in promyelocytic leukemia]. The diagnosis of cutaneous myelogenous leukemia requires a high degree of suspicion as the cytoplasmic granules critical for diagnosis are not seen with H & E staining because they do not survive routine processing.

Differential diagnoses

Lymphomatoid papulosis (types A and B)	31.1
Anaplastic large cell CD30 (Ki-1+) lymphoma	31.2
Mycosis fungoides	31.3
Adult T-cell lymphoma / leukemia	31.4
Small lymphocytic lymphoma / chronic lymphocytic leukemia (B-cell)	31.5
Lymphoplasmacytoid B-cell lymphoma (SALToma; immunocytoma)	31.6

31.1 Lymphomatoid papulosis (LyP)

♦ lymphoproliferative lesion of T cells characterized by a dense and often top-heavy, wedge-shaped, dermal, lymphoid, cellular infiltrate

♦ the epidermis seen here (first picture) is hyperplastic, but some lesions ulcerate

♦ recurrent crops of erythematous to violaceous papulo-nodules that may ulcerate

♦ individual lesions last for weeks to months, and often heal with postinflammatory hyperpigmentation

♦ often persists for years before burning itself out

♦ usually benign, but 10–20% progress to lymphoma (usually Ki-1+ anaplastic large cell lymphoma and, less commonly, mycosis fungoides and Hodgkin's disease)

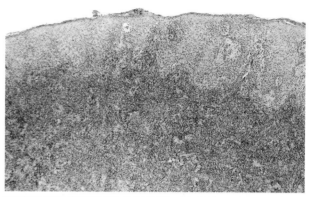

♦ **type A LyP**, in which larger histiocytic cells predominate, is shown under higher magnification (second picture)

♦ atypical cells have moderately faint basophilic cytoplasm and vesicular nuclei with prominent nucleoli, giving a histiocytic appearance (arrow)

♦ occasional multinucleated Reed–Sternberg-like cells are seen; these atypical cells are CD30 (Ki-1+)

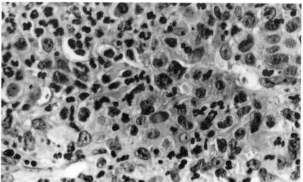

♦ **type B LyP** (third picture), in which epidermotropic, small, atypical CD30– lymphocytes with cerebriform nuclei similar to those in mycosis fungoides are seen in the epidermal cell layers

♦ infrequent mitoses, and fewer eosinophils and neutrophils

♦ CD30+ large cells are inconspicuous, but are found when specifically looked for (large arrow)

♦ atypical CD30– lymphocytes (fourth picture; small arrows) have hyperchromatic nuclei when seen under higher magnification

♦ type A lesions are more common than type B, and both types may be seen in the same patient

♦ both histologic types are a chronic recurrence of necrotic skin papules and nodules that spontaneously regress

♦ patients are otherwise in good health, and the disease may last for years

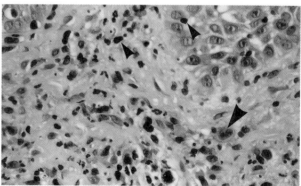

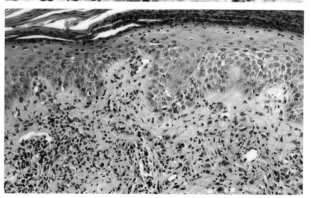

31.2 Anaplastic large cell CD30 (Ki-1+) lymphoma

- histologic appearance similar to that of lymphomatoid papulosis
- atypical lymphocytes are more numerous (>50% of the cellular infiltrate) and arranged in sheets
- Reed–Sternberg-like, 'embryo' and wreath-like cells are more numerous
- mitoses typically numerous
- inflammatory infiltrate relatively inconspicuous in contrast to LyP
- Epstein–Barr virus infection is associated with disease in some Asian and immunosuppressed patients
- most common cutaneous lymphoma in HIV+ patients
- may be primary cutaneous or primary nodal
- **primary nodal disease** has a less favorable prognosis, is common in childhood and adolescence, and associated with t(2;5) chromosomal translocation
- **primary cutaneous disease** often shows partial and occasionally complete spontaneous regression, usually occurs in adults, and is not associated with the t(2;5) chromosomal translocation
- larger and fewer persistent lesions than seen in lymphomatoid papulosis

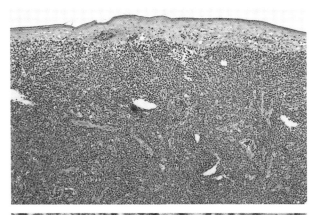

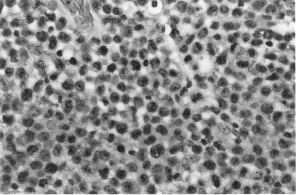

31.3 Mycosis fungoides (MF)

- plaque lesion with a thick band of lymphoid cellular infiltrate distributed along the upper dermis (upper picture)
- spongiosis is slight, but superimposed dermatitis and impetiginization, as seen here, give rise to marked spongiosis and neutrophilic exocytosis that may be misleading
- degree and extent of infiltrate are not typical of lichen planus or banal dermatitis
- very dense, broad band of lymphoid cellular infiltration should raise suspicion for MF
- higher magnification (lower picture) shows epidermotropic lymphocytes with enlarged hyperchromatic nuclei
- sometimes, irregularities in the nuclear membrane may be visualized in 4–5-μ-thick, well-stained, H & E tissue sections
- aggregates of these epidermotropic lymphocytes in the epidermis form the so-called Pautrier's microabscesses (arrow)

(continued next page)

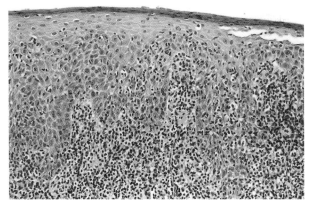

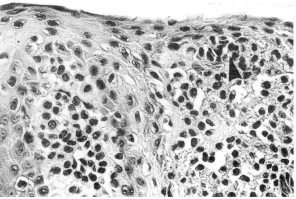

- patch and plaque stages clinically resemble chronic persistent refractory dermatitis
- tumor stage of MF (seen here) shows heavy neoplastic lymphocytic infiltration of the entire dermis and possibly the subcutaneum as well
- cells with cerebriform nuclei, and others with large vesicular nuclei and prominent nucleoli (blastic transformation) are seen under high magnification as are mitotic figures (arrow)
- Reed–Sternberg-like cells are common
- in contrast to the patch and plaque stages, epidermotropism may be minimal
- often a long history of patch and plaque stages
- tumor formation may arise *de novo* or in preexisting plaques
- reddish-brown to violaceous nodules that may ulcerate
- tumors may occur anywhere on the body, but have a predilection for the face and intertriginous areas
- clinical differential diagnosis: metastatic lymphoma; leukemia cutis; lymphocytoma cutis; sarcoid; deep fungal infections; and mycobacterial infections

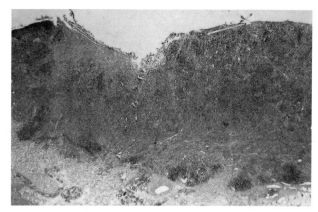

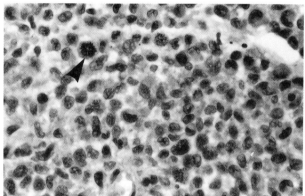

31.4 Adult T-cell lymphoma/leukemia (ATLL)

- usually a dense papillary dermal infiltrate which may extend to the epidermis, deep dermis, and subcutis
- histologic appearance (upper picture) is not unlike that of mycosis fungoides
- under higher magnification (lower picture), the malignant cells show moderately large vesicular nuclei with scant cytoplasm
- the occasional cerebriform nucleus may be seen
- associated with human T-cell lymphotropic virus type 1 (HTLV-1), and is endemic in southern Japan and Southeast Asia
- acute onset with rapid, fulminant, clinical course
- skin lesions, lymphadenopathy, hepatosplenomegaly, and interstitial pulmonary infiltrates are common
- hypercalcemia, osteolytic bone lesions, T-cell leukemia, and skin involvement (HOTS)

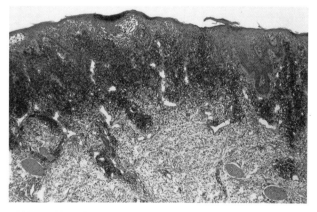

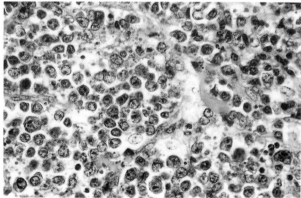

31.5 Small lymphocytic lymphoma (SLL)/ chronic lymphocytic leukemia (CLL)

♦ usually B-cell malignancies with virtually indistinguishable microscopic features

♦ variably dense dermal infiltrate of cells with small round nuclei, inconspicuous nucleoli, and scant cytoplasm

♦ cells may align along collagen bundles

♦ although true follicles are absent, pseudofollicles or 'proliferation centers' of prolymphocytes are often seen (pale under low power and no tingible body macrophages)

♦ macules, papules, plaques, nodules which may be purpuric, and ulcerated and bullous lesions may be seen in CLL

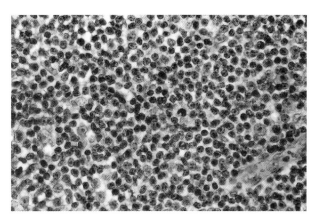

31.6 Lymphoplasmacytoid B-cell lymphoma [skin-associated lymphoid tissue (SALT) or marginal cell-like lymphoma; immunocytoma]

♦ Grenz-zone is present; may be top-heavy, unlike most B-cell lymphomas

♦ cellular infiltrate is mixed with eosinophils, plasmacytoid lymphocytes, and small lymphocytes showing indented nuclei and clear cytoplasm

♦ non-neoplastic lymphoid follicles may be seen, resulting in a follicular histologic appearance

♦ often invades hair follicles; heavy infitration of the pilosebaceous units is characteristic

♦ demonstration of light chain restriction on immunohistochemistry; monoclonal rearrangement of JH gene using PCR in atypical lymphocytes helps to confirm the diagnosis

♦ primary cutaneous disease manifested clinically as solitary or regionally clustered erythematous to violaceous papules and nodules particularly on the trunk

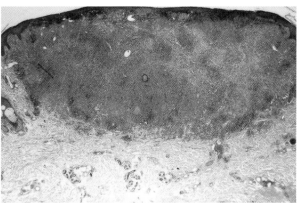

31.7 Diffuse large cell lymphoma

♦ not an single entity, but a final high-grade pathway for many nodal lymphomas with cutaneous involvement

♦ thus, many immunophenotypic subtypes are seen on light microscopy

♦ 50% are B-cell, 10% are T-cell, and 40% are null type

♦ all show abundant large cells with pleomorphic nuclei and prominent nucleoli

♦ large cleaved and non-cleaved cells are present in most cases

♦ erythematous to violaceous papulonodules are seen in patients with nodal disease

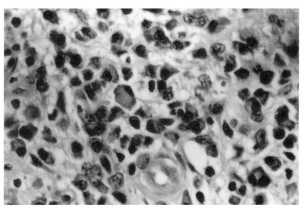

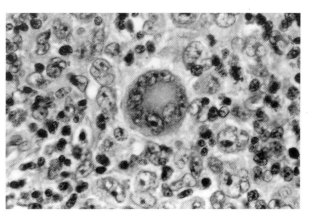

31.8 Cutaneous Hodgkin's disease (HD)

♦ primary HD is rare; most lymphomas of the skin are non-Hodgkin's

♦ cutaneous HD occasionally occurs as a consequence of nodal HD; its presence indicates a poor prognosis

♦ four subtypes: lymphocyte-predominant and -depleted; nodular sclerosis; and mixed cellularity

♦ characterized by Reed–Sternberg cells, which are large bilobed cells with large vesicular nuclei, large acidophilic nucleoli, and abundant, pale, eosinophilic cytoplasm

♦ usually CD30 and CD15 (LeuM1) are expressed by Reed– Sternberg cells

♦ epidermis is usually spared

♦ papulonodules that may ulcerate

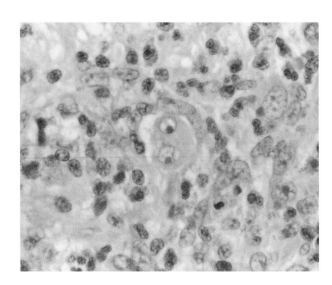

31.9 Leukemia cutis (myelogenous)

♦ cutaneous lesion of myelocytic leukemia (upper picture)

♦ as discussed in Chapter 24, cells are of small epithelioid type that may suggest lymphoid, melanocytic, or epithelial origin

♦ some degree of cytologic atypia is usually evident to suggest a neoplastic process; often KP-1+

♦ positive staining with Leder's stain, and absence of leukocyte common antigen, S100 protein, and cytokeratin support a myelocytic leukemic infiltrate

♦ leukemic cells in the skin frequently, but not always, have a morphology similar to those in bone marrow and peripheral blood [lymphoblasts in **acute lymphocytic leukemia** (ALL), small cells in **chronic lymphocytic leukemia** (CLL), and immature myelocytes in **acute** and **chronic myelocytic leukemia** (AML, CML)]

♦ subtyping is usually not possible with routine stains

♦ typing should not be based on skin biopsy findings alone

♦ bone marrow and peripheral blood smear cytochemical and cytomorphologic studies are more reliable in determining the type of leukemia

♦ **granulocytic sarcoma** refers to a collection of granulocytic leukemic cells which form a mass

♦ rarely, skin involvement is the initial manifestation of leukemia

♦ macules, papules, plaques, and nodules which may be purpuric and ulcerated

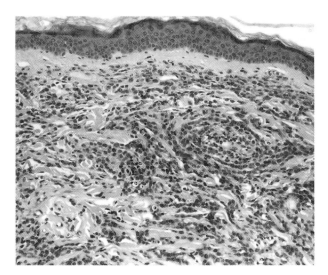

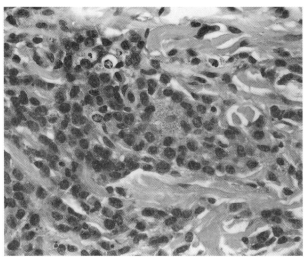

CONNECTIVE TISSUE TUMORS

Tumors of the various types of connective tissue found in the dermis and subcutaneum (fibrous, adipose, neurogenous, vascular, and smooth muscle tissues) are discussed in this chapter. Fibrous, neurogenous, and smooth muscle tumors are spindle cell tumors. Lipomatous and vascular tumors, especially if benign, are easily recognizable by their histopathologic appearances as the normal fat cells and vascular channels are usually duplicated. In general, deeply infiltrative neoplasms involving the fascia and showing cytologic atypia are usually locally aggressive, if not frankly malignant.

Most of the commonly encountered connective tissue skin tumors (dermatofibromas, lipomas, neuromas and hemangiomas) are benign. Some tumors are locally aggressive (dermatofibrosarcoma protuberans and atypical fibroxanthoma of the skin) or frankly malignant (malignant fibrous histiocytoma, the most common soft tissue tumor of the body). Kaposi's sarcoma, a malignancy of vascular tissue, is frequently associated with HIV infection. Liposarcoma, leiomyosarcoma from arrector pili smooth muscle of the vessel wall, and malignant nerve tumors (malignant schwannoma, which is also called neurofibrosarcoma) are exceedingly rare tumors of the skin and subcutaneum.

Differential diagnoses

Predominantly spindle cells

Fibrous tumors

Trichodiscoma (perifollicular fibroma)	32.1
Benign fibrous papule of the face	32.2
Dermatofibroma (fibrous type)	32.3
Dermatofibroma (cellular type)	32.4
Dermatofibroma (deep penetrating type)	32.5
Dermatofibrosarcoma protuberans	32.6
Atypical fibroxanthoma	32.7
Malignant fibrous histiocytoma	32.8

Neurogenous tumors

Traumatic (Morton's) neuroma	32.9
Encapsulated and palisaded neuroma	32.10
Neurilemmoma (schwannoma)	32.11
Solitary neurofibroma	32.12
Plexiform neurofibroma	32.13
Neurothekeoma (myxoma of nerve sheath)	32.14
Malignant schwannoma	32.15

Leiomyomatous tumors

Angioleiomyoma	32.16
Piloleiomyosarcoma	32.17

Predominantly vacuolated fat cells

Adipose tumors

Lipoma	32.18
Hibernoma	32.19
Pleomorphic lipoma	32.20
Liposarcoma	32.21

Predominantly vascular

Vascular tumors

PREDOMINANTLY SPINDLE CELLS

Fibrous tumors

32.1 Trichodiscoma (perifollicular fibroma)
♦ small, well-demarcated, but non-encapsulated, fibrous tumor in the superficial dermis originating from the touch receptor (Haarscheibe)
♦ normal-looking fibroblast nuclei and capillaries among the collagen tissue; no hyaline change
♦ may contain a small amount of mucin; a lesion showing follicular epithelial proliferation is called a fibrofolliculoma (see 26.6)
♦ multiple flesh-colored papules 1–5 mm in diameter, on the face, trunk, and extremities
♦ may be part of **Birt–Hogg–Dubé syndrome**

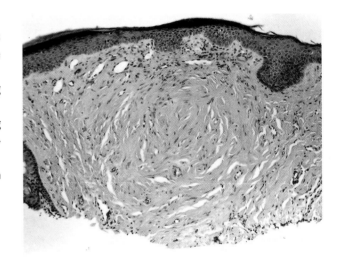

32.2 Benign fibrous papule of the face
♦ increased number of dilated vessels in the dermis
♦ perivascular fibrosis and stellate-shaped fibroblasts are present
♦ overlying epidermis is stretched over this papule; a slight degree of melanocytic hyperplasia may be seen
♦ very common flesh-colored papule on the nose and surrounding facial skin
♦ solitary lesion seen in adults
♦ histopathologically identical to angiofibroma; multiple lesions in a young person with mental retardation and epilepsy should raise the possibility of tuberous sclerosis

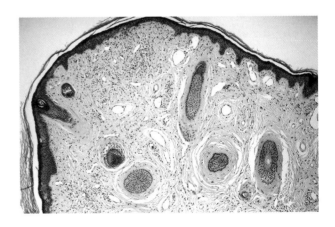

32.3 Dermatofibroma (fibrous type)

♦ spindle-shaped fibroblasts infiltrating the dermis
♦ phagocytosis of lipid material is not obvious
♦ infrequent histiocytes with foamy cytoplasm and Touton giant cells
♦ birefringent normal collagen fibers trapped in the center of the lesion
♦ epidermal acanthosis and hyperpigmentation with a Grenz-zone
♦ single or multiple, firm, reddish-brown papule(s) with ill-defined borders that fade into the surrounding skin usually on the extremities

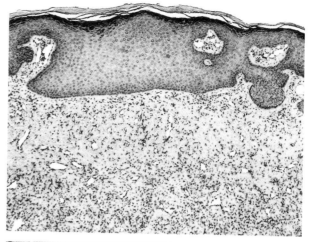

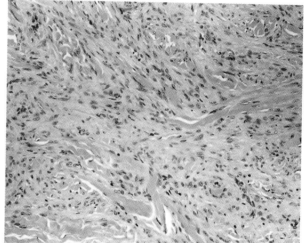

32.4 Dermatofibroma (cellular type)

♦ the term **cellular dermatofibroma** is best used to indicate the significant presence of foamy histiocytic cells in addition to the usual spindle fibrous cells, as in a fibrous histiocytoma of the skin
♦ diagnosis of cellular dermatofibroma does not indicate greater aggressiveness or malignancy
♦ cells in the lesion are postulated to have fibroblastic and phagocytic properties; a dual population of spindle cells and foamy histiocytes is seen
♦ some lesions are vascular and heavily laden with hemosiderin pigment (**siderotic type**)
♦ histologic features to differentiate from juvenile xanthogranuloma include epidermal acanthosis and pigmentation, copious amounts of hemosiderin pigment, storiform spindle cell proliferation and, usually, less intense inflammation and eosinophilic infiltration in cellular dermatofibroma

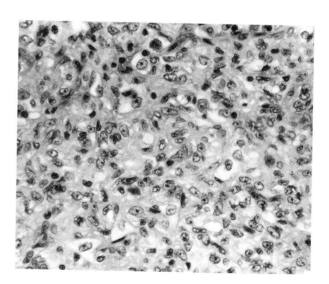

213

32.5 Dermatofibroma (deep penetrating type)

♦ also known as **atypical benign** and **pseudosarcomatous fibrous histiocytoma**

♦ these larger and more cellular dermatofibromas may extend into subcutaneous fat

♦ overlying epidermis may be atrophic and the Grenz-zone is sometimes absent

♦ a varying degree of cellular atypia and the occasional mitosis are seen more often in this type, but fibrohistiocytic tumors confined to the dermis and superficial subcutaneous fat are seldom malignant

♦ look for trapped normal collagen fibers in the center of the lesion, frequent foamy histiocytes, histiocytic giant cells, vascularity, and easily demonstrable hemosiderin pigment and CD34 reactivity to differentiate from dermatofibrosarcoma protuberans

♦ deep margin may be infiltrative or pushing, but layering or honeycomb appearance typical of dermatofibrosarcoma protuberans (see 32.6) is not seen in benign dermatofibroma

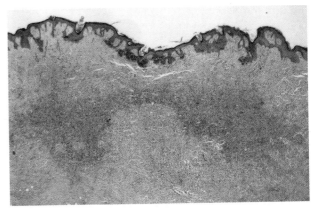

32.6 Dermatofibrosarcoma protuberans (DFSP)

♦ atrophic epidermis with no Grenz-zone (upper picture)

♦ epidermis may ulcerate in some lesions

♦ monotonous, spindle cell proliferation in dermis; normal-looking birefringent collagen fibers are not seen trapped in the center of the tumor

♦ prominent storiform ('cartwheel') pattern of spindle cells (lower picture)

♦ foamy histiocytes and Touton giant cells are rare

♦ no hemosiderin pigment

(continued next page)

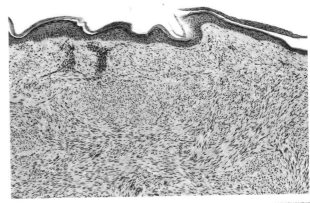

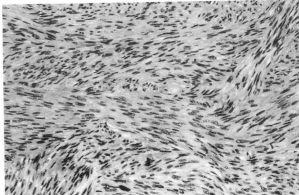

♦ cellular infiltration of subcutaneous fat gives a multi-layered and honeycomb effect, as seen here

♦ usually slight to moderate degree of cytologic atypia with the occasional mitotic figure

♦ presence of markedly atypical sarcomatous cells should suggest other spindle cell tumors, such as atypical fibroxanthoma, spindle cell carcinoma, and spindle cell melanoma

♦ large, firm, reddish-brown plaque with surface papules and nodules and, sometimes, focal ulceration typically on the trunk in men

♦ locally aggressive, frequently recurrent, but rarely metastasizing

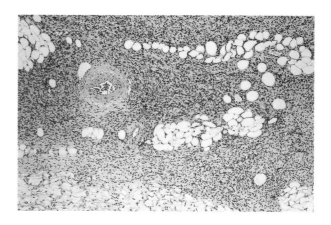

32.7 Atypical fibroxanthoma (AFX)

♦ atrophic epidermis and no Grenz-zone

♦ markedly pleomorphic, sarcomatous tumor cells

♦ frequent tumor giant cells with bizarre nuclei

♦ numerous mitotic figures including abnormal forms

♦ differential diagnosis: spindle squamous cell carcinoma (SCC); and melanoma (look for squamous features and atypical melanocytes along the basal epidermis; cytokeratin-positive in SCC; S100 protein-positive in melanoma, and CD68-positive in AFX)

♦ correct diagnosis is assured by the presence of numerous pleomorphic sarcomatous cells in the superficial dermis (lower picture)

♦ superfical dermal location of AFX is perhaps the only difference between this lesion and malignant fibrous histiocytoma, which involves the subcutis, fascia, and deep soft tissue

♦ low malignant potential and metastatic risk are related to its skin location

♦ typically exophytic and noduloulcerative tumor on the head and neck in areas with actinic or radiation damage in the elderly, but may occur on the trunk and extremities in younger people

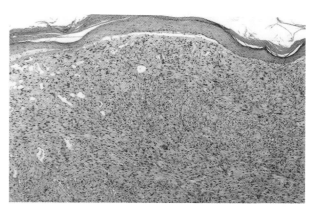

32.8 Malignant fibrous histiocytoma (MFH)

♦ usually a fascial and subcutaneous location

♦ secondary involvement of the skin

♦ various histologic subtypes, including myxoid, pleomorphic, inflammatory, vascular, and giant cells

♦ inflammatory type with epithelioid tumor cells, tumor giant cells, and mitoses, as seen here

(continued next page)

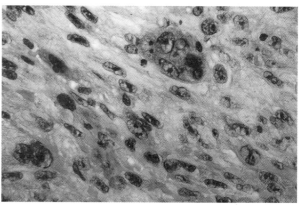

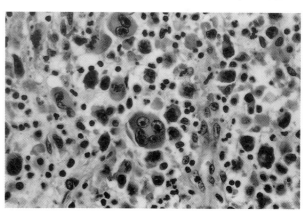

♦ storiform cellular proliferative pattern is common, but usually a mixture of different tumor cells, including histiocytic cells with foamy cytoplasm

♦ usually on the extremities or in the retroperitoneum in younger people than seen with atypical fibroxanthoma

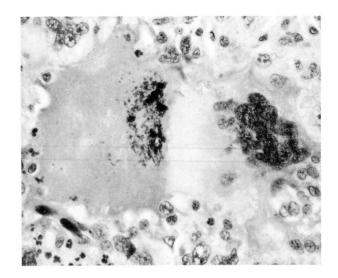

Neurogenous tumors

32.9 Traumatic (Morton's) neuroma

♦ not a true neoplasm; basically, a fibrous scar along the course of a nerve bundle

♦ proliferating Schwann cells and axons are seen with haphazardly arranged fibrous scar tissue

♦ tender and painful lesions found in scars and on amputation stumps

♦ **Morton's neuroma** is the term used for a small traumatic neuroma of the digital nerve between the heads of metatarsal bones

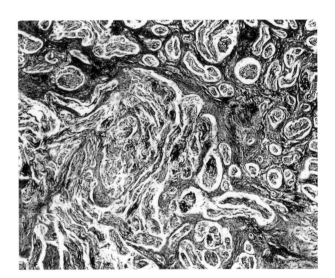

32.10 Encapsulated and palisaded neuroma

♦ this includes most smaller encapsulated neuromas seen in the dermis

♦ broad, interlacing, compact bundles and fascicles of spindle cells

♦ alignment of spindle cells and their nuclei may be seen

♦ axonal fibers in the tumor, unlike neurilemmoma

♦ solitary, asymptomatic, firm, flesh-colored papule on the face in young and middle-aged adults

♦ clinical differential diagnosis: intradermal nevus; and basal cell carcinoma

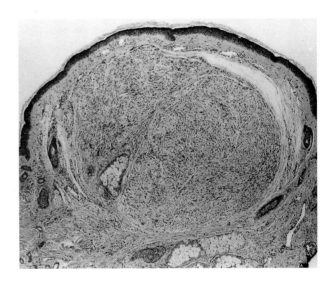

32.11 Neurilemmoma (schwannoma)

♦ large encapsulated tumor seen more commonly in subcutaneous fat and fascial tissue
♦ benign tumor of proliferating Schwann cells; no axonal fibers in the tumor (unlike neurofibroma)
♦ spindle cells may have a parallel arrangement; alignment of nuclei forms the Verocay body; cellular area is Antoni type A tissue and myxomatous area is Antoni type B
♦ usually contains mast cells (as do most neurogenous and myxoid tumors)
♦ usually solitary, often painful, tumor along the course of peripheral or cranial nerves
♦ multiple lesions have a predilection for the trunk and may be associated with neurilemmomas elsewhere (for example, spinal cord, cranial nerves, viscera, bones), meningiomas, gliomas, and astrocytomas

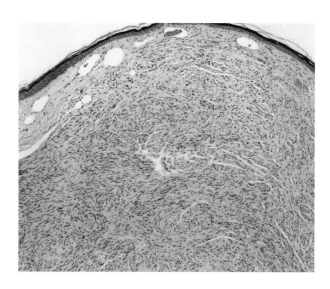

32.12 Solitary neurofibroma

♦ non-encapsulated infiltrative margin
♦ wavy fibers with elongated nuclei
♦ frequently contains mast cells
♦ Bodian staining of neurofilaments reveals axonal fibers not seen in the center of a neurilemmoma
♦ soft or firm, flesh- to tan-colored, smooth, polypoid papules
♦ solitary lesions usually arise in adulthood
♦ multiple lesions arising in late adolescence and associated with ≥6 café au lait patches suggests **neurofibromatosis (von Recklinghausen's disease)**

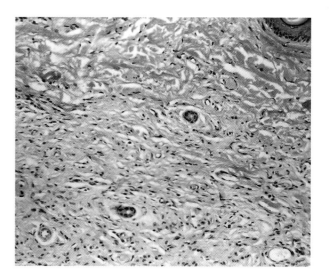

32.13 Plexiform neurofibroma

♦ only found in patients with neurofibromatosis
♦ segments of dermal and subcutaneous nerve bundles are transformed into thickened cords
♦ proliferating perineural fibroblasts and Schwann cells are surrounded by a myxoid stroma, as seen here
♦ feels like a bag of worms and may cause disfigurement
♦ most commonly found on the head, neck, and chest

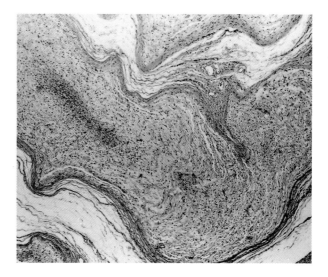

32.14 Neurothekeoma (myxoma of nerve sheath)

♦ deep dermal and subcutaneous tumor a few centimeters in size

♦ well-demarcated mass of myxoid tissue compartmentalized by invaginating fibrous septa (upper picture)

♦ wavy spindle-shaped cells with uniform nuclei are seen as well as a few mast cells

♦ some of these spindle cells may be S100 protein-positive and are considered to have Schwann cell origin

♦ higher magnification (lower picture) shows a mixed population of spindle and epithelioid cells

♦ lesions with predominantly epithelioid cells have been described and are considered to be less mature than predominantly spindle cell myxoid lesions

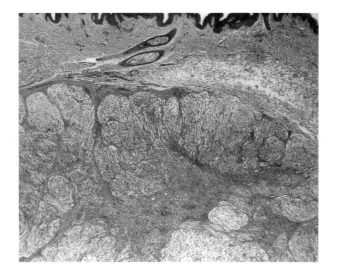

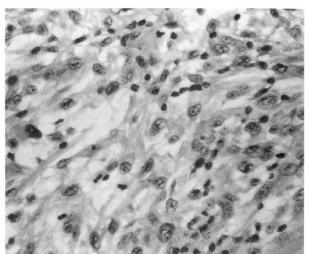

32.15 Malignant schwannoma

♦ most are high-grade spindle cell sarcomas with malignant cytologic features

♦ neurogenous origin is usually difficult to document

♦ recognizing schwannoma-like areas by the presence of Verocay bodies, S100 protein reactivity, type IV collagen staining of basal lamina around cells (which may also be seen ultrastructurally), and complex finger-like villi of the cell membrane help to make the diagnosis of malignant nerve tumor

♦ rare tumor of the subcutaneous and soft tissue

♦ high incidence in patients with neurofibromatosis

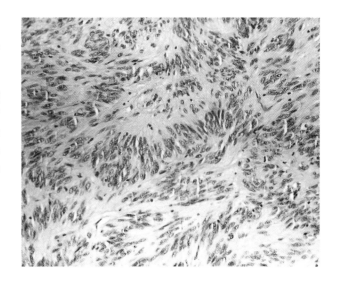

Leiomyomatous tumors

32.16 Angioleiomyoma

- primary cutaneous tumor of smooth muscle origin which may originate from arrector pili muscle (pilo-leiomyoma), nipple and genital smooth muscle (dartoic leiomyoma), or smooth muscle of the tunica media of vessels in the subcutis (angioleiomyoma)
- **angioleiomyoma** (upper picture), a well-circumscribed tumor in the subcutaneum typically on the legs of women
- **piloleiomyomas** are often multiple and tender to touch whereas others are usually solitary and seldom painful; reddish-brown tumors on the extremities, trunk, face, and neck
- higher power (lower picture) shows fibers that are eosinophilic on H&E staining
- elongated nuclei with blunted ends (boxcar appearance) are typical of smooth muscle cells
- immunohistochemistry to demonstrate actin may be helpful
- piloleiomyoma is dermal in location and, unlike angioleiomyoma, is non-encapsulated; margins are infiltrative even if the lesion is benign

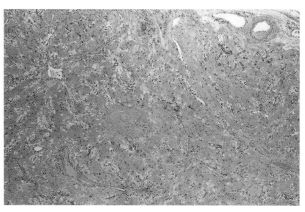

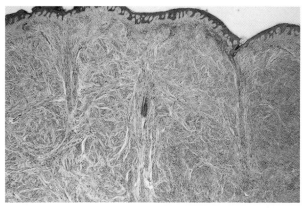

32.17 Piloleiomyosarcoma

- lesions >2 cm demonstrating some degree of cellular pleomorphism and a mitotic count of >1–2 figures/10 high-power (×400) fields should be considered a low-grade sarcoma (**piloleiomyosarcoma**)
- local recurrence (upper picture) after 2 years despite apparently complete excision
- higher power (lower picture) shows slightly enlarged cells, hyperchromatic nuclei, and several mitoses
- multiple leiomyosarcomas may be secondary to primary leiomyosarcoma in the retroperitoneum

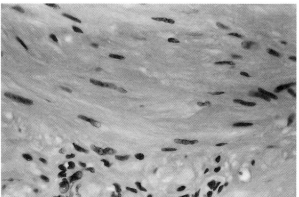

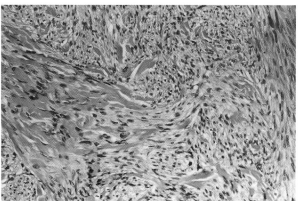

PREDOMINANTLY VACUOLATED FAT CELLS

Adipose tumors

32.18 Lipoma

♦ tumor of normal-looking adipocytes; an angiolipoma is seen here

♦ loss of fat during tissue processing produces the clear appearance of the cytoplasm

♦ benign adipocytes have small, pyknotic, shrunken nuclei lying along the cell membrane

♦ depending on the content of other tissues in a lipoma, prefixes such as angio-, fibro-, and myelo- may be added

♦ single or multiple, often lobulated, compressible, sub-cutaneous masses commonly found on the trunk and forearms

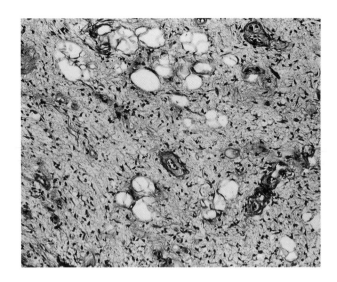

32.19 Hibernoma

♦ benign tumor of fetal fat

♦ so-called brown fat because of its color when seen grossly, the fat cells have a microvesicular rather than clear cytoplasm ('mulberry' cells)

♦ cell nuclei are centrally located and not displaced to the inner surface of the cell membrane, as seen in normal fat cells

♦ solitary subcutaneous mass most commonly on the upper back

♦ clinically indistinguishable from lipoma

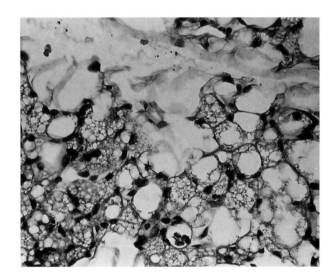

32.20 Pleomorphic lipoma

♦ occasionally, lipomas may contain adipose cells with enlarged and pleomorphic nuclei

♦ multinucleated tumor giant cells may be seen ('floret' cells)

♦ pleomorphic lipoma is a descriptive term for such tumors; almost all lipomas of superficial subcuta-neous tissue are benign despite the sometimes marked cytologic atypia

♦ lipomas with a high content of spindle cells are called **spindle cell lipoma**, and mast cells are usually prominent

♦ in both pleomorphic and spindle cell variants, the key to the diagnosis is identification of lipoblasts (arrow)

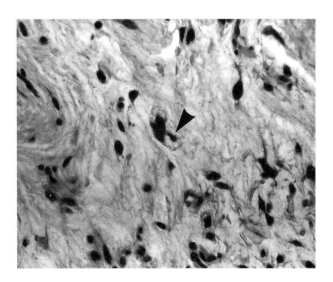

32.21 Liposarcoma

♦ second most common sarcoma of soft tissue
♦ usually originates in intermuscular fascial planes on the leg, buttock, and shoulder in middle-aged men
♦ extremely rare in superficial subcutaneous tissue
♦ tumors previously termed 'well-differentiated liposarcoma of subcutaneous tissue' are most probably pleomorphic lipomas
♦ tumor giant cells and sarcomatous cells are highly pleomorphic
♦ differentiation from malignant fibrous histiocytoma may be difficult; myxomatous forms of the two most common sarcomas are probably indistinguishable and have similar patterns of behavior
♦ liposarcomas may be S100 protein-positive
♦ search for lipoblasts with light and electron microscopy

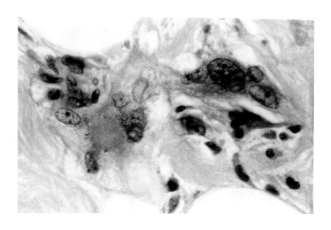

PREDOMINANTLY VASCULAR

Vascular tumors

32.22 Capillary hemangioma

♦ papillary proliferation of capillaries lined by endothelial cells with prominent nuclei; usually an exophytic lesion, but vascular channels may extend into the reticular dermis
♦ cytologic atypia and mitotic figures are not uncommon in proliferative lesions in children
♦ sometimes satellite nodules and ulcerated surface
♦ histologically similar lesions, but with an ulcerated epidermis and acute inflammation, are **pyogenic granuloma** and **benign lobular hemangioma**
♦ may occur at any age and during pregnancy

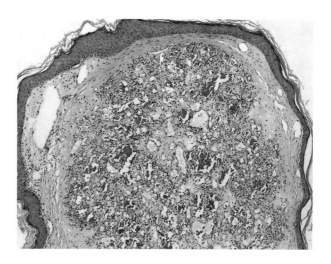

32.23 Glomus tumor

♦ benign tumor of pericytes, specialized contractile cells lining special arteriovenous shunts (Sucquet–Hoyer canal) important for temperature control in certain anatomic locations (nail beds and extremities)
♦ they surround dilated blood vessels, and some lesions appear angiomatous
♦ lesional cells have uniform, round, central nuclei and slight pale-staining cytoplasm, as seen here
♦ usually solitary, bluish-red, painful nodule(s) often involving the nail bed, but may occur anywhere
♦ multiple lesions are called **glomangiomas** and may have autosomal-dominant inheritance; they are less often painful

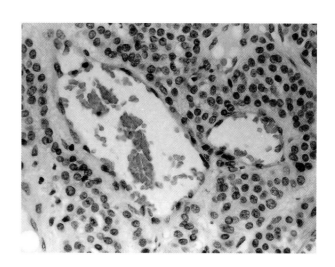

32.24 Intravascular papillary hemangioendothelioma

♦ benign soft tissue tumor of circumscribed vascular proliferation in the dermis or subcutaneous tissue
♦ most lesions are intravascular and associated with an organizing thrombus
♦ proliferating endothelial cells form complex papillary structures
♦ non-specific clinical findings
♦ most occur on the extremities, especially the fingers

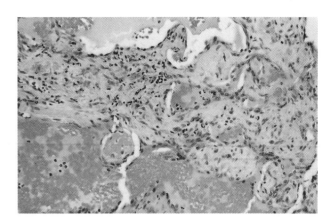

32.25 Angiokeratoma

♦ thin-walled capillaries are present in the papillary dermis and intimately associated with the overlying hyperplastic epidermis
♦ lesions of **angiokeratoma corporis diffusum (Fabry's disease)** usually have capillaries lined by endothelial cells, which contain abnormal phospholipids that may be demonstrated by PAS or lipid stains, and extend into the deep dermis
♦ small, red to purple, keratotic papules which may present at birth as a linear warty growth (**angiokeratoma circumscriptum**) OR develop as a solitary lesion on the limbs in childhood or adolescence, OR develop in adolescence on the hands and feet in association with cold intolerance (**angiokeratoma of Mibelli**), OR as multiple lesions on the scrotum or vulva (**angiokeratoma of Fordyce**), OR as part of **Fabry's syndrome** (X-linked recessive condition of defective α-D-galactosidase A, characterized by multiple angiokeratomas primarily on the trunk and thighs, episodic severe pain, and constant discomfort in the extremities, hypohidrosis, corneal and lenticular opacities, myocardial ischemia and infarction, strokes, and renal failure), OR as part of **fucosidosis** (mental retardation and multiple angiokeratomas on the trunk and upper legs which develop during early childhood)

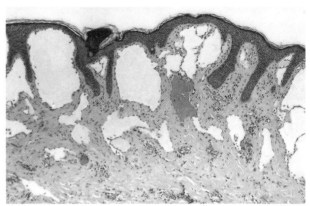

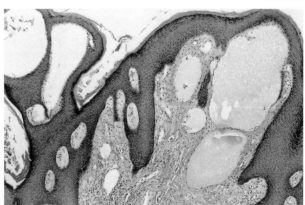

32.26 Venous hemangioma

♦ thin-walled venous channels in dermis
♦ endothelial cells are uniform and have flattened nuclei
♦ red cells in lumina help to differentiate from lymphangioma, although clinical appearance is diagnostic
♦ solitary, dark-red papule or nodule on the face or extremities
♦ biopsy usually carried out to differentiate from other pigmented lesions

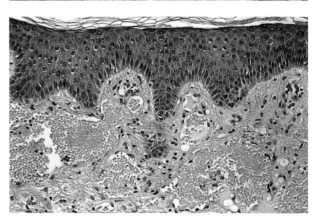

32.27 Kaposi's sarcoma (KS)

♦ irregularly shaped vascular channels in the superficial dermis (upper picture)

♦ in earlier patch lesions, spindle cell proliferation and malignant cell features may be difficult to appreciate

♦ some extravasation of red cells and focal hemosiderin pigmentation

♦ marked spindle endothelial cellular proliferation in later stages resulting in plaques and tumors

♦ histologic diagnosis is not difficult with plaque and tumor KS lesions (middle picture); resemblance to pyogenic granuloma is superficial and only with low magnification

♦ unlike pyogenic granuloma and hemangioma, the lesional cells have vacuolated cytoplasm containing eosinophilic inclusions, which are fragments of red cells (lower picture)

♦ associated with herpesvirus type 8

♦ patch lesion is a bruise-like macule which is often linear

♦ purple papules, plaques, and nodules

♦ KS may be endemic (African), classic (sporadic), or associated with AIDS or immunosuppression (transplant patients)

♦ in the classic form, lesions commonly occur on the legs of older men and the patch lesions may resemble stasis dermatitis

♦ endemic form may be nodular, florid, infiltrative, or lymphadenopathic, and usually occurs in children

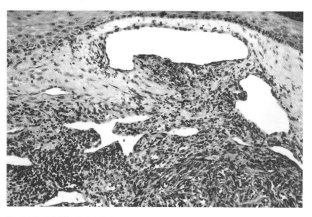
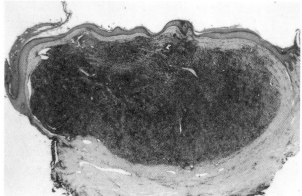
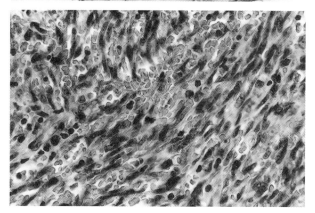

32.28 Angiosarcoma

♦ neoplastic cells are most commonly spindle-shaped, although a few tumors are composed almost entirely of epithelioid tumor cells

♦ highly infiltrative tumor involving the dermis and subcutaneous tissue

♦ marked cytologic atypia and mitotic activity, although pleomorphic sarcomatous tumor giant cells such as those in atypical fibroxanthoma are not seen in angiosarcoma

♦ vascular nature is reflected by tumor cells lining cleft-like spaces as they attempt angiogenesis

(continued next page)

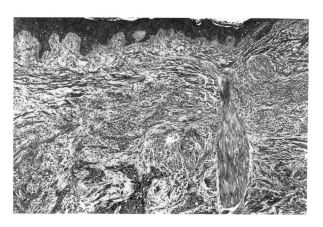

◆ higher magnification shows spindle-shaped tumor cells with cytoplasmic lumina (arrow)
◆ cellular groupings and growth pattern are reminiscent of branching vessels in the dermis
◆ typically a dark-red plaque with small satellite nodules on the scalp and face of the elderly

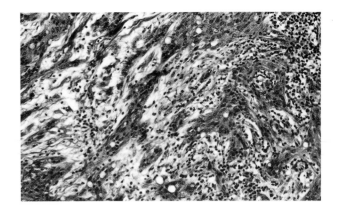

CYSTS

True cysts are epithelium-lined space-occupying lesions in the dermis or subcutaneous tissue. Clinically firm to fluctuant papules and nodules, their cystic nature is usually more apparent in superficial lesions. Some cysts are fluid-filled whereas others have a solid center. Keratinous cysts include epidermal and pilar cysts, proliferating pilar tumor, dermoid, first branchial and most second branchial cysts, eruptive vellus hair cyst, and steatocytoma. Non-keratinous cysts include cutaneous ciliated and genital perineal raphe cysts, mucinous cyst of the vulva, cutaneous endometriosis, thyroglossal duct, omphalomesenteric and bronchogenic cysts, 4% of second branchial cysts, and hidrocystoma. Ciliated epithelium is not commonly found in the skin, but may be seen in bronchogenic and branchial cleft cysts, mucinous cyst of the vulva, cutaneous endometriosis, and cutaneous ciliated cyst. Sequestration and cell migration during embryonic development, transplantation after trauma, or *via* the lymphatics or bloodstream, and metaplasia of pluripotential cells in the skin are potential mechanisms which may explain the presence of ciliated epithelium within the skin.

Cysts may or may not be neoplastic; non-neoplastic cysts may be acquired or congenital. Attention to the type of epithelial lining and whether there is an associated cellular proliferative activity are important for the correct diagnosis of these lesions. Differentiating a simple cyst from a cystic neoplasm, however, is seldom difficult.

Differential diagnoses

Cysts with simple squamous epithelium

Epidermal cyst	33.1
Pilar (trichilemmal) cyst	33.2
Dermoid cyst	33.3
Eruptive vellus hair cyst	33.4
Steatocystoma simplex / multiplex	33.5

Cysts with simple glandular epithelium

Cutaneous ciliated / median raphe cyst	33.6

Cysts with complex proliferative epithelium

Proliferating trichilemmal (pilar) tumor	33.7
Syringocystadenoma papilliferum	33.8
Cystic basal cell carcinoma	33.9

CYSTS WITH SIMPLE SQUAMOUS EPITHELIUM

33.1 Epidermal cyst
♦ most common cutaneous cyst
♦ center of the cyst is filled with laminated keratin; hairs are not present
♦ squamous epithelial lining has a granular layer, but is devoid of adnexal structures
♦ epidermal cysts are follicular in origin and the follicular infundibulum forms the cyst wall
♦ so-called epidermal inclusion cyst is due to proliferative cystic enlargement of implanted squamous cell nests during trauma
♦ cyst rupture always excites a foreign body-type granulomatous reaction to the keratinaceous content; eosinophilic fibrils in bipointed spaces in the cytoplasm of giant cells are typical of keratin
♦ clinically, a cystic nodule with a central punctum which usually onsets after puberty; may occur anywhere on the body, but has a predilection for the postauricular area and upper back
♦ **Gardner's syndrome** (epidermal cysts, multiple intestinal polyposis, colonic adenocarcinoma, osteomas of the skull, fibromas, and dermoid tumors) should be suspected if epidermal cysts occur before puberty, or if there is a family history of epidermal cysts or intestinal polyposis
♦ a **milium** (lower picture) is a papule 1–2 mm in diameter which is histologically identical to an epidermal cyst
♦ milia are often multiple and commonly found on the cheeks, forehead, eyelids, and at sites of trauma

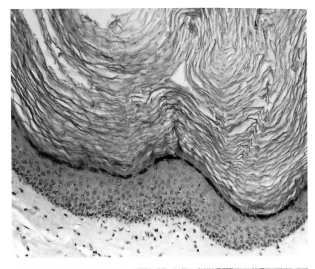

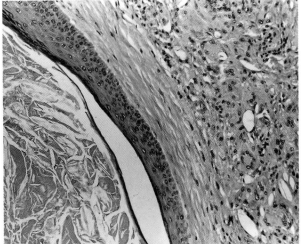

33.2 Pilar (trichilemmal) cyst
♦ pilar cysts are often deep and subcutaneously located
♦ overlying epidermis is stretched over the cyst, as seen here
♦ as with epidermal cysts, origin is follicular, but with epithelium of the isthmus and inferior segment of the terminal follicles forming the cyst wall; trichilemmal type of keratinization is observed

(continued next page)

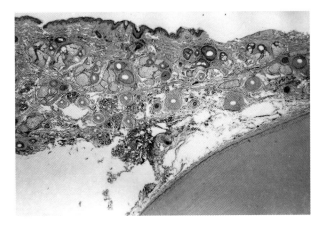

♦ squamous epithelium shows a trichilemmal type of keratinization with absent granular layer

♦ amorphous, eosinophilic, sebaceous material containing lipid, such as cholesterol, within the cyst

♦ calcification in approximately 25% of cases

♦ common at locations with terminal hairs, such as the scalp

♦ dome-shaped nodules without the central punctum seen in epidermal cysts

♦ multiple cysts usually have an autosomal-dominant inheritance

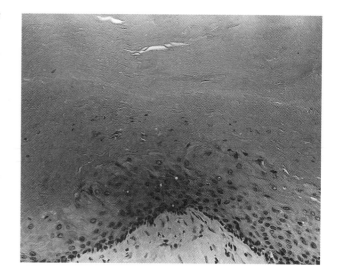

33.3 Dermoid cyst

♦ true congenital cyst developing from displaced germinative cells of skin

♦ squamous cyst lining has numerous adnexal structures, including hairs (arrow)

♦ occurs along the embryonic fusion lines

♦ most commonly seen on the head and neck

♦ present at birth and clinically apparent by age 4–8 years

♦ may have bony defects and be connected to the central nervous system

♦ **first branchial cyst** is a dermoid cyst with cartilage found anterior to the external auditory canal

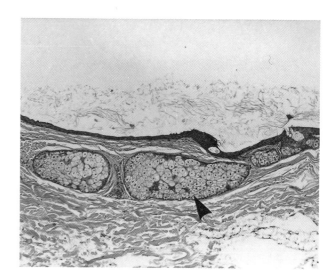

33.4 Eruptive vellus hair cyst

♦ vellus hair (arrow; diameter <0.03 mm) is present in the laminated keratin within the cyst

♦ hairs emerge from invaginations in cyst wall, but well-developed hair bulbs or sebaceous glands are not seen

♦ developmental abnormality of vellus follicle

♦ umbilicated and non-umbilicated, multiple, acneform papules 1–4 mm in diameter, typically on the central chest in children or young adults

♦ may be familial and may spontaneously remit

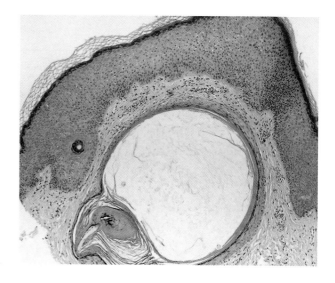

33.5 Steatocystoma

♦ similar to dermoid cysts, sebaceous gland lobules and follicular structures are seen in the cyst wall

♦ cyst wall may show folds; cysts are often partially collapsed

♦ onsets at birth, or during childhood or early adulthood

♦ predilection for the anterior chest, but common in the axillae and on the face, scalp, arms, back, groin, and thighs

♦ may be solitary (**simplex**), but almost always multiple (**multiplex**)

♦ multiple lesions may have autosomal-dominant inheritance

♦ may be associated with acrokeratosis verruciformis of Hopf, pachyonychia congenita, natal teeth, koilonychia, hypohidrosis, hypotrichosis, hypothyroidism, hidradenitis suppurativa, and hypertrophic lichen planus

♦ clinical differential diagnosis: epidermal cyst; eruptive vellus hair cyst; cystic acne; hidradenitis suppurativa; lipoma; cylindroma; and xanthoma

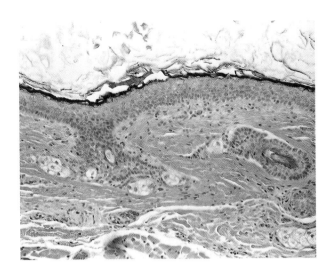

CYSTS WITH SIMPLE GLANDULAR EPITHELIUM

33.6 Cutaneous ciliated cyst

♦ cilia (arrow) along surface of the epithelium; usually multilocular on the lower extremities in women aged 15–30 years

♦ other columnar (glandular) epithelium-lined cysts include **eccrine** and **apocrine hidrocystoma**; **bronchogenic cyst**; **cyst of the genital perineal raphe**; **mucinous cyst of the vulva**; **cutaneous endometriosis**; **thyroglossal duct cyst**; and **omphalomesenteric cyst**, which is found by the umbilicus

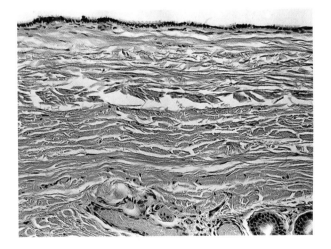

CYSTS WITH COMPLEX PROLIFERATIVE EPITHELIUM

33.7 Proliferating trichilemmal (pilar) tumor

♦ nodular, deep, dermal or subcutaneous encapsulated cystic tumor
♦ squamous epithelial lining is thick and cellular with complex folds
♦ solid islands of cells and focal calcification are common
♦ peripheral cells of these islands have abundant basophilic cytoplasm whereas necrotic 'ghost' cells without nuclei are seen in the center
♦ cytologic atypia and complex squamous cell masses suggest squamous cell carcinoma (SCC); the central shadow cells, calcification, encapsulated margin, and trichilemmal type of keratinization (without the granular layer) allow differentiation from SCC
♦ majority of lesions (90%) are on the scalp in elderly women
♦ solitary, lobulated, scalp nodule ± ulceration
♦ may be associated with other pilar cysts

33.8 Syringocystadenoma papilliferum (SCP)

♦ many benign adnexal tumors, such as hidradenoma, syringocystadenoma papilliferum, and apocrine cystadenoma, are often partially or totally cystic
♦ cystic lumina is lined by hyperplastic, papillary, double-layered epithelium, as seen here
♦ check for apocrine secretion and cytologic atypia
♦ remember: most adnexal glandular tumors are benign neoplasms

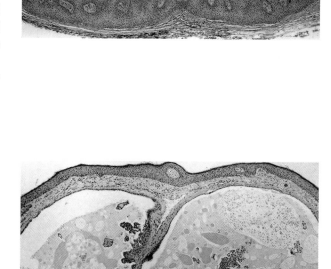

33.9 Cystic basal cell carcinoma (BCC)

♦ squamous cell carcinomas arising in epidermal and pilar cysts are extremely rare
♦ cystic basal cell and squamous cell carcinomas are common, but tumors are rarely completely cystic on microscopy
♦ typical micronodular masses of BCC are seen here in the periphery of the cystic cavity
♦ pleomorphic infiltrating squamous or basal cells are usually apparent on multiple sections of the tumor

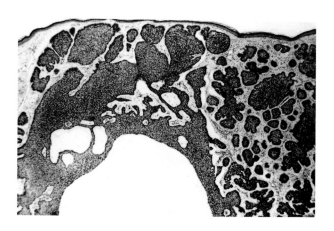

SUBCUTIS

PANNICULITIS

The subcutaneum is organized into lobules of fat cells divided into compartments by thin fibrous septa that are richly supplied by vascular and lymphatic channels. Subcutaneous fat serves as an energy reserve as well as an insulating mechanical cushion for the body.

Panniculitis is inflammation of subcutaneous fat. Clinically, it is manifested by tender and non-tender erythematous nodules or plaques with or without ulceration. To arrive at an appropriate diagnosis, a thorough history, including a systems review and clinicopathologic correlation, is essential. In cases of suspected panniculitis, a deep biopsy with ample subcutaneous tissue should be taken. A wedge incisional biopsy is usually required as a shave biopsy is too shallow, and a small punch biopsy does not usually yield sufficient tissue. Part of the specimen should be submitted for tissue culture to rule out an infectious etiology.

On the basis of histopathology, panniculitis is divided into three groups according to the distribution of inflammatory cells within the tissue. In the first group, the inflammation is angiocentric. The primary abnormality is large-vessel vasculitis and the subcutaneous fat is secondarily affected. Polyarteritis nodosa, migratory thrombophlebitis, and nodular vasculitis (erythema induratum) are examples of angiocentric inflammation.

In polyarteritis nodosa, there is vasculitis of the medium-sized arteries in the subcutaneous tissue whereas, in superficial migratory thrombophlebitis, venous thrombosis occurs. Erythema induratum was classically described as a hypersensitivity reaction to tuberculosis ('tuberculid'), although it is now known that this condition may develop due to a variety of antigenic stimuli. However, all patients suspected of having erythema induratum should be questioned for exposure to tuberculosis and undergo a purified protein derivative (tuberculin; PPD) skin test. Patients with erythema induratum associated with tuberculosis require treatment of the infection to resolve the panniculitis. Erythema induratum usually affects women in the fourth to seventh decades. Tender erythematous nodules which may ulcerate and heal with scarring (in contrast to erythema nodosum) are most often seen on the calf. The lesions are often chronic and may be unilateral, involving the thighs, buttocks, feet, and upper extremities.

In **septal panniculitis**, the second histopathologic group, the fibrous septa are the foci of inflammation. The fat in the lobules is secondarily involved by overflow of inflammation from the fibrous partitions in the subcutaneum. Septal inflammation is seen in erythema nodosum, the most common type of panniculitis, which is a reaction pattern seen in response to a number of different stimuli. It has been associated with drugs, infections, inflammatory bowel disease, sarcoidosis, Behçet's syndrome, cancer, and pregnancy. Clinically, tender, warm, erythematous nodules are typically present on the pretibial surfaces. The nodules do not ulcerate, but involute with bruise-like discoloration without scarring after 3–6 weeks. Fever, malaise, and arthralgia may be associated.

The third group is **lobular panniculitis**, where the inflammation is centered primarily in the subcutaneous fat lobules. Fat necrosis is a prominent histologic feature. Lobular panniculitis is seen in pancreatitic fat necrosis, traumatic panniculitis, cold panniculitis, subcutaneous fat necrosis of the newborn, sclerema neonatorum, poststeroid panniculitis, lupus erythematosus profundus, α_1-antitrypsin deficiency, histiocytic cytophagic panniculitis, and lipodystrophy. Malignant cellular infiltrates (from metastatic carcinomas, lymphoma, or leukemia) may invade the subcutaneum and give rise to a histologic picture similar to lobular panniculitis. At low power, an inflammatory process may be suggested but, at higher power, examination of cell morphology should reveal the malignant nature of the infiltrating cells. In addition, these cells may be found in vessels, around nerves, and between collagen bundles in the dermis.

Pancreatic fat necrosis may occur in association with pancreatitis, pancreatic cancer, and pancreatic pseudocyst. Fever, multiple nodules, arthritis, and abdominal pain (particularly with pancreatitis) are seen clinically. The nodules typically drain an oily substance, and are most commonly located on the trunk, buttocks, and legs. The foci of fat necrosis in the subcutaneous lobules are thought to be due to the release of lipases. The amylase level is usually elevated in pancreatitis.

Panniculitis may be the result of injection of foreign material such as oil, silica, talc, and starch. In **oil granulomas**, clear, round to oval spaces of varying size or needle-shaped clefts are seen. Similar, but smaller, clefts may be seen in **sclerema neonatorum**.

Cold panniculitis is a rare condition. It has been observed in children after prolonged direct contact with cold (for example, on the cheek after eating a Popsicle®) or on the thighs in young women after horseback riding.

Subcutaneous fat necrosis of the newborn and sclerema neonatorum are seen in newly born infants. In the former condition, the child is healthy and full-term, the nodules are discrete and non-tender, and the prognosis is favorable. In contrast, with sclerema neonatorum, the infant is usually premature or ill with diffuse hardening of the skin. Poststeroid panniculitis is a rare complication of sudden steroid withdrawal in children in which erythematous, firm, warm nodules develop within 2 weeks of discontinuation of high doses of steroids. The cheeks are characteristically involved and the lesions resolve without scarring over a period of months. Poststeroid panniculitis has the same histologic picture as subcutaneous fat necrosis of the newborn.

Lupus erythematosus profundus is most commonly seen in association with discoid lupus erythematosus (DLE) and less commonly with systemic lupus erythematosus (SLE) or as an isolated event. It typically occurs in women in the third to seventh decades as subcutaneous nodules or plaques on the thighs, buttocks, upper arms, breasts, or face. In contrast to other forms of panniculitis, the lower leg is usually not involved. The overlying skin may show the typical features of DLE (erythema, hyperpigmentation, telangiectasia, atrophy, hyperkeratosis) or ulceration. Healing may be associated with lipoatrophy and a large skin depression.

Only a small number of patients with α_1-**antitrypsin deficiency** develop panniculitis. In the event, recurrent, tender, erythematous nodules, which may be fluctuant and ulcerate, develop most commonly on the trunk and proximal extremities. α_1-Antitrypsin deficiency should be suspected where there is a personal or family history of emphysema, especially in non-smokers at a young age. Hepatitis and cirrhosis are other common clinical manifestations of the deficiency. Serum α_1-antitrypsin levels are easily ascertained. The homozygous form is the most severe and affects 1 in 2500 people whereas the heterozygous form affects only 1 in 50.

Histiocytic cytophagic panniculitis is a rare condition seen in association with infections (including Epstein–Barr virus, mycobacteria, spirochetes, and fungi) or malignancy (typically T-cell lymphoma). Non-tender widespread erythematous nodules and plaques become ecchymotic and may ulcerate. Fever, hepatosplenomegaly, lymphadenopathy, pancytopenia, and coagulation abnormalities may be associated.

Lipodystrophy resulting from steroid or insulin injection ultimately results in loss of subcutaneous fat. The fat cells shrink and are replaced by capillaries in a loose myxomatous stroma.

Lobular and septal changes may be seen in **lipodermatosclerosis**, which is usually seen in older women with chronic venous insufficiency. It starts as an erythematous indurated plaque on the lower leg. Over time, the leg becomes woody and resembles an inverted champagne bottle.

Eosinophilic panniculitis is characterized by infiltration of the subcutis with eosinophils. It is thought to be a reactive process as most patients have an associated condition, such as arthropod bite, atopic and contact dermatitis, gnathostomiasis, streptococcal and other bacterial infections, leukocytoclastic vasculitis, erythema nodosum, eosinophilic cellulitis, hematologic disorders, or malignancy. Clinically, nodules, plaques, and vesicles are seen.

A number of other conditions may also have subcutaneous fat involvement but, in these conditions, the inflammation is usually centered outside of the fat; for example, granulomas such as sarcoidosis, deep fungal and mycobacterial infections, granuloma annulare and necrobiosis lipoidica, cellulitis, and ruptured cysts have a greater involvement in the dermis than in subcutaneous fat. In addition, the characteristic histologic features (giant cells and granulomas in sarcoid, and deep fungal and mycobacterial infections, necrobiosis in granuloma annulare and necrobiosis lipoidica, and cyst walls in ruptured cysts) are usually present. These conditions may, however, clinically mimic the three types of panniculitides discussed above. Brown recluse spider bites may have widespread inflammation, necrosis, and marked involvement of the subcutis. Eosinophilic fasciitis and nodular fasciitis are centered in the fascia, but may have septal subcutaneous involvement.

Normal subcutaneous fat — 34.1

Differential diagnoses

Angiocentric inflammation / vasculitis

Cutaneous polyarteritis nodosa — 34.2
Superficial migratory thrombophlebitis — 34.3
Nodular vasculitis (erythema induratum) — 34.4

Septal inflammation

Erythema nodosum — 34.5

Lobular panniculitis

Pancreatic fat necrosis — 34.6
Traumatic panniculitis — 34.7
Subcutaneous fat necrosis of the newborn — 34.8
Sclerema neonatorum — 34.9
α_1-Antitrypsin deficiency — 34.10
Lipodermatosclerosis — 34.11

Other

Subcutaneous (Darier–Roussy) sarcoid — 34.12
Lymphomatous infiltration — 34.13

34.1 Normal subcutaneous fat
♦ square-shaped compartments of adipocytes
♦ individual cells have vacuolated cytoplasm and small nuclei along the cell border

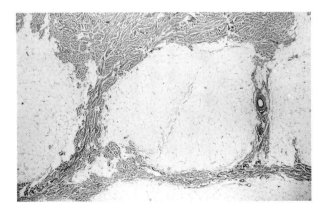

ANGIOCENTRIC INFLAMMATION / VASCULITIS

34.2 Cutaneous polyarteritis nodosa (PAN)

♦ confirmation of the diagnosis hinges on finding an inflamed muscular-type artery in the deep dermis or subcutis (arrow; upper picture); serial sections may be required as the vasculitis is often focal and segmental

♦ arterial inflammation is easily discernible by the heavy angiocentric neutrophilic infiltration; leukocytoclasis is common and eosinophils are usually present

♦ higher power (lower picture) shows fibrinoid necrosis of the vessel wall, perivascular hemorrhage, and inflammation extending to the surrounding fat

♦ grouped nodules along the course of superficial arteries, especially on the lower leg; may have systemic involvement, including renal disease, coronary thrombosis, pericarditis, mesenteric thrombosis, and mononeuritis multiplex

♦ may have preceding streptococcal infection or hepatitis

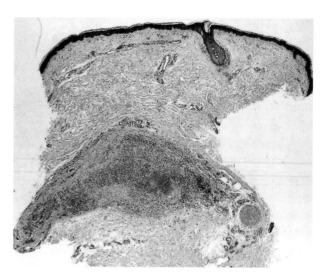

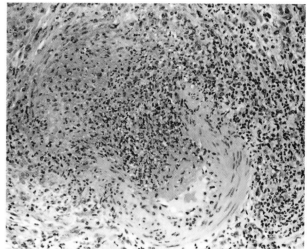

34.3 Superficial migratory thrombophlebitis

♦ a larger vein is involved by an occluding thrombus, which is the initiating event

♦ inflammation is usually confined to the perivenous tissue, and neutrophilis are seen in the acute phase

♦ with time, the inflammation becomes lymphohistiocytic and granulomatous

♦ organization of the thrombus is associated with infiltration of lymphocytes and macrophages

♦ erythematous nodules along the superficial veins

♦ may be associated with Behçet's disease or visceral carcinoma, especially pancreatic cancer (**Trousseau's syndrome**)

♦ patients with this condition should be investigated for underlying malignancy

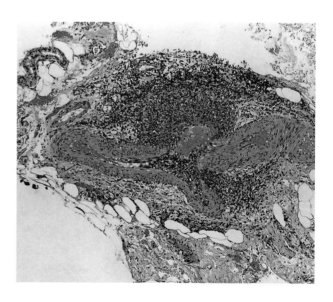

34.4 Nodular vasculitis (erythema induratum)

- low-power view (upper picture) demonstrates juxtaposition of the necrotizing granuloma to inflamed vessel
- high-power view (lower picture) shows heavy lymphocytic infiltration of the veins and arteries
- instead of fibrinoid necrosis, there is fibrous thickening of the vessel wall with perivascular granulomatous inflammation (arrow)
- swollen endothelial cells and thrombi in vascular lumina
- lobular fat necrosis and inflammation are secondary to thrombotic occlusion of vessels and ischemia
- classically, a hypersensitivity reaction to tuberculosis, but Ziehl–Neelsen staining almost always negative
- usually affects women in the fourth to seventh decades with chronic, tender, erythematous nodules on the calf which may ulcerate and heal with scarring (in contrast to erythema nodosum)
- may be unilateral and involve the thighs, buttocks, feet, and arms

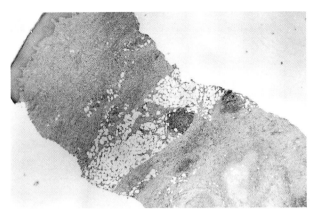

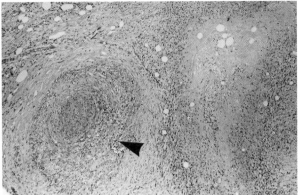

SEPTAL INFLAMMATION

34.5 Erythema nodosum (EN)

- edema and neutrophilic infiltration of edematous and thickened fibrous septa; fat cells in the center of the lobules are preserved and there is no fat necrosis
- Miescher's nodule (upper picture) is an aggregate of lymphocytes and macrophages
- lesions of longer duration are granulomatous with multinucleated giant cells and fewer neutrophils
- small vessels in the septa may be infiltrated by lymphocytes, but fibrinoid necrosis of vessel walls is not seen
- may be associated with drugs, infections, inflammatory bowel disease, sarcoidosis, Behçet's syndrome, cancers, and pregnancy
- tender, warm, erythematous nodules are typically present on the pretibial surfaces; nodules do not ulcerate, but involve with bruise-like discoloration without scarring after 3–6 weeks
- fever, malaise, and arthralgia may be associated

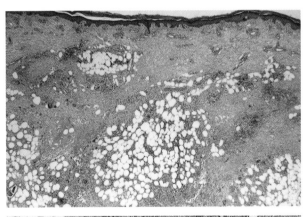

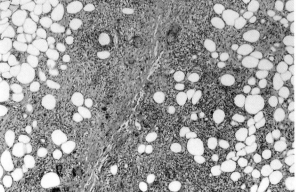

LOBULAR PANNICULITIS

34.6 Pancreatic fat necrosis
♦ necrotic fat cells resemble ghost cells with faintly basophilic peripheral cell borders and no nuclei
♦ extravasated red cells may be seen
♦ necrotic cell debris attracts neutrophils
♦ dystrophic calcification of necrotic fat is characteristic
♦ similar histologic appearance is seen in traumatic panniculitis, but fat necrosis is widespread in pancreatic
disease
♦ fever, multiple nodules, arthritis, and abdominal pain
(particularly with pancreatitis) are seen clinically
♦ nodules typically drain an oily substance, and are most
commonly located on the trunk, buttocks, and legs

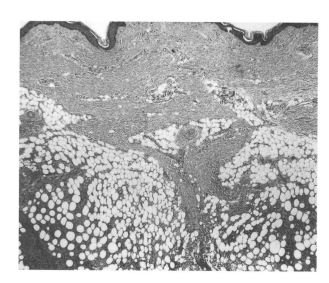

34.7 Traumatic panniculitis
♦ fat necrosis is often focal with a few ghost cells
♦ inflammation and fibrous reaction are limited to the
local area of trauma
♦ in **oil granulomas**, clear, round to oval spaces of
varying size or needle-shaped clefts are seen; similar,
but smaller, clefts may be seen in sclerema neonatorum
♦ may be due to physical trauma-induced fat necrosis in
female breasts (in these cases, focal fat necrosis and
inflammation may mimic a mass lesion), or injections
of foreign material (for example, drugs such as
steroids, oil, silica, talc, and starch)

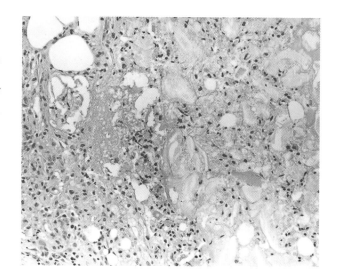

34.8 Subcutaneous fat necrosis of the newborn
♦ lobular fat necrosis associated with an infiltrate of
lymphocytes, histiocytes, and foreign body-type giant
cells
♦ intracytoplasmic, radiating, bipointed crystalline material is seen in adipocytes, macrophages, and giant cells,
but these lipid inclusions are non-specific and may
be present in sclerema or other forms of lobular
fat necrosis
♦ focal calcification may be seen
♦ occurs in full-term infants as symmetric, firm, erythematous to violaceous, freely movable nodules on the
trunk, legs, and cheeks

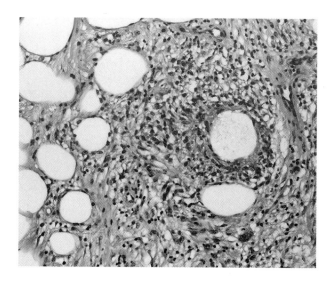

34.9 Sclerema neonatorum

♦ minimal inflammation (unlike subcutaneous fat necrosis) in the presence of abnormal thickened fibrotic subcutaneous fat is characteristic

♦ cleft-like spaces, some in rosettes, may be seen in fat cells and macrophages, but not in giant cells

♦ no fat necrosis

♦ occurs suddenly in premature or debilitated infants as an induration of the subcutaneous fat in most of the body except the palms, soles, and scrotum

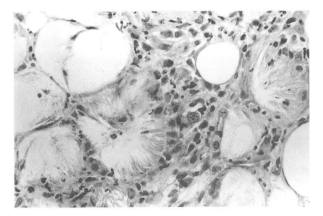

34.10 α_1-Antitrypsin deficiency

♦ neutrophilic inflammation within lobules

♦ hemorrhage, foci of fat necrosis, foam cells and fat microcysts

♦ may start as a septal panniculitis, but lobular changes often predominate

♦ stains for acid-fast bacilli and fungi rule out infectious panniculitis

♦ recurrent, tender, erythematous nodules, which may be fluctuant and frequently ulcerate, often develop after minor trauma most commonly on the trunk and proximal extremities

♦ personal or family history of emphysema, especially in non-smokers at a young age, hepatitis, and cirrhosis

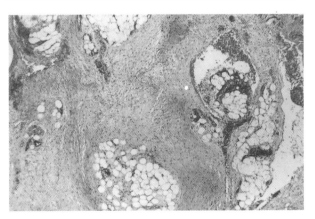

34.11 Lipodermatosclerosis

♦ early lesions show central ischemic necrosis in fat lobules, capillary congestion, hemorrhage, and hemosiderin deposition

♦ fat-microcyst formation and membranous fat necrosis

♦ septa become thickened and fibrotic with time

♦ fibroplasia and hemosiderin deposition in the dermis

♦ usually seen in older women with chronic venous insufficiency

♦ starts as an erythematous indurated plaque on the lower leg which, with time, becomes woody and resembles an inverted champagne bottle

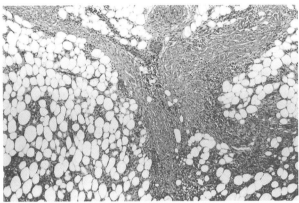

OTHER

34.12 Subcutaneous (Darier–Roussy) sarcoid

♦ non-caseating granulomatous inflammation of fat

♦ granulomata are well developed and fat inflammation is usually slight

♦ subcutaneous nodules with normal overlying skin

♦ rare form of sarcoid

♦ persistent, immobile, often painful nodules

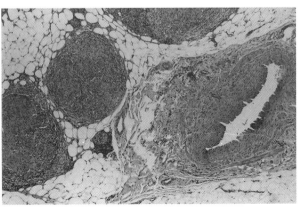

34.13 Lymphomatous infiltration

- malignant cellular infiltration may involve both the septa and lobules
- diagnosis requires positive identification of atypical neoplastic cells
- malignant lymphocytes appear monotonous with larger vesicular nuclei and nucleoli
- erythematous to violaceous papules and nodules

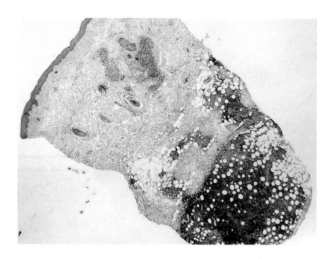

HAIR AND ALOPECIA

Understanding alopecia requires basic knowledge of the histology of the hair follicle and physiology of the hair cycle. There are approximately 100 000 hair follicles on the scalp. The base of the hair follicle is invaginated by the dermal papilla, which contains highly vascularized connective tissue. Above the papilla are the germinative or hair matrical cells that differentiate into concentrically arranged layers. The innermost cells form the medulla and cortex of the hair. Peripheral to the hair cortex is the hair cuticle, a single layer of cells that interlocks with another cuticle layer of the inner root sheath. Matrical cells in the periphery produce cells for the inner Huxley layer and the outermost Henle cell layer of the inner root sheath. Melanocytes are seen with the basal layer of the hair matrical cells, and melanin pigment is transferred to the innermost matrical cells that form the hair medulla and cortex. The inner root sheath does not contain melanin pigment. The outer root sheath is a continuation of the surface epidermis and is thinnest at the level of the hair follicle. The cells of the outer root sheath have clear cytoplasm because of their glycogen cytoplasmic content. The infundibulum refers to that portion of the hair shaft between the epidermis and sebaceous duct. The follicular isthmus is the region between the sebaceous duct and arrector pili muscle insertion. It is in this region that the inner root sheath cells disintegrate and the hair shaft loses its connection with the outer root sheath. Beneath the arrector pili insertion is the inferior segment, a transient structure that is only present in growing hair.

The **hair cycle** is composed of three distinct, but overlapping, phases: anagen (growth); catagen (involutional); and telogen (resting). The papilla ascends during catagen to the superficial dermis and the hair shaft is discharged in telogen. When the follicle resumes anagen, there is a downgrowth of papilla and matrix to the deep subcutaneum. At any given time, approximately 90% of scalp hair shafts are in anagen. During this time, the hair grows 1 cm / day. The duration of anagen is under strict genetic control, but generally lasts between 2–6 years. Normally, the distribution of hair follicles in anagen, catagen, and telogen is random in any given area. Thus, physiologic hair loss (telogen) is inconspicuous in humans in contrast to some mammals which shed hair from relatively circumscribed regions. This is because the hair follicles in any given area tend to be in the same phase of the hair cycle.

Alopecia refers to a greater than normally expected loss of hair from a skin surface. Histopathologically, alopecia is subdivided into inflammatory and non-inflammatory categories. Non-inflammatory causes of alopecia include telogen effluvium, anagen arrest due to cancer chemotherapeutic agents, poisoning (arsenic, bismuth, boric acid, thallium) or radiation, androgenetic alopecia, trichotillomania, pseudopelade of Brocq, developmental abnormalities (cutis aplasia congenita), and neoplasia.

Inflammatory alopecia may occur as a consequence of direct lymphocyte-mediated destruction of hair follicles, as in lichen planopilaris. Alternatively, hair follicle epithelium may be destroyed as an 'innocent bystander' as in hidradenitis suppurativa and acne conglobata. These latter conditions are rarely biopsied because they have highly typical clinical features. Inflammatory alopecia includes noninfectious causes such as alopecia areata, alopecia mucinosa, lupus erythematosus, dermatomyositis, scleroderma, lichen planopilaris, acne keloidalis, folliculitis decalvans, perifolliculitis capitis abscedens et suffodiens (dissecting folliculitis of the scalp), and sarcoid. Discoid lupus erythematosus and lichen planopilaris each account for approximately one-third of cases of inflammatory scarring alopecia. In systemic lupus erythematosus, a telogen or, occasionally, anagen effluvium is usually seen rather than inflammatory scarring alopecia. Infectious causes may be bacterial (*Staphylococcus aureus*, syphilis), fungal, viral (herpesvirus), or protozoal (leishmaniasis).

Inflammatory alopecia is often associated with scarring. It is important to identify scarring as its presence indicates irreversible alopecia. Scarring is seen histologically as areas of vertically oriented collagen and elastic fibers. Destruction of the bulge area with middermal scarring or hyalinization is a hallmark of permanent alopecia. In addition, in contrast to a hyalinizing process, such as scleroderma, in a true scar, elastin is absent in the upper dermis. Scarring alopecia may also be the result of physical injury (burns).

An accurate diagnosis for a given case of alopecia requires clinical correlation and a deep punch biopsy at least 4 mm in diameter. In straight-haired persons, the punch should be placed tangential to the skin surface so that it follows the direction of the hair. In curly-haired individuals, the punch should be placed perpendicular to the skin surface. The biopsy should be taken from an active area of hair destruction and not from inactive scarred areas. If quantitative analysis of the number of the hair follicles in anagen, catagen, and telogen is required, the biopsy should be embedded transversely. The usual vertically oriented biopsy demonstrates only 10% of the hair follicles in the tissue whereas transverse sections maximize the number of hair follicles examined.

Elastic tissue and PAS stains, and direct immunofluorescence may be helpful. The absence of elastin in the upper dermis indicates a true scar whereas PAS highlights fungi in tinea capitis, basement membrane thickening in lupus erythematosus, and apoptotic cells in catagen follicles in trichotillomania. Direct immunofluorescence may demonstrate IgG and C3, seen at the dermoepidermal junction in lupus erythematosus, and globular IgM, adjacent to follicular epithelium in lichen planopilaris.

Differential diagnoses

Normal anagen follicle	35.1
Catagen follicle	35.2
Telogen follicle	35.3
Cross-section of inferior segment of anagen hair	35.4

Non-inflammatory alopecia

Androgenetic alopecia	35.5
Trichotillomania	35.6
Pseudopelade of Brocq	35.7

Inflammatory alopecia

Alopecia areata	35.8
Discoid lupus erythematosus	35.9

35.1 Normal anagen follicle

- vertical section showing a dermal papilla during the active-growth phase of the a (anagen) follicle
- hair matrical cells differentiating into hair and inner root sheath
- follicular papilla (arrow) is an invagination of the dermis where capillaries gain entrance to the matrical cells
- melanophages with their cytoplasmic melanin pigment are present in the follicular papilla
- melanogenesis ceases with the onset of catagen
- anagen phase lasts around 3 years; a normal pull test should consist of > 80% anagen hair

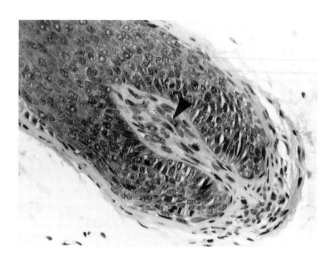

35.2 Catagen follicle

- involuting follicle, where shrinkage of follicular epithelium is accomplished by apoptosis
- numerous apoptotic bodies (small arrows) are seen
- shrunken hair bulb (large arrow)
- basophilic matrical cells are no longer present; the entire inferior segment has been reduced to a thin epithelial cord surrounded by a prominent vitreous layer
- catagen phase lasts around 3 weeks, and catagen hairs account for < 2%

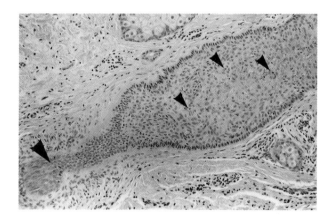

35.3 Telogen follicle

- resting phase of the follicular structure; both mitotic and apoptotic activities are at minimum
- involution of the inferior segment of the follicle is complete, and the follicle is now reduced to around one-third of its original size
- the small protrusion of basal cells (arrow) will become the hair bulb when the follicle is ready to cycle into anagen phase again
- formation of new anagen hair pushes the old club hair out of the follicle

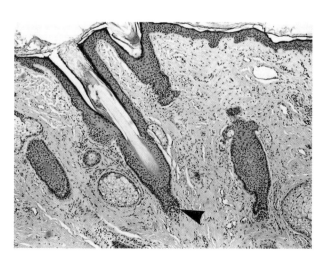

35.4 Cross-section of inferior segment of anagen hair

♦ layers of the inferior segment of an anagen hair from the outermost layer in: vitreous or glassy membrane; outer root sheath with clear glycogen-rich cells (multilayers); one-cell-thick Henle layer (large arrow); Huxley layer (two cells thick and identified by its eosinophilic keratohyaline granules); and inner root sheath cuticle (one cell thick) that interlocks with the hair cuticle, which points upwards (small arrow)

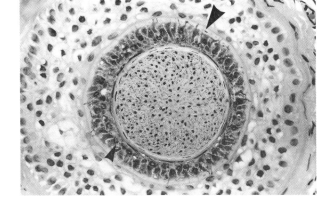

NON-INFLAMMATORY ALOPECIA

35.5 Androgenetic alopecia

♦ also known as 'male-pattern baldness', although it may occur in females as well
♦ transverse section through the level of the inferior segment of hair shows a decreased follicular density and follicular atrophy
♦ reduction in number and size of anagen follicles with increased numbers of telogen follicles
♦ bifrontal recession and thinning over the vertex in men
♦ thinning over the crown in women

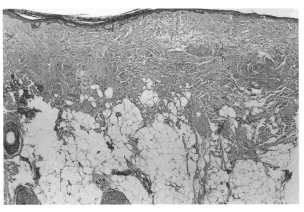

35.6 Trichotillomania

♦ increase in catagen hair follicles without an increase in small follicles; look for apoptotic bodies in follicular epithelium
♦ anagen follicles without hair shafts (recent avulsion); intrafollicular hemorrhage in an empty follicle (upper picture)
♦ follicular epithelium looks folded and distorted probably as a result of traction
♦ pigment hair casts are commonly seen (arrow; lower picture)
♦ lack of significant inflammatory infiltrate
♦ results from frequent, often subconscious, manipulation (such as twisting, rubbing, or plucking) of hair, thereby causing a patch of alopecia; however, the process may be diffuse
♦ may be seen in patients with psychiatric disorders
♦ biopsy may be necessary to differentiate from alopecia areata and tinea capitis

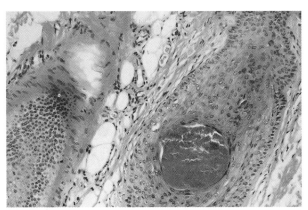

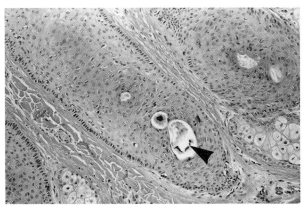

35.7 Pseudopelade of Brocq

♦ follicular structures replaced by vertically oriented scar tissue

♦ atrophic epidermis in long-standing disease

♦ early in the disease, a lymphocytic infiltrate may be seen in the upper two-thirds of the hair follicle

♦ true pseudopelade of Brocq is not associated with other causes of inflammatory alopecia (it is idiopathic)

♦ slowly progressive (usually over 2 years), often self-limiting, non-inflammatory, well-defined, patchy scarring alopecia resembling footprints in the snow

♦ more common in women; usually starts in the third or fourth decade; parietal and vertex primarily affected

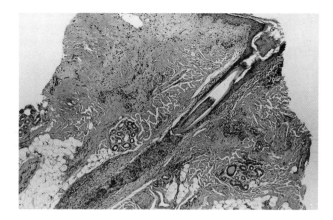

INFLAMMATORY ALOPECIA

35.8 Alopecia areata

♦ most important histologic feature is the presence of T lymphocytes in and around anagen or early catagen follicles

♦ diminished size and superficially located follicles

♦ depletion of lymphocytes with hair recovery

♦ non-scarring, often transient, alopecia with well-demarcated non-scarring patches of hair loss and short tapered 'exclamation mark' hairs

♦ may affect any hair-bearing area, but the scalp, eyebrows, and beard are most commonly involved

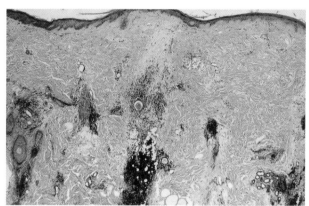

♦ may have associated nail abnormalities

♦ hair loss may be extensive and involve all hair on the body

♦ diagnosis is usually made clinically, and a biopsy is often not needed

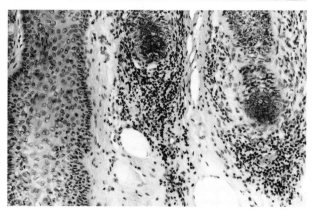

35.9 Discoid lupus erythematosus

♦ epidermal atrophy, follicular plugging, and a slight degree of perivascular and periadnexal lymphocytic infiltration are seen here

♦ other changes of LE: basement membrane thickening; hyperkeratosis; increased dermal mucin

♦ PAS staining may show basement membrane thickening in chronic lesions

♦ IgG and IgC at the dermoepidermal junction are demonstrated by direct immunofluorescence

♦ erythematous to violaceous atrophic patches with areas of hyper- and hypopigmentation, follicular plugging, telangiectasia, and atrophy

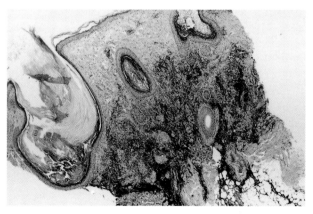

(continued next page)

♦ marked inflammatory damage to the inferior segment of an anagen follicle in an acute lesion, as seen here

♦ anagen hairs may be pulled out of active areas

♦ carpet-tack appearance of scale that has been removed

♦ face and scalp are commonly involved, although lesions may occur at any site

♦ this is a trichologic emergency as early intervention may arrest or prevent scarring alopecia

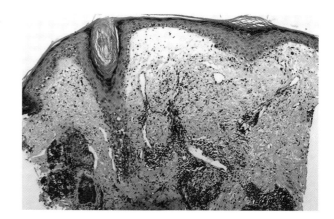

35.10 Lichen planopilaris

♦ lymphocytic infiltration, which may be band-like, obscures the dermoepidermal and dermofollicular junctions

♦ apoptotic keratinocytes, colloid bodies, and pigmentary incontinence seen on high power (second picture)

♦ colloid bodies may stain positively for IgM or IgG

♦ perifollicular fibrosis with degeneration of hair structures

♦ no basement membrane thickening, unlike LE

♦ atrophic, smooth, well-demarcated patches of alopecia with perifollicular erythema, follicular papules, or hyperkeratosis particularly at the margins of bald areas; typical lichen planus (LP) papules (pruritic, polygonal, planar, purple papules) are not seen on the scalp

♦ usually affects adults, especially women

♦ results in atrophy and scarring alopecia

♦ usually occurs with foci of LP elsewhere

♦ **Graham Little syndrome** refers to scalp scarring alopecia, loss of pubic and / or axillary hair, and keratosis pilaris

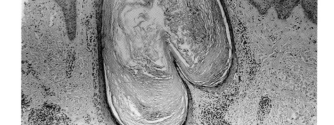

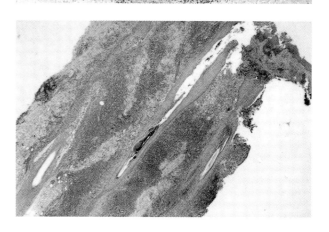

35.11 Alopecia mucinosa (follicular mucinosis)

♦ exocytosis of lymphocytes with reticular degeneration of follicular structures

♦ accumulation of mucin within pilosebaceous units

♦ presence of atypical lymphocytes strongly suggests cutaneous T-cell lymphoma

♦ primary (idiopathic) and secondary forms

♦ secondary form associated most often with lymphoma, usually mycosis fungoides

(continued next page)

- secondary form may precede or coexist with lymphoma
- well-demarcated erythematous plaque with follicular accentuation and alopecia
- may be benign and self-limiting, resolving within 2 months to 2 years, chronic and relapsing, or persistent and associated with cutaneous T-cell lymphoma

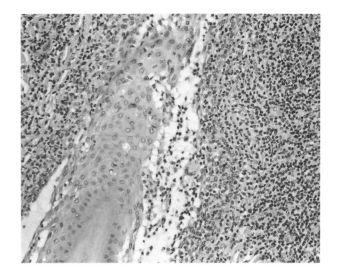

35.12 Folliculitis decalvans

- follicular plugging, suppurative neutrophilic folliculitis, perifollicular neutrophilic abscesses, foreign-body giant cells, and granulomas
- fibrosis and loss of follicles with time
- **folliculitis decalvans** presents with patches of alopecia showing crops of follicular pustules; crusting, scaling, and erosions may be present
- **dissecting folliculitis** has similar features on microscopy; part of the follicular occlusion triad which also includes acne conglobata and hidradenitis suppurativa; presents with deep inflammatory, boggy, nodules and plaques ± sinus tracts

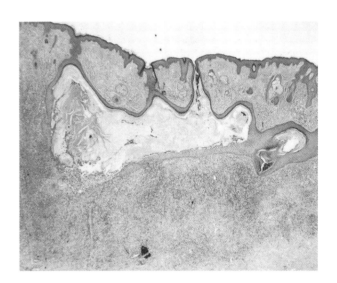

35.13 Tinea capitis

- hyphae may be in the epidermis and follicular wall (exothrix), or in the hair shaft (endothrix); may be highlighted with PAS staining
- perifollicular lymphocytic infiltrate
- foreign-body giant cells if follicular wall is disrupted
- usually seen in children prior to puberty as hair loss with short broken-off hairs (black dots) and scaling, or as an erythematous pustular nodule (**kerion**), which may cause scarring
- neutrophilic dermal and follicular abscesses in kerions
- usually a clinical diagnosis based on positive KOH and / or fungal culture
- clinical differential diagnosis of scaly tinea capitis: psoriasis, seborrheic dermatitis, atopic dermatitis; of black-dot ringworm: alopecia areata, trichotillomania; of kerion: folliculitis decalvans, folliculitis

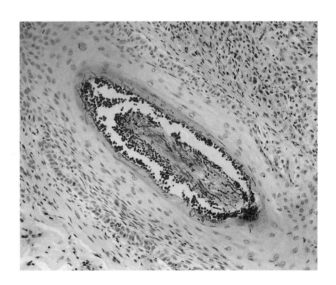

ORGANISMS

BACTERIA, FUNGI, VIRUSES, AND PARASITES

Certain bacterial, fungal, viral, protozoal, and parasitic organisms have a highly characteristic microscopic appearance. Finding these organisms in tissue sections is virtually diagnostic. Microscopic identification of infectious agents is usually much quicker than culture but, in contrast to the latter, does not permit differentiation of the species subtypes of most bacteria and fungi.

Bacteria demonstrable with Gram, silver, or acid-fast stains

Cocci (bacterial folliculitis)	36.1
Staphylocccus aureus (botryomycosis)	36.2
Mycobacterium (lepromatous leprosy)	6.3
Mycobacterium (tuberculoid leprosy)	36.4
Mycobacterium avium–intracellulare (MAI)	36.5
Spirochetes (syphilis) / Lyme disease	36.6

Fungi demonstrable with silver or PAS stains

Dermatophytes	36.7
Candida (candidiasis)	36.8
Pityrosporum ovale	36.9
Sporothrix (sporotrichosis)	36.10
Paracoccidioides (North American blastomycosis)	36.11
Paracoccidioides (South American blastomycosis; paracoccidioidal granuloma)	36.12
Cryptococcus neoformans (cryptococcosis)	36.13
Coccidioides (coccidioidomycosis)	36.14
Histoplasma (histoplasmosis)	36.15
Aspergillus (aspergillosis)	36.16
Mucor (mucomycosis, zygomycosis, phycomycosis)	36.17

Viruses

Poxvirus (molluscum contagiosum)	36.18
Cytomegalovirus (CMV inclusion disease)	36.19
Herpes simplex / varicella–zoster virus	36.20
Human papillomavirus	36.21
Parapoxvirus (orf)	36.22

Parasites / protozoa

Sarcoptes (scabies)	36.23
Pediculus (pediculosis capitis)	36.24
Phthirus (pediculosis pubis)	36.25
Demodex folliculorum	36.26
Amoeba	36.27

BACTERIA DEMONSTRABLE WITH GRAM, SILVER, OR ACID-FAST STAINS

36.1 Cocci (bacterial folliculitis)

♦ bacteria seen on the skin surface may not be significant unless associated with an inflammatory exudate, but bacteria seen within an inflamed follicle, as seen here, is probably indicative of a bacterial folliculitis

♦ clump of cocci (arrow) in an inflamed follicle

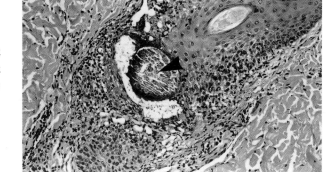

36.2 *Staphylococcus aureus* (botryomycosis)

♦ eosinophilic granules composed of colonies of bacteria are seen in the suppurative foci

♦ Gram staining highlights the cocci (usually *S. aureus*), although Gram-negative organisms such as *Pseudomonas* and *Proteus* are also described

♦ dermal abscesses and warty plaques on the extremities

♦ usually occurs in immunologically compromised individuals (as in **Job syndrome**), or in patients with ulcerative colitis, arthritis, or leukemia

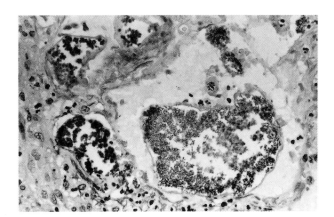

36.3 *Mycobacterium* (lepromatous leprosy)

♦ well-demarcated clear zone immediately beneath the acanthotic epidermis (upper picture)

♦ extensive infiltration of the dermis by epithelioid histiocytes with faintly eosinophilic and microvesicular cytoplasm

♦ higher magnification (lower picture) shows the lepra or Virchow cells (arrows), histiocytes that are distended by clumps of bacilli within their cell bodies

♦ presence of *Mycobacterium leprae* may be confirmed by Fite–Faraco staining

♦ note the complete absence of granulomas in lepromatous leprosy due to complete anergy and incompetent cell-mediated hypersensitivity

♦ numerous organisms are readily seen in lepromatous leprosy whereas they may be difficult to find in tuberculous leprosy (see 36.4)

♦ usually multiple erythematous macules, papules, nodules, or diffuse infiltration in lepromatous leprosy

♦ a solitary skin lesion is rare

♦ leonine facies and loss of eyebrows with facial skin lesions

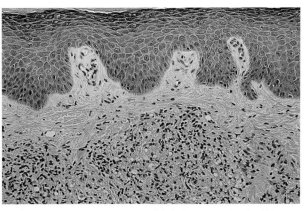

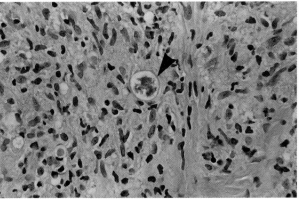

36.4 *Mycobacterium* (tuberculoid leprosy)

♦ reaction is granulomatous (arrow) with Langhans' giant cells and nerve involvement

♦ bacilli are difficult to find as they are destroyed by the high cell immunity and activation of macrophages

♦ heavy lymphocytic infiltration of the dermal nerves is commonly seen

♦ hypopigmented lesions with impaired sensation in tuberculous leprosy

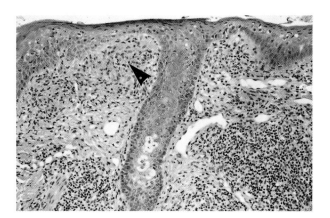

36.5 *Mycobacterium avium–intracellulare* (MAI)

♦ as with other infectious mycobacterial and deep fungal skin lesions, epidermal hyperplasia is present; a peri-anal skin lesion from a patient with HIV infection is shown here

♦ a suppurative area in the dermis (upper picture) is surrounded by epithelioid histiocytes and lymphocytes

♦ depending on the history, special stains may include Gram, Ziehl–Neelsen (Z-N) or Fite, Grocott–methenamine–silver, and periodic acid–Schiff (PAS) with diastase

♦ MAI infection is usually seen in patients with T-cell immunodeficiency, especially AIDS

♦ numerous acid-fast bacilli (arrows; lower picture) are stained red by Z-N staining

♦ transformation of macrophages to spindle cells similar to a histoid reaction in leprosy has been described

♦ disseminated MAI infection usually affects the lungs, bone marrow, and lymph nodes; skin involvement is rare

♦ may have cutaneous abscesses, necrotic lesions, and disseminated pustules with varioliform scarring

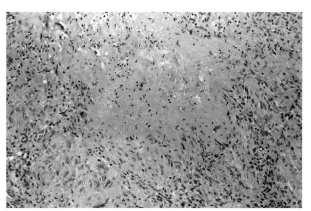

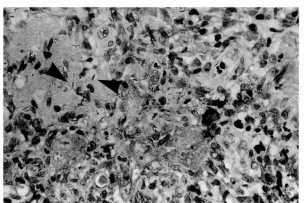

36.6 Spirochetes (syphilis)

♦ chancre is the prototypical skin lesion and is caused by *Treponema*

♦ inflammatory infiltrate is plasma cell-rich (see 22.4)

♦ lesions are highly vascular; a striking degree of endothelial cell swelling and intimal proliferation is seen

♦ spirochetes are almost always present in primary lesions, and may be demonstrated in approximately 30% of secondary lesions

♦ *Treponema pallidum*, the cause of syphilis, is demonstrated by silver staining (Steiner), as seen here

♦ **Lyme disease** is caused by a spirochete that may also be seen by silver staining

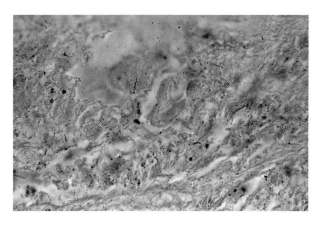

FUNGI DEMONSTRABLE WITH SILVER OR PAS STAINS

36.7 Dermatophytes

♦ hyphae (arrow) in the stratum corneum are visible with routine H&E staining, but PAS staining after diastase highlights the organisms

♦ dermatophytes may cause infection of the skin, nails, and hair

♦ the three genera are indistinguishable histopathologically

♦ biopsy is usually necessary if KOH and fungal culture are negative, or if the patient does not respond to treatment

♦ biopsy should be taken from the advancing edge of the lesion

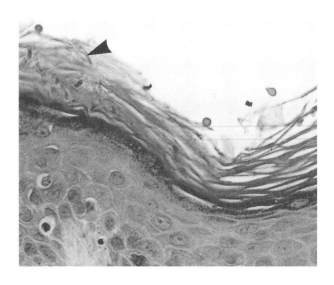

36.8 *Candida* (candidiasis)

♦ round or oval yeast cells and pseudohyphae (arrow) may be difficult to distinguish from dermatophytes

♦ may cause a marked degree of squamous epithelial hyperplasia

♦ mucocutaneous disease includes prelèche (erythematous, macerated, fissured angles of the mouth), paronychia, thrush, genital and intertriginous infection (erythematous, macerated patch with a gray-white pseudomembrane associated with satellite erythematous papules and pustules), and generalized disease (multiple erythematous and purpuric macules, papules, and pustules; usually in debilitated or very young patients)

♦ triad of fever, myalgias, and erythematous skin lesions in a septic patient unresponsive to oral antibiotics is suggestive of disseminated candidiasis

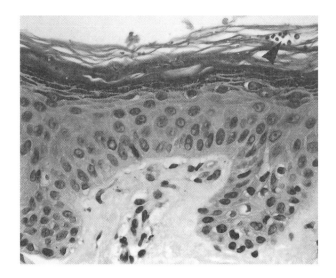

36.9 *Pityrosporum ovale*

♦ small budding yeast cells, 2–3 μ in size, are seen among keratin fragments and bacteria at a follicular opening

♦ overgrowth of these commensal yeast cells is typically seen with many hyperkeratotic lesions, including actinic keratosis and seborrheic keratosis

♦ *Pityrosporum ovale* and *P. orbiculare* are among the resident flora of the skin and hair follicles

♦ *Pityrosporum* may cause tinea versicolor, folliculitis, blepharitis, and seborrheic dermatitis

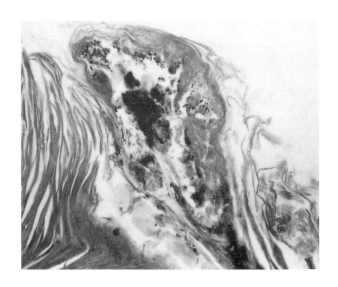

36.10 Sporothrix (sporotrichosis)

♦ spores are 4–6 μ in size and may show single buds; PAS staining is almost always required to demonstrate the organisms

♦ cigar and asteroid bodies are infrequent; rarely, spores and non-septate pseudohyphae may be seen in the keratin layer

♦ saprophyte in soil and on vegetation; usually through a skin abrasion, forestry workers and horticulturists acquire the infection from sphagnum moss, old timbers, roses, and other plants

♦ in the cutaneous lymphatic variant, the most common form, a crusted ulcerated nodule develops on the hand and, within a few days, multiple linear nodules appear up the arm

♦ fixed cutaneous form typically occurs on the face or trunk as an ulcerative, warty, acneform or erythematous, scaly plaque

♦ disseminated cutaneous disease and systemic disease are rare, and are usually seen in immunosuppressed patients

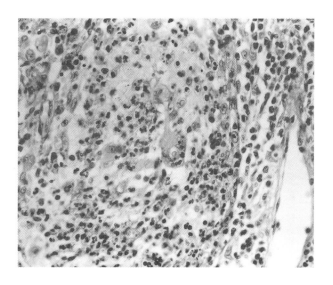

36.11 *Paracoccidioides* (North American blastomycosis)

♦ an individual fungal cell is round to oval, and around 10 μ in diameter with a thick refractile wall

♦ sporing cells appear as a pair of unequal-sized spores, often seen in the cytoplasm of giant cells

♦ pseudoepitheliomatous hyperplasia, intraepidermal and dermal microabscesses

♦ primary infections are extremely rare

♦ infection is usually acquired by inhalation with skin involvement secondary to dissemination

♦ skin lesions occur in up to 80% of disseminated cases

♦ typical lesion is a solitary papule or nodule that may ulcerate and drain purulent material; as the lesion enlarges, the border becomes warty and the center clears

♦ clinical differential diagnosis: squamous cell carcinoma; cutaneous tuberculosis; tertiary syphilis; and leprosy

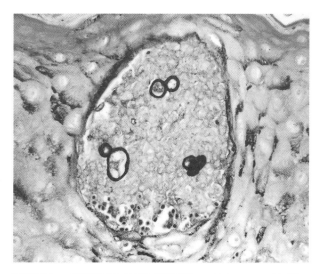

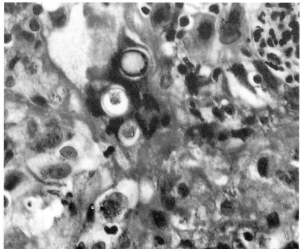

36.12 *Paracoccidioides* (South American blastomycosis; paracoccidioidal granuloma)

- mature cells may be large, with an average diameter of 30 μ
- budding may be single or multiple
- smaller buds around the larger central mother cell has been compared to a marine pilot's wheel
- endemic in countries from Mexico to Argentina
- more common in men
- infection is usually acquired through inhalation, and the lung is the primary site of infection
- skin lesions have a predilection for the extremities and face, and may be acneform
- oral lesions are commonly seen, and are granulomatous and ulcerative, with ill-defined borders and small hemorrhagic dots (mullberry-like lesions)

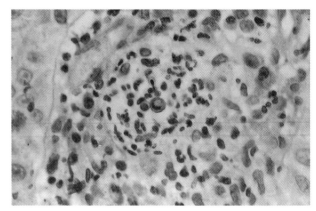

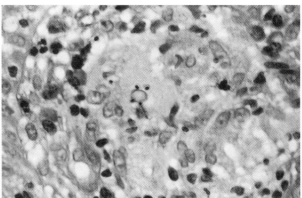

36.13 *Cryptococcus neoformans* (cryptococcosis)

- tissue reaction often varies from gelatinous areas with minimal inflammatory cell infiltrate (upper picture) to a marked granulomatous reaction
- each fungus cell is round to oval and small (2–4 μ) in the presence of granulomatous inflammation
- spores may be larger, up to 20 μ, in mucoid areas
- budding is single; pairs of unequal-sized spores may resemble North American blastomycosis
- special stains, such as mucicarmine, highlight the mucinous capsule of the organism (lower picture)
- found in soil, dust, and bird droppings
- airborne infection with a predilection for the central nervous system; cutaneous lesions are encountered in 10–15% of systemic disease
- common infection in immunocompromised patients with defective cell-mediated immunity
- spectrum of cutaneous disease includes cellulitis, acneform papules and pustules, abscesses, molluscum contagiosum-like lesions, herpetiform lesions, panniculitis, and indurated oral ulcer
- head and neck are preferentially affected

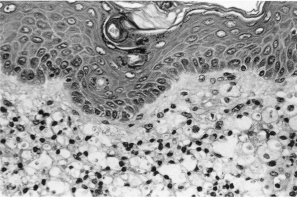

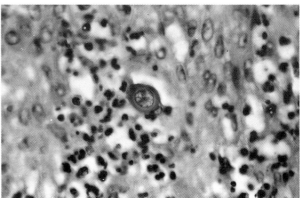

36.14 *Coccidioides* (coccidioidomycosis)

♦ thick-walled sporangia contain sporangiospores (arrow)
♦ sporangia, but not sporangiospores, are demonstrated by H & E staining
♦ sporangiospores are seen by PAS staining
♦ granulomas and / or suppuration around sporangia
♦ present in soil in Argentina, Paraguay, Venezuela, Central America, Mexico, and in the southwestern United States
♦ infection results from inhalation and is usually limited to the lungs
♦ dissemination of pulmonary disease almost always involves the skin; papules, pustules, nodules, abscesses, warty granulomas, and ulcers with sinus tracts may be seen clinically; most characteristic lesion is a warty nodule on the nasolabial fold
♦ primary cutaneous disease is extremely rare

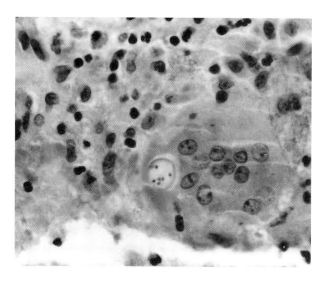

36.15 *Histoplasma* (histoplasmosis)

♦ small (1–4 μ) round to oval fungus often found in the cytoplasm of macrophages, but may be free in tissue
♦ single cells with or without a solitary bud
♦ special stains are needed to visualize the organism
♦ found in soil, the infection is airborne
♦ similar to cryptococcosis, cutaneous lesions occur in a minority (< 6%) of systemic cases, although oral mucosal lesions are common (> 50%)
♦ clinical manifestations include a widespread erythematous and purpuric maculopapular eruption, cellulitis, and erythematous nodules

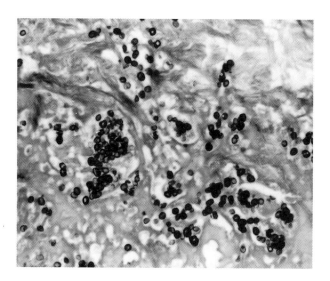

36.16 *Aspergillus* (aspergillosis)

♦ hyphae are septate, 2–4 μ in diameter, and branch at acute angles; spores are absent
♦ tend to invade blood vessels, producing thrombosis
♦ wide distribution in soil, dust, and decomposing vegetation
♦ infection primarily in immunocompromised patients
♦ most patients are neutropenic or taking high-dose corticosteroids
♦ cutaneous aspergillosis is rare; may be secondary to hematogenous dissemination or primary in burn wounds (seen here), ischemic ulcers, and at sites of trauma or near intravenous catheters (especially in patients with leukemia)
♦ necrotic, often ulcerated macules, papules, plaques, nodules or hemorrhagic bullae; primary cutaneous disease may disseminate

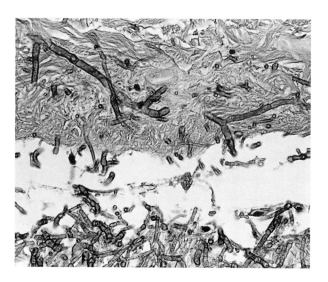

36.17 *Mucor* (mucormycosis, zygomycosis, phycomycosis)

♦ hyphae are broad (diameter up to 30 μ), non-septate, larger, and longer than those of *Aspergillus,* and typically branch at 90° angles; spores are absent

♦ invasion of blood vessel walls, causing thrombosis and infarction of the surrounding tissue

♦ may cause rhinocerebral, pulmonary, gastrointestinal, cutaneous, and disseminated disease; in common with aspergillosis, cutaneous disease is rare, usually seen in compromised patients, and may be secondary to disseminated infection or primary

♦ acute, often fatal, rapidly progressive infection seen primarily in ketoacidotic diabetics, patients with hematologic malignancies, burns patients, and severely malnourished children

♦ erythematous, tender plaques with black, necrotic centers

♦ clinical differential diagnosis: ecthyma gangrenosa, which is usually caused by *Pseudomonas aeruginosa*

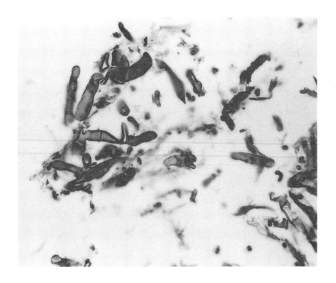

VIRUSES

36.18 Poxvirus (molluscum contagiosum)

♦ numerous intracytoplasmic inclusion bodies (molluscum bodies), which are eosinophilic inclusions that grow in size from the parabasal to the superficial epidermal cell layers

♦ in the granular and keratin layers, the molluscum bodies are more basophilic and fill the entire cell; the cell nuclei become displaced to the periphery of cells and appear as hyperchromatic crescents

♦ pearly papules with central umbilication

♦ common infection in children and HIV-infected patients

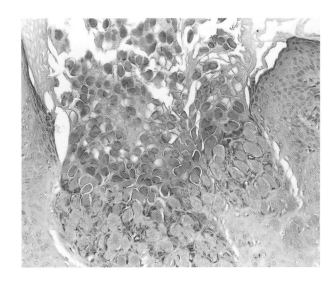

36.19 Cytomegalovirus (CMV inclusion disease)

♦ affects endothelial cells; viral inclusions are found in the enlarged cells lining dilated vessels

♦ basophilic intranuclear inclusions are seen here, and some are surrounded by a clear halo (arrows)

♦ usually widespread papulomacular eruption in immunologically compromised individuals

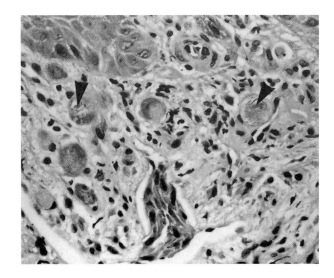

36.20 Herpes simplex virus

♦ ballooning degeneration of keratinocytes, which show 'washed-out' nuclei with empty steel-gray centers and thickened nuclear membranes

♦ multinucleated keratinocytes with prominent nuclear molding

♦ herpes simplex virus and **herpes varicella–zoster virus** cannot be differentiated histologically, but require monoclonal antibody testing and viral culture

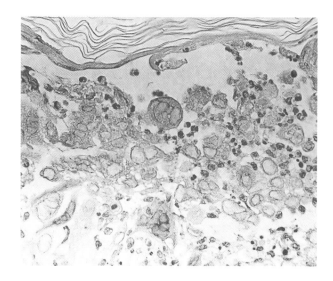

36.21 Human papillomavirus

♦ warts are classified by their gross appearances, location, or genotype of causal virus

♦ clinical appearance and site differentiate the common wart (verruca vulgaris), flat wart (verruca plana), palmoplantar wart, and genital wart (condyloma acuminatum)

♦ the histopathologic change common to most papillomavirus lesions is koilocytosis (shown here)

♦ affected keratinocytes have slightly enlarged nuclei with vacuolated cytoplasm; they are commonly seen in the superficial epidermis with parakeratosis

♦ eosinophilic inclusions are seen in palmoplantar warts (see 6.9)

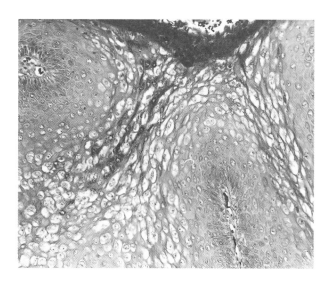

36.22 Parapoxvirus (orf)

♦ skin lesions are on the finger and due to infection by a parapoxvirus from sheep

♦ over a 6-week period, the typical lesion progresses through six stages: maculopapular; target lesions as in erythema multiforme; acute weeping; nodular; papillomatous; and regressive

♦ lesion in acute weeping stage shows extensive reticular degeneration and necrosis of epidermal cells, as seen here

♦ lymphocytic infiltration and a few keratinocytes still have eosinophilic inclusions

♦ intranuclear inclusions have also been described, but are not seen in this example

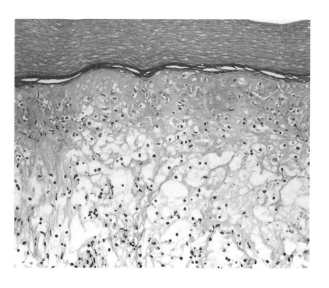

PARASITES / PROTOZOA

36.23 *Sarcoptes* (scabies)

♦ parts of a *Sarcoptes scabiei* female mite (upper picture) inside the keratin layer burrow

♦ eosinophilic spongiosis and inflammation are seen around the burrow

♦ itchy, erythematous, excoriated papules in the inter-digital spaces, flexor aspects of the wrists, elbows, anterior axillary folds, nipples, around the umbilicus, penis, scrotum, and buttocks

♦ an imaginary circle intersecting the main sites of infestation (axillae, flexures of elbow, wrists, hands, and crotch) has long been called the 'circle of Hebra'

♦ burrows may be seen on the palms

♦ bullae and pustules may occur on the hands and feet in children

♦ adult female *S. scabiei* (lower picture)

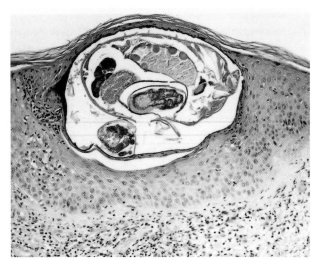

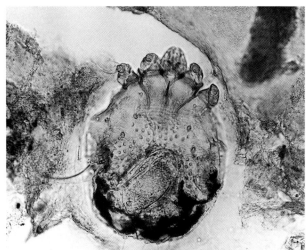

36.24 *Pediculus* (pediculosis capitis)

♦ a nit (shown here) is the casing of an ovum of *Pediculus humanus capitis*

♦ pediculosis is an infestation by three species of lice: *P. humanus capitis*, the head louse; *Phthirus pubis*, the pubic louse; and *P. humanus corporis*, the body louse

♦ in **pediculosis capitis**, adult organisms may not be as easy to find as nits, which are attached to hair shafts

♦ may mimic hair casts or nodes of trichorrhexis nodosa, but microscopic examination reveals ovum within a capsule

♦ itchy head

♦ body louse is the only louse to spend most of its time off the body; it lives on clothes and returns to the body only to feed; bites appear along clothing seams

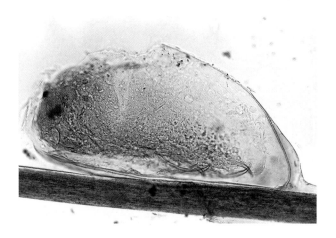

36.25 *Phthirus* (pediculosis pubis)

♦ caused by *Phthirus pubis*, the crab louse, which is 0.8–1.2 mm long (seen here)
♦ pubic lice spend most of their time hanging onto hairs
♦ intense itching in the involved area
♦ perianal and axillae are commonly infested
♦ pubic lice may move up or down the body if the host is hairy
♦ eyelashes may become infested by manual transmission

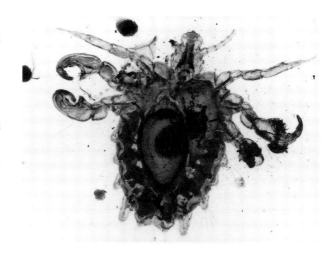

36.26 *Demodex folliculorum*

♦ another common mite frequently found in sebaceous hair follicles of the head and neck region
♦ usually does not cause problems, but may cause follicular papules, and an appearance similar to that of rosacea and perioral dermatitis

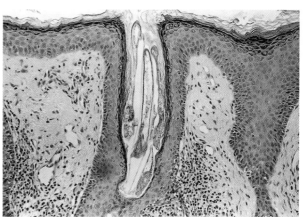

36.27 *Amoeba*

♦ round to oval and around 20 μ in diameter
♦ central round nucleus and single dense nucleolus
♦ amoebae (arrow) may easily be overlooked as they resemble macrophages
♦ granulomatous or suppurative inflammation
♦ *Acanthamoeba* is an ubiquitous protozoan found in soil and water
♦ cutaneous *Acanthamoeba* infection is rare, but may be seen in patients with the acquired immunodeficiency syndrome (AIDS) and in immunosuppressed patients after transplantation
♦ skin lesions may be the only manifestation of disseminated disease
♦ cutaneous disease occurs in 75% of patients with AIDS and *Acanthamoeba* infection
♦ pustules, indurated papules and plaques, cellulitis, nodules, non-healing ulcers with rolled borders, and eschar may be seen, preferentially on the arms, legs, and face
♦ ulceration of the palate may occur
♦ clinical differential diagnosis: furunculosis; varicella; and deep fungal and *Mycobacteria* infections

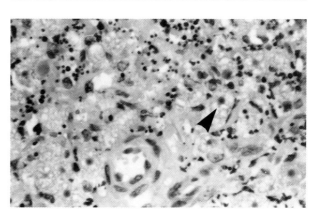

Index